The Mediterranean Diet
Health and Science

The Mediterranean Diet
Health and Science

Richard Hoffman PhD, FRSA
Senior Lecturer, University of Hertfordshire, Hatfield,
Herts, UK

and

Mariette Gerber MD, PhD
Former INSERM Senior Scientist, Cancer Research Institute,
Montpellier, France

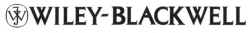

WILEY-BLACKWELL
A John Wiley & Sons, Ltd., Publication

Blackwell Publishing was acquired by John Wiley & Sons in February 2007. Blackwell's publishing program has been merged with Wiley's global Scientific, Technical and Medical business to form Wiley-Blackwell.

Registered Office
John Wiley & Sons, Ltd, The Atrium, Southern Gate, Chichester, West Sussex, PO19 8SQ, UK

Editorial Offices
9600 Garsington Road, Oxford, OX4 2DQ, UK
The Atrium, Southern Gate, Chichester, West Sussex, PO19 8SQ, UK
2121 State Avenue, Ames, Iowa 50014-8300, USA

For details of our global editorial offices, for customer services and for information about how to apply for permission to reuse the copyright material in this book please see our website at www.wiley.com/wiley-blackwell.

Library of Congress Cataloging-in-Publication Data

Hoffman, Richard, 1957-
  The Mediterranean diet : health and science / Richard Hoffman and Mariette Gerber.
    p. cm.
  Includes bibliographical references and index.
  ISBN-13: 978-1-4443-3002-1 (pbk.)
  ISBN-10: 1-4443-3002-0 (pbk.)
1. Nutrition. 2. Cooking, Mediterranean–Health aspects. 3. Biochemistry.
I. Gerber, Mariette. II. Title.
  RM216.H685 2012
  613.2–dc23

                                          2011021992

A catalogue record for this book is available from the British Library.

Set in 10/12 pt Sabon by SPi Publisher Services, Pondicherry, India
Printed and bound in Malaysia by Vivar Printing Sdn Bhd

1 2012

Contents

Preface

This book is an introduction to the health benefits of the Mediterranean diet (MedDiet), and the epidemiological and experimental evidence that underpins these benefits. The book is mainly intended for dietitians and nutritionists, and will also be of interest to other health workers, food scientists, and students taking courses in biomedical sciences.

The MedDiet is best known for helping prevent cardiovascular diseases (CVDs) and, to a lesser extent, cancers, and these are discussed in detail. In addition, we discuss the increasing evidence that the MedDiet can help prevent other chronic degenerative diseases such as neurodegenerative disorders and metabolic syndrome. With the ageing of populations, these diseases have become the major cause of morbidity and mortality in both developed countries and many less-developed countries. This highlights the growing importance of nutrition in helping prevent these diseases, and the book concludes with a discussion of public health strategies that can facilitate implementing a MedDiet in the community, and so help increase the number of years that people live in good health.

Several chapters in the book discuss experimental evidence that contributes to understanding how the MedDiet works. In particular, we have discussed common disease mechanisms that underlie many chronic diseases, and how, by targeting these mechanisms, key nutrients in the MedDiet can help prevent a broad range of diseases. These key nutrients probably include various plant chemicals (phytochemicals), some vitamins, fibre and fatty acids. The levels of these nutrients – in Mediterranean foods as elsewhere – are influenced by many steps of the food chain, from food production to metabolic effects in the body. Hence, we have highlighted features of the food chain that can have a significant impact on levels of these nutrients and hence impact on the overall health benefits of a MedDiet. For example, phytochemical levels are influenced all along the food chain from decisions regarding plant cultivar selection, to the growth conditions of the plant, food preparation and metabolic effects in the body. Similarly, the feed of land animals and fish has a major impact on their fatty acid composition and hence this impacts on human nutrition as well.

Throughout the book we have emphasised the importance of considering the composition of the MedDiet in its totality, i.e. as a Mediterranean "dietary pattern", rather than as a collection of individual foodstuffs. This is because both epidemiological evidence and – increasingly – underlying experimental studies, support the notion that the food groups (such as plant foods, fish and olive oil) comprising the totality of a MedDiet interact for optimum health. In fact, even this perspective is probably insufficient, since many other aspects associated with a traditional Mediterranean lifestyle can influence health. Best recognised of these is physical activity, but other features such as social eating, regular meal structure, sunlight, and even taking a siesta, may contribute to the benefits of a MedDiet. By discussing these aspects, we hope to provide something of a counter-balance to some current nutritional trends which are promoting individual "superfoods" or "nutraceuticals" as strategies for reducing chronic degenerative disorders.

Research on the MedDiet is proceeding at a very rapid pace, and we have highlighted promising new areas of experimental research, some of which may in the future lead to a deeper understanding of the scientific basis of the MedDiet. What is evident even now is that the MedDiet is very much a diet for our times, both through its potential for improving the health and well-being of an ageing society, and its low environmental impact by eschewing the consumption of large amounts of meat from intensively raised animals and instead favouring foods, both plant and animal, produced under more natural conditions. These features promote a healthy attitude towards food, and help make the MedDiet very appealing to a large number of people. And its delicious tastes help ensure high levels of compliance amongst consumers.

1 Overview

Summary

- Olive oil is the main dietary fat in the Mediterranean diet (MedDiet), and there is high consumption of fruits, vegetables, unrefined cereals and legumes, moderate consumption of fish, dairy products and wine, and low consumption of meat.
- There are many variations of the MedDiet reflecting influences of culture and landscape.
- Factors such as social eating and physical activity are also important, so the MedDiet represents a whole lifestyle.
- There is strong epidemiological evidence for a protective effect by the MedDiet against cardiovascular diseases and also protection against cancers and neurological disorders. Many biologically plausible mechanisms have been developed to explain these health benefits.
- There is increasing evidence that the health benefits are best explained by considering the overall dietary pattern.
- Consumption of the MedDiet is decreasing in some Mediterranean countries, whereas consumption of Mediterranean foods in some North European countries is increasing.

1.1 Development of the MedDiet

The Mediterranean diet (MedDiet) is tasty, easy to prepare and extremely healthy. The ability of the MedDiet to help prevent a wide range of today's most common ailments has been confirmed in numerous studies, and more widespread implementation of a MedDiet would undoubtedly result in significant public health benefits. How has this cuisine become one of the healthiest in the world? Probably part of the answer lies in the enlightened understanding in the Mediterranean of the link between food and health. From the Ancient Greeks to the Moors onwards, the MedDiet has been developed not only for its gastronomic virtues, but also as a synonym for a complete system of life. Another important aspect of the MedDiet is related to climate. The long growing season in the Mediterranean reduces the need for complex preservation techniques, and this has permitted an emphasis on natural, seasonal ingredients. The reliance on fresh ingredients cooked from raw is probably the single most important factor in Mediterranean cuisine that helps to ensure the consumption of a balanced intake of nutrients. Many traditional cooking pots, such as the *tagine*, *paella* and *plancha*, are still widely used in Mediterranean countries

The Mediterranean Diet: Health and Science, First Edition. Richard Hoffman and Mariette Gerber.
© 2012 Richard Hoffman and Mariette Gerber. Published 2012 by Blackwell Publishing Ltd.

and have given their names to classic Mediterranean dishes. Although originally developed to enhance flavour, these vessels are employed in cooking techniques that help enhance the health benefits of the food. Indeed, flavour and health are closely interlinked in any cuisine based on natural ingredients. A third factor is the dominance of the olive and the eschewing of animal products rich in saturated fat. Cooking vegetables with olive oil is the quintessential Mediterranean way of obtaining the benefits of both taste and health. Hence, the MedDiet represents a legacy of the link between Man and the Mediterranean environment that has existed since the time of the last Ice Age.

1.1.1   A brief history of the MedDiet

The land surrounding the Mediterranean sea has been the cradle for many civilisations and cultures, and the MedDiet represents one of the most significant achievements of these civilisations. Agriculture itself began with the cultivation of cereals and pulses in the Levant, a region which comprises the Eastern Mediterranean countries of Lebanon, Israel, Palestine, Syria, Jordan and Iraq. Later, the Phoenicians, Greeks and Romans cultivated the three basic elements of the MedDiet: olive trees for producing olives and olive oil, wheat for making bread, and grapes for fermenting into wine. These colonisers of the Mediterranean basin then spread olives and grapes to the Western Mediterranean. A wide range of vegetables were already being consumed by the time of the Romans including onions, leeks, lettuce, carrots, asparagus, turnips, cabbage, celery and artichokes. Among the fruits consumed by this time were figs, apples, pears, cherries, plums, peaches, apricots and citrons (a type of citrus fruit). Chestnuts, almonds and walnuts were also eaten [1, 2].

Important developments in the MedDiet occurred from the 8th century when the Moors occupied much of the Iberian peninsula (calling the region al-Andalus). The Moors introduced rice, lemons, aubergines (American: egg plants), saffron and other spices, and these products then spread, to varying extents, throughout the Mediterranean basin. The Moors had a particularly enlightened awareness of the importance of diet for general health. For them, 'diet was a synonym for a system of life. It included the practice of eating correctly, of choosing the best places for staying healthy and lengthening one's life, of bathing and washing correctly, of sleeping and staying awake, of expelling useless substances from one's body and of dealing with the ups and downs of the spirit' [3]. The occupation by the Moors ended in 1492, and this was the same year that Christopher Columbus arrived in the New World. Columbus returned to Spain with tomatoes and bell peppers, and these are now an integral part of the MedDiet.

1.1.2   The traditional MedDiet and present day MedDiets

The term 'Mediterranean diet' was originally coined in the 1950s by Ancel Keys, the epidemiologist who first recognised the health benefits of this way of eating. Since then, the MedDiet has undergone many changes, and it is now convention to use the term 'traditional' MedDiet to indicate the type of diet that could be found in rural communities in the 1950s and early 1960s, especially in Southern Italy and Greece (and rural Crete in particular), and before the impacts of migrations to the towns, rising wealth and modern food technologies. The traditional MedDiet was shaped by terrain and climate. Cereals and vegetables were grown in the flatter, low-lying areas, vines and olive trees on the slopes, and higher ground was left for grazing sheep and goats. The Cretan diet up until the 1960s has been described as 'olives, cereals, grains, pulses, wild greens, herbs and fruits, together with limited quantities of goat meat and milk and fish ... no meal was complete without bread ... olives and olive oil contributed heavily to the energy intake ... food seemed to be "swimming' in oil"' [4].

There are various formulations of what is meant by the term 'traditional MedDiet', and the following list is taken from a statement issued by a working group at the MedDiet 2004 International Conference [5]:

- Olive oil as added lipid
- Daily consumption of vegetables
- Daily consumption of fruits
- Daily consumption of unrefined cereals
- Bi-weekly consumption of legumes
- Nuts and olives as snacks (generally eaten just before a meal)
- Bi-weekly consumption of fish
- Daily consumption of cheese or yogurt
- Monthly or weekly consumption of meat or meat products
- Daily moderate consumption of wine, if it is accepted by religion and social grounds

Although this list sums up most of the important aspects of a traditional MedDiet, other versions include consumption of herbs and spices, herbal teas, and wild greens gathered from the countryside, and also the importance of significant levels of physical activity.

The traditional MedDiet is a rich source of macronutrients and micronutrients. It is not possible to define the precise amounts of various beneficial nutrients in the MedDiet because of significant variations between countries (see below). However, one set of figures, based on an analysis of a traditional Greek diet, is shown in Table 1.1.

Fats are an important component of the traditional MedDiet, and account for about 30% of total calories in Spain, and up to about 40% of total calories in Greece [7] This compares with about 34% in the American diet [8]. Hence, the traditional MedDiet is not a low fat diet. There are, however, significant differences in the fatty acid composition compared to a North European or a North American diet. This is mainly due to the fairly low level of saturated fats in the MedDiet (7–8% of total calories), and relatively high consumption of monounsaturated fatty acids (MUFAs) (>20% of total calories), which is mostly oleic acid derived from olive oil. Not only are total saturated fats relatively low in a traditional MedDiet, but the types of saturated fatty acids (SFAs) consumed are quantitatively different to those in a North European diet. This is partly because consumption of SFAs from meat and cow's milk is relatively low, and consumption of SFAs from cheese and yogurt made from goat and sheep milk can be quite high. Goat and sheep milk contain a relatively high percentage of medium chain fatty acids (MCFAs) compared to cow's milk, and these are not as strongly associated with adverse effects on plasma cholesterol levels as some longer chain SFAs. The Greeks have one of the highest consumption of cheese in the world – at 26 kg per person per year (2005 figures) it is even higher than for the French! But about half of this is feta, a cheese traditionally made with ewe's milk and up to 30% goat milk.

Table 1.1 Estimated daily intake of macro- and micronutrients in a Greek MedDiet [6]. Reproduced with permission. © 2006 Elsevier.

Component	Daily intake
Macronutrients	
Protein	74.5 g
Carbohydrates	255.8 g
Dietary fibre	29.8 g
Ethanol	14 g
Total lipids	110.7 g
SFA	29.8 g
MUFA	63.8 g
PUFA	9.9 g
TFA	1.4 g
Phytochemicals	
Flavonoids	118.6 mg
Carotenoids	65.7 mg
Sterols	256.8 mg
α-tocopherol	4.3 mg
Inorganic constituents	
K	1774 mg
Fe	14.9 mg
Na	2632 mg
Ca	696 mg
Mg	234 mg
Zn	10.3 mg
Cu	3.8 mg
Mn	3.5 mg
Total energy value	2473 Kcal

SFA, saturated fatty acids; MUFA, monounsaturated fatty acids; PUFA, polyunsaturated fatty acids; TFA, trans fatty acids.
Note: There were no data on vitamins in this analysis.

The traditional MedDiet is also a good source of polyunsaturated fats (PUFAs). Fish is the main contributor of the long chain (LC) *n*-3 FAs eicosapentaenoic acid (EPA) (20:5 *n*-3) and docosahexaenoic acid (DHA) (22:6 *n*-3). There is a modest intake of the *n*-6 fatty acid linoleic acid from nuts and sunflower seeds and pumpkin seeds, and these are popular aperitif foods in some Mediterranean countries. Linoleic acid is the predominant fatty acid in many seeds such as sunflower seeds and corn, and hence in oils made from these seeds. Seed oils are not a significant part of the traditional MedDiet and, as a consequence, *n*-6 fatty acid consumption is lower than in North Europe and North America. However, it should be mentioned that corn oil and sunflower oil are now increasingly replacing olive oil for cooking in some Mediterranean countries due to their lower cost.

Fats in the MedDiet

- High consumption of MUFAs, particularly oleic acid from olive oil
- High consumption of LC *n*-3 PUFAs (α-linolenic acid – ALA, EPA and DHA)
- Relatively low consumption of *n*-6 PUFAs
- Relatively high consumption of SCFAs and MCFAs from goat and sheep milk

Table 1.2 Estimate of the macronutrient composition of a typical MedDiet and a typical western diet (data from [9]).

Macronutrients	Mediterranean diet (%)	Western diet (%)
Carbohydrates	47	42
Proteins	15	20
Saturated fats	10	17
Monounsaturated fats	22	14
Polyunsaturated fats	6	7

Besides its typical fat composition, the MedDiet is also a rich source of a variety of carbohydrates, and these are discussed in Chapter 2. One estimate of how the overall proportions of macronutrients in a 'typical' western diet compare with those in a 'typical' MedDiet is shown in Table 1.2 [9]. This estimates MUFA intake in the MedDiet at 22% compared to 14% in a typical 'Western' diet. Although this analysis estimates that total PUFA intake between the two diets is similar, it should be noted that this analysis did not distinguish between n-6 and n-3 PUFAs.

Due to the high consumption of plants foods, the traditional MedDiet is a particularly rich source of plant chemicals (phytochemicals) and some vitamins and minerals (see Table 1.1). One aspect of particular relevance here is that plasma folate levels have been found to be a good biomarker for adherence to the MedDiet [10]. This mainly reflects the high consumption of green leafy vegetables in the MedDiet. Folate consumption is linked to a wide range of beneficial effects in the body, including prevention of neural tube defects in early pregnancy, and protection against cancers of the pancreas, oesophagus and colon-rectum [11]. By contrast, folic acid given in supplements has been shown to promote the progression of pre-malignant colorectal lesions [12]. This illustrates the increasing evidence that micronutrient supplements may not always afford the same protective effects attributed to dietary sources. This is an important point in the debate between whole diets and the use of supplements, and is discussed further in later chapters.

Although a traditional MedDiet is still widely consumed, especially by more elderly people, the diet is now increasingly under threat. Protecting healthy traditional diets against the encroaching uniformity of food, particularly the influence of fast food, is now recognised as a high priority [6]. Consequently, there was an initiative by Spain, Italy, Greece and Morocco to help protect the traditional MedDiet by applying for it to be adopted by UNESCO's Intergovernmental Committee for the Safeguarding of the Intangible Cultural Heritage of Humanity [13]. The MedDiet achieved this recognition in November 2010. The box below gives the statement issued by UNESCO at the time of this recognition, and emphasises how much the MedDiet represents an overall lifestyle rather than just the consumption of food.

UNESCO DECLARATION ON THE MEDITERRANEAN DIET AS AN INTANGIBLE CULTURAL HERITAGE OF HUMANITY

http://www.unesco.org/culture/ich/index.php?lg=en&pg=00011&RL=00394

The Mediterranean diet constitutes a set of skills, knowledge, practices and traditions ranging from the landscape to the table, including the crops, harvesting, fishing, conservation, processing, preparation and, particularly, consumption of food. The Mediterranean diet is characterized by a nutritional model that has remained constant over time and space, consisting mainly of olive oil, cereals, fresh or dried fruit and vegetables, a moderate amount of fish, dairy and meat, and many condiments and spices, all accompanied by wine or infusions, always respecting beliefs of each community. However, the Mediterranean diet (from the Greek diaita, or way of life) encompasses more than just food. It promotes social interaction, since communal meals are the cornerstone of social customs and festive events. It has given rise to a considerable body of knowledge, songs, maxims, tales and legends. The system is rooted in respect for the territory and biodiversity, and ensures the conservation and development of traditional activities and crafts linked to fishing and farming in the Mediterranean communities which Soria in Spain, Koroni in Greece, Cilento in Italy and Chefchaouen in Morocco are examples. Women play a particularly vital role in the transmission of expertise, as well as knowledge of rituals, traditional gestures and celebrations, and the safeguarding of techniques.

The current widespread interest in the MedDiet has necessitated the development of various definitions of what constitutes a 'modern' MedDiet. Such a definition is particularly important for epidemiologists in order to be able to assess the adherence of individuals to a MedDiet [14]. Many of these epidemiological studies have been conducted in European Mediterranean countries, and hence the definitions of the MedDiet tend to reflect the traditional MedDiet of these countries [10]. One widely-used definition of the relative consumption of nine key food groups is as follows:

1. high consumption of olive oil and low consumption of lipids of animal origin (resulting in a high ratio of monounsaturated to saturated fat)
2. high consumption of vegetables
3. high consumption of fruit
4. high consumption of legumes
5. high consumption of cereals (including bread)
6. moderate to high consumption of fish
7. low to moderate consumption of milk and dairy products (mainly cheese and yogurt from goats and sheep milk)
8. low consumption of meat and meat products
9. moderate consumption of wine

The use of current definitions of the MedDiet is discussed in Chapter 8, and the application of these assessments to disease prevention is considered in Chapters 10–13.

It is important to recognise that the MedDiet not only defines foods whose consumption *is* desirable, but should also encompass foods whose consumption is *not* desirable. This includes the absence of industrial processed foods, and is one reason for the relatively low levels of salt, saturated fat, trans fats and sugar in the MedDiet compared to the standard Western diet.

1.1.3 International differences

Despite some similarities between MedDiets, it is generally agreed that there is no one MedDiet. This is not surprising in view of the fact that Mediterranean countries are located in three different continents, namely Europe, Asia and Africa. These continents have major cultural differences, not least of which is religion: European Mediterranean countries are Christian and those in Asia and Africa are Muslim. Hence wine consumption, a cornerstone of the European MedDiet, is absent in Muslim countries where alcohol consumption is prohibited. There are many other differences throughout the Mediterranean basin that can influence dietary habits, and these range from climate and geography, to socio-economic factors, culture and history. These can be regional as well as international. For example, consumption of fish within a country tends to vary depending on proximity to the sea, and, at the international level, low consumption in some countries is also due to the relative scarcity of fish in some parts of the Mediterranean. Even olive oil consumption – considered another cornerstone of the MedDiet – can vary widely between Mediterranean countries. Hence, the overall types of foods can vary quite widely between various Mediterranean regions as is illustrated in Table 1.3.

The geographical boundaries within which a 'MedDiet' is eaten are not precisely defined. Twenty-one countries border the Mediterranean sea (although this number varies according to the definition of a national state) (Figure 1.1). The climates of these countries can vary widely from region to region, and parts of many countries that border the Mediterranean sea do not have a 'Mediterranean' climate in its precise climatological definition. (This is defined by climatologists as the Cs climactic region, i.e. having warm to hot, dry summers and cool, wet winters.) Even bordering the Mediterranean sea itself does not guarantee a MedDiet since parts of the coasts of Libya and Egypt do not have a Mediterranean climate. Northern Italy is another region that does not have a Mediterranean climate and correspondingly the traditional diet here is quite different to that found in Mediterranean Southern Italy. In France, only the regions of Provence, Languedoc and part of Roussillon have a Mediterranean climate, and the cuisines of other regions are quite different. By contrast, many parts of Portugal do have a Mediterranean climate, although this country is on the Atlantic seaboard and has no border with the Mediterranean sea.

A poetic, yet very useful, definition of the Mediterranean is that of the French writer Georges Duhamel who wrote: 'The Mediterranean ends where the olive tree no longer grows'. This can be used to delineate the northern limits of 'Mediterranean' cuisine and is shown in Figure 1.2.

The Mediterranean climate, as defined by climatologists, is not restricted to countries of the Mediterranean region but includes parts of California, the Western Cape in South Africa, central Chile, southern Western Australia and the coastal areas of central and south-east Australia (Figure 1.3). For cultural and historical reasons, these countries did not develop a traditional MedDiet. However, their climates have allowed the production of traditional Mediterranean foods, especially grapes, and, increasingly, olives, and levels of production of traditional Mediterranean foods are increasing in these countries.

1.1.4   National representations of the MedDiet

Efforts to promote the MedDiet have led to the development of various pictorial representations. These graphics aim to convey the essentials of the MedDiet in a single glance without recourse to lengthy text, as it is considered that this could be off-putting to some people. The design of the graphic is often angled in order to appeal to the populace of a particular country.

Perhaps the best known of these pictorial representations is the food pyramid developed by the American organisation Oldways (Figure 1.4). This structure is

Table 1.3 Important food groups in Mediterranean regions (from [15]). With permission from Elsevier.

Mediterranean region	Cereals	Dairy	Olive oil consumption	Meat	Other
Western (Spain, France, Italy, Malta)	Bread, rice, pasta	Cheeses	High in Italy and Spain	Pork	Potato
Adriatic (Croatia, Bosnia, Albania)	White wheat flour as bread and pitta	High (butter, buttermilk, ricotta, cheese, sour cream)	Low to moderate	Beef	
Eastern (Greece, Lebanon, Cyprus, Turkey, Egypt)	White flour products	Various cheeses	Very high in Greece, negligible in Egypt	Chicken*	Okra in summer, herbs (dill, parsley, oregano)
North Africa (Libya, Algeria, Morocco, Tunisia)	Bread made from whole meal flour and barley flour Couscous		Wide range	Lamb	Potato, pumpkin, chickpeas, dates, date molasses

*Lamb is also popular, especially in Greece.

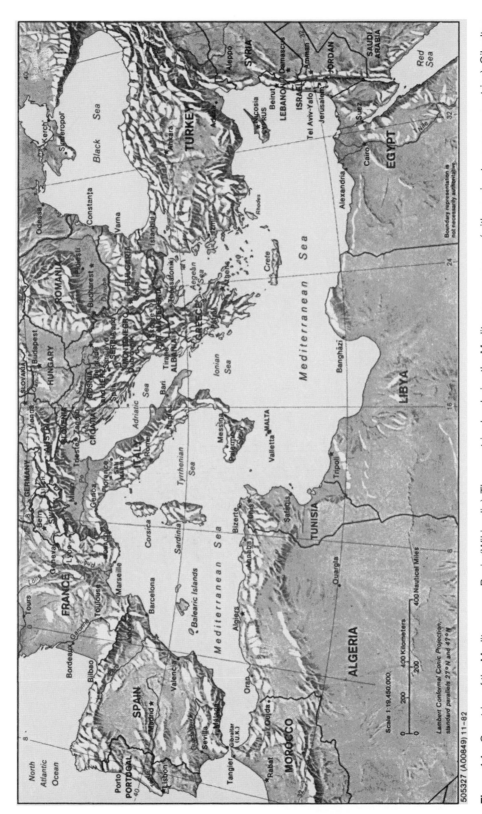

Figure 1.1 Countries of the Mediterranean Basin (Wikipedia). The countries bordering the Mediterranean sea are (with semi-autonomous countries): Gibraltar, Spain, France, Monaco, Italy, Slovenia, Croatia, Bosnia & Herzegovina, Albania, Greece, Turkey, Cyprus, Syria, Israel, Lebanon, Egypt, Libya, Malta, Tunisia, Algeria, Morocco.

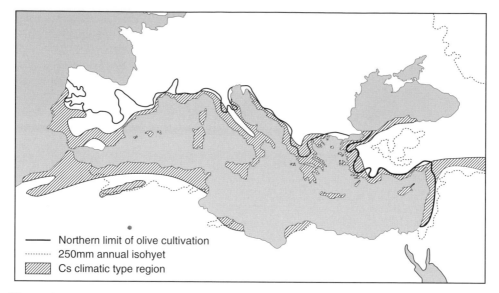

Figure 1.2 The Mediterranean region as defined by the northern limits of olive cultivation (black line) and climate (hashed areas) [1]. With permission from John Wiley & Sons.

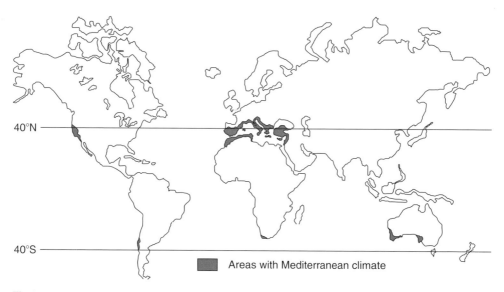

Figure 1.3 Regions of the world with a Mediterranean climate (Wikipedia).

similar to the US Food Guide Pyramid developed by the USDA. The Oldways pyramid has been refined over several versions. The base of the pyramid depicts physical activity and enjoying food with others. The remainder of the pyramid depicts the relative proportions of various foodstuffs that should be consumed, with the largest portion of the pyramid being devoted to plant foods. In addition, this 2009 version includes herbs and spices for the first time, although wild greens are not included, perhaps because their collection is not a traditional part of food culture in industrialised countries such as the US. Fish and shellfish have a prominent

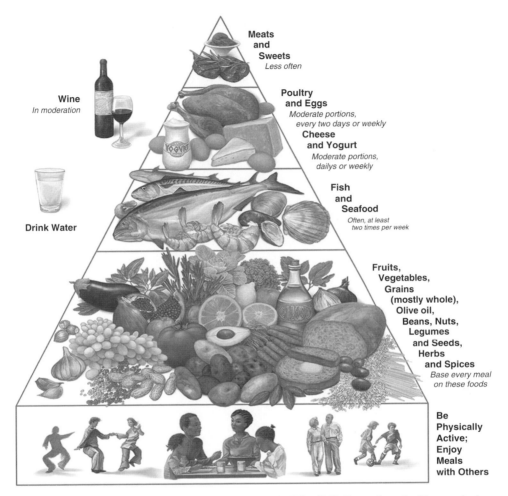

Mediterranean diet pyramid

A contemporary approach to delicious, healthy eating

Meats
and
Sweets
Less often

Wine
In moderation

Poultry
and Eggs
*Moderate portions,
every two days or weekly*

Cheese
and Yogurt
*Moderate portions,
dailys or weekly*

Fish
and
Seafood
*Often, at least
two times per week*

Drink Water

Fruits,
Vegetables,
Grains
(mostly whole),
Olive oil,
Beans, Nuts,
Legumes
and Seeds,
Herbs
and Spices
*Base every meal
on these foods*

Be
Physically
Active;
Enjoy
Meals
with Others

Figure 1.4 The Oldways' pyramid depiction of a MedDiet [16]. Reproduced with permission. © 2009 Oldways Preservation & Exchange Trust, www.oldwayspt.org

position, with lesser amounts of poultry and dairy produce. No distinction is made between dairy produce from cow milk (uncommon in the traditional MedDiet) and milk from goats and sheep, although cheese and yogurt are depicted and milk is excluded, and this is consistent with a traditional MedDiet. Meats and sweets are simply advised to be eaten 'less often'. Wine in moderation and water are also shown.

Nutritionists in Mediterranean countries may not necessarily consider (Egyptian) pyramids to be the most appealing depiction of the MedDiet for their populaces, so they have developed images more representative of their own countries. Greek nutritionists have come up with the idea of seven Greek columns, each column showing the food to be consumed – in words rather than images – on one day of the

The eatwell plate

Use the eatwell plate to help you get the balance right. It shows how
much of what you eat should come from each food group.

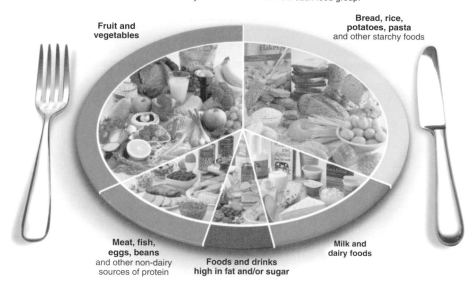

Figure 1.5 The Food Standards Agency Eatwell plate (http://www.eatwell.gov.uk/healthydiet/
eatwellplate/). © Crown copyright material 2007, with permission from the Controller of HMSO and
Queen's Printer for Scotland.

week [17]. The basic principles of a healthy way of life, 'moderation, variety and
proportionality', are also mentioned, together with having a correct energy balance.
Italian nutritionists have developed the historical theme by turning the Greek column
into a Greco-Roman temple, an apparent attempt to capitalise on the idea that a
temple symbolises 'healthiness, spirituality and self-improvement' [18]. In this Italian
model, the steps of the temple convey a healthy lifestyle, the need for adequate exercise, and to use virgin olive oil and to drink wine in moderation. The columns of the
temple represent desirable food groups, and foods that should only be consumed in
limited amounts are shown at the top of the temple. A practical weekly guide has also
been developed for French consumers [19] and this is discussed fully in Chapter 14.

It is interesting to compare these representations of the MedDiet with a current
pictorial representation of UK dietary guidelines as promoted by the UK Food
Standards Agency (FSA) – the so-called 'Eatwell Plate' (Figure 1.5). Although there
are some similarities, there are also significant differences. Fruits, vegetables and
carbohydrates all feature prominently on the Eatwell Plate, and this is similar to the
representations of the MedDiet. Dairy products (from cow milk) are a more
prominent feature on the Eatwell Plate than on the MedDiet depictions, reflecting a
long tradition of dairy farming and dairy consumption in the UK. No distinction is
made on the Eatwell Plate between the relative proportions of meat and fish to be
consumed. Cakes and biscuits represent a relatively large slice of the Eatwell plate.
Although these are also depicted on some of the MedDiet graphics, in the MedDiet
these products are likely to be based on fruit, honey, nuts and olive oil, whereas in

the UK there will be a far higher content of refined sugar and saturated fat. Olive oil and wine are absent from the Eatwell Plate.

1.1.5   Sources of information for the general public

Mediterranean restaurants and cookery books

Tourism has had a major impact on the appreciation by North Europeans of Mediterranean cuisine, not to mention Mediterranean wines. There are now a plethora of Mediterranean restaurants in most towns. Elizabeth David pioneered home cooking of Mediterranean food in the UK with the publication of her book *A Book of Mediterranean Food* in 1950. It remains in print to this day. Many other Mediterranean cookery books are now available and some, such as those by Claudia Roden on Middle Eastern cookery and those by Clifford A. Wright, are scholarly works and include authentic recipes. There is, however, very little information on whether or not cookery books promote a healthier lifestyle. In the case of Mediterranean cookery books, most do not give a clear indication of the relative proportions of different foods that should be eaten – a fundamental aspect of healthy eating. Some books emphasise recipes using ingredients readily available to the non-Mediterranean cook rather than being truly representative of local Mediterranean cooking. In particular, MedDiet cookery books often include a relatively high proportion of recipes that contain meat, and this is not representative of a traditional MedDiet.

MedDiet organisations

There are several organisations that promote the MedDiet, and these have useful websites. The Mediterranean Diet Foundation (La Fundación Dieta Mediterránea, FDM) is a non-profit organisation based in Barcelona, Spain which promotes the investigation and dissemination of the MedDiet and the Mediterranean lifestyle. It organises conferences, runs courses, and organises a range of workshops with a particular focus on children and the elderly. Its website is at http://www.fdmed.org. Oldways is an American non-profit organisation that was responsible for developing the best-known of the Mediterranean diet food pyramids (see above). It promotes the MedDiet through conferences, events and has introduced the 'Med Mark' in the US to help guide consumers in choosing traditional Mediterranean foods, drinks and other products. They have a website at http://www.oldwayspt.org.

1.2   Lifestyle factors

"We do not sit at table only to eat, but to eat together."

(Plutarch)

The traditional MedDiet, and its health benefits, cannot be fully understood without considering its cultural context. The 'Mediterranean food culture' (or 'Mediterranean lifestyle' as it is sometimes known) includes factors such as fixed meal times, eating as part of a social gathering and – in some countries – taking a siesta after the midday meal. Other lifestyle factors such as physical activity, not smoking, and low

Table 1.4 Breakfast ingredients in Mediterranean countries (adapted from [23]). With permission from Elsevier.

Country	Typical breakfast ingredients
Greece (rural)	bread, cheese, coffee, goat's milk, fruits, olives
Greece (urban)	coffee, milk, pastries, fruit juices, preserved fruits, eggs with ham and sausages, cheese, butter
Spain	coffee, pastries (*churros*)
Egypt (rural)	coffee or tea, bread, onion, salt
Egypt (Cairo)	coffee or tea, goat cheese, bread, broad beans (in a stew accompanied with eggs or smoked meat)
Italy	cappuccino, wheat biscuits, fruit
Turkey	Turkish coffee or tea, cheese, raw vegetables, olives

levels of stress have also been found to contribute to the overall health benefits of a MedDiet [20–22]. If one considers 'diet' in terms of its original meaning of 'a mode of living' from the Greek *diaita*, then the term 'Mediterranean diet' is completely congruous when implying the overall Mediterranean lifestyle.

The central part played by food in daily Mediterranean life is reflected in the care with which local, seasonal ingredients are sourced from respected producers and the care given to preparation and cooking. Producers themselves often sell their produce at local Mediterranean markets, and this promotes a close relationship between the consumer and the producer. This relationship helps maintain the quality of the produce and ensures that good agricultural practices are used, practices that can have a major impact on the nutritional value of the food (see Chapter 3).

1.2.1   Meal patterns

Meals are still an integral part of daily society in most Mediterranean countries, and the main meal is an important opportunity for bringing family members together. Lunch is still the main meal for many Mediterranean people, and many go home for lunch whenever possible, especially in Southern and Eastern countries [23]. However, the evening meal is increasingly becoming the main meal in regions where people work through the day or who work too far away from home to return there for lunch [23]. Breakfasts tend to be light compared to North European countries (Table 1.4), both in terms of quantity and in the low consumption of produce with high levels of saturated fats such as butter, sausages and bacon that typify the traditional English breakfast.

There is evidence that eating at fixed times during the day, and the associated periods when meals are not consumed, is important for inducing satiety which discourages excessive calorie intake [24]. This does not exclude the occasional consumption of snacks in traditional MedDiets (see Table 1.5), but whereas snacks in Northern Europe are a major source of salt, sugars, and saturated and trans fats [25], snacks in Mediterranean countries mostly consist of either fruit, nuts or home-made delicacies.

Table 1.5 shows a weekly food pattern collated from Cretans eating a traditional diet. During the week, the meal that included the main daily source of protein was mostly lunch, and this may particularly benefit physically active people, since studies have shown that optimal muscle building occurs when protein is eaten immediately after exercise [26]. By contrast, dinners were mainly based on easily digested cooked vegetables.

Table 1.5 Typical foods in a traditional Cretan Mediterranean diet consumed over a week [27]. With permission from Elsevier.

	Breakfast	Mid-morning	Lunch	Mid-afternoon	Dinner
Monday	ksinohontros[1], rusk, orange	pear	broad beans, onion, salad (cucumber, tomato, purslane, olives, olive oil), whole-wheat bread, apple, red wine	walnuts, dry figs	boiled vegetables, potatoes, olive oil, boiled egg, melon, red wine
Tuesday	rusk, cheese, apple	orange	snails, potatoes and vegetables, salad (tomato, cucumber, onion, olive oil), whole-wheat bread, red wine, longan	halva[2] (home-made)	rice with spinach, yogurt, whole-wheat bread, longan
Wednesday	doughnuts (homemade) with honey, apple, herbal tea	pear	chickpeas, herring, salad (tomato, cucumber, onion, olive oil), whole wheat bread, red wine	walnuts, figs, *raki*	stuffed tomatoes, whole wheat bread, salad (tomato, cucumber, onion), melon
Thursday	fresh whole milk boiled with ground wheat	melon	fish, broad beans (puree), oil, lemon juice, whole-wheat rusk, salad (tomato, cucumber, onion, olives, olive oil), pear, red wine	halva (home-made)	lentils, salad (tomato, cucumber, onion, olives, olive oil), apple, red wine, cheese, whole wheat bread
Friday	rusk, olives, herbal tea, apple	apple	beans, potatoes, whole-wheat bread, olives, orange	walnuts, dry figs, raki	broad beans, artichoke, olive oil, rusk, red wine, melon
Saturday	milk and whole wheat, melon	apple	chicken, okra, potatoes, salad (lettuce, cucumber, olives, olive oil)	home-made cheese pie, honey, coffee	boiled vegetables with olive oil, rusk, red wine, melon
Sunday	homemade cheese pie with honey, melon		rabbit, pasta, salad (tomato, cucumber, onion, olives, olive oil), rusk, wine, orange	coffee, halva	fish, fish soup with vegetables, rusk, red wine, apple

[1]Ksinohontros = yogurt, wheat; [2]halva = semolina, olive oil, sugar, walnuts.

1.2.2   Siestas

A siesta after a midday meal is still common in many Mediterranean countries. In Spain, most siestas were found to last for less than an hour. In a large study of healthy Greek men and women, working men who took a siesta were found to have fewer coronary deaths than those who did not nap [28].[1] The authors of this study suggested that regular siestas acted as a stress-reducing habit, which lowered the risk for CVD [28]. Not all studies, however, have found an inverse association between siestas and coronary deaths; indeed some studies have found a positive association. Taking a siesta is not conducted in a vacuum, and interpreting the data from some of these studies is subject to possible confounding factors. For example, people taking a siesta may take less physical exercise, which is a protective factor against CVD, and hence could give rise to a positive association between taking a siesta and CVD. Also, some individuals sleep during the day due to nightly sleep disturbances, which could be associated with underlying health problems. The Greek study did attempt to control for these possible confounding factors, although more studies examining the possible benefits of a siesta would be useful.

1.2.3   Physical activity

The high level of physical activity of the traditional Mediterranean peasant contrasts with the far more sedentary lifestyle of most present-day Mediterranean people. Despite this modern trend, the clement Mediterranean climate does still favour an outdoor lifestyle and more physical activity than is the case for many people living in more northern climates. In the HALE project, which evaluated the effects of a Mediterranean diet and lifestyle factors on mortality in elderly European men and women, physical activity was associated with a lower risk of all-cause mortality [22]. Increasing evidence is demonstrating that the health benefits of diet interact with other lifestyle factors, and physical exercise is now widely accepted to be an important factor that reduces the risk of age-related diseases such as CVD and some cancers [29]. A detailed study of Spanish children found that physical fitness is very important to reduce the risk of CVD and other diseases in later life, a point emphasised in the title of the paper: 'A Mediterranean diet is not enough for health' [30].

1.2.4   Sunshine

That Mediterranean countries are sunny is accepted almost without thought. But it has been argued that by inducing endogenous synthesis of vitamin D, sunlight is an important contributor to the health of Mediterranean people [31]. This proposal is based on recent evidence that the role of vitamin D in the body extends well beyond its role in bone health by preventing rickets and osteoporosis, and may also include a reduction in the risk for some cancers, hypertension and some immunological disorders (see Chapter 2).

1.3   Health benefits

There is a substantial body of epidemiological evidence for the health benefits of the MedDiet, and this is discussed fully in Chapters 10–13. A useful meta-analysis of a number of epidemiological studies generated the following estimates for the protective value of the MedDiet [32]:

---

[1] This analysis was not possible for women due to their lower incidence of coronary deaths.

- overall mortality reduced by 9%
- mortality from CVD reduced by 9%
- incidence of or mortality from cancers reduced by 6%
- incidence of Parkinson's disease and Alzheimer's disease by 13%

Other epidemiological studies show that there is some protection from other disorders including obesity, diabetes and metabolic syndrome [33], and these studies are also discussed in later chapters. Protection against CVD and cancers is the most significant in terms of reducing overall mortality.

The precise composition of the MedDiet that contribute to these protective effects continues to be an area of intense research interest. Key nutrients of the MedDiet that are thought to contribute to its beneficial effects include:

- high levels of MUFAs provided by olive oil
- high levels of PUFAs, especially *n*-3 fatty acids
- low levels of SFAs, and no TFAs from industrial sources
- high levels of plant-derived substances (including fibre, phytochemicals and vitamins)

A wide range of biologically plausible mechanisms has been elucidated that can explain how particular nutrients in the MedDiet may be protective against various disorders. This is a major theme of this book, and the evidence is discussed in later chapters.

1.3.1 Mediterranean dietary patterns

There is currently much interest in the relative health benefits of whole dietary patterns compared to individual dietary components [34, 35]. Although epidemiological studies can in some cases identify health benefits for individual foodstuffs, these studies do not give the complete picture. Rather, epidemiological evidence suggests that whole dietary patterns, such as a Mediterranean dietary pattern, should be considered for disease prevention, and that any one component is by itself insufficient to provide optimal health benefits [36–38]. For example, analysis of the Greek EPIC cohort found that adherence to a traditional Mediterranean diet was associated with a significantly reduced incidence of overall cancer, although there was not a statistically significant benefit simply from high consumption of fruits and vegetables [36]. This suggests that the overall dietary pattern was important in this study.

Figure 1.6 shows a comparison between the dietary patterns of Greece and the UK [39]. Compared to the UK, the Greek diet had a higher average consumption of olive oil, fruits, nuts and vegetables (although potatoes and red meat were also relatively high indicating a move away from a traditional MedDiet by the time of this 1999 analysis).

Clearly, the importance of the effect associated with a dietary pattern means that many dietary foodstuffs in this pattern may interact in a positive manner. In relation to CVD, this perspective has been summed up as follows: 'It is very likely that the ideal combination of the different dietary components with all the possible interactions and synergy is able to produce a maximum beneficial effect on all or, at least, the majority of mechanisms linking diet and cardiovascular disease, resulting in an enhanced reduction of cardiovascular disease risk' [40].

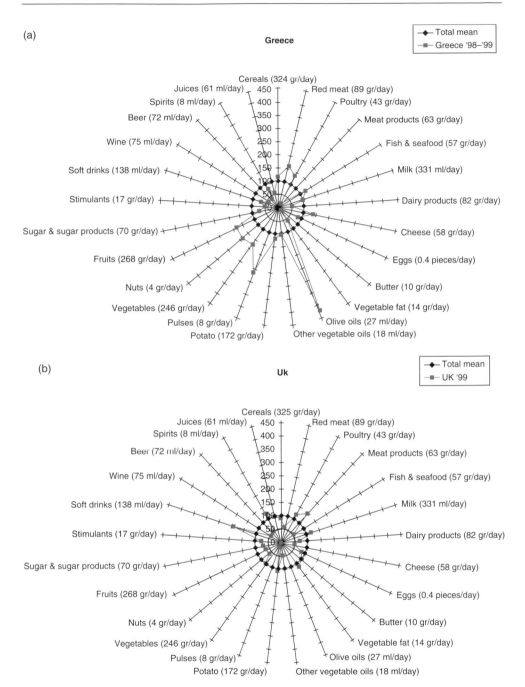

Figure 1.6   Dietary patterns of (a) Greece and (b) the UK in 1999 [39]. The reference circle of radius 100% indicates the mean for the Data Food Networking project (DAFNE) (absolute values are shown in brackets), and the second set of points indicates the % deviation of the food group from the reference DAFNE mean. Reprinted with permission from Macmillan Publishers Ltd, copyright 2006 Nature.

There are a plethora of candidate molecules that could contribute to the overall benefit of a traditional Mediterranean dietary pattern. However, establishing which molecules are involved is no trivial matter. A good illustration of the challenges that must be confronted is the estimate that up to 10,000 phytochemicals and their breakdown products may be consumed as part of a diet rich in vegetables [41]. Elucidating the underlying mechanistic basis for synergistic protection between such a large number of potentially active dietary components represents a major challenge as there are clearly many potential opportunities for synergistic interactions between these phytochemicals [42]. An illustration of the possible complexities is that over 1600 compounds have been identified in grapes, of which only a fraction have been studied in any detail [43]. Extending this to the overall MedDiet greatly amplifies the possible number of interactions between constituents in the different foods and their metabolic products.

1.3.2 Endorsements

Several health bodies have now endorsed the MedDiet. These endorsements have been prompted not only because of the well-established health benefits of the MedDiet, but also because people enjoy eating a MedDiet and so show a high degree of compliance when asked to maintain this dietary pattern over a period of time. In relation to CVD, there is evidence that the MedDiet is useful not only for primary prevention, but may also be beneficial for secondary prevention (i.e. after a first episode) of CVD [40]. Both the American Heart Association (AHA) and British Heart Foundation (BHF) have given endorsements of the MedDiet. The AHA Science Advisory and Coordinating Committee stated that 'it would be short-sighted not to recognize the enormous public health benefits that the Mediterranean-style diet could confer' [44]. The British Heart Foundation in one of its leaflets (2/99) states that 'Positive advice to eat more fish, fruit and vegetables or to eat a more Mediterranean diet rather than simply recommending a reduction in saturated fat may be more effective at reducing mortality in patients with existing coronary heart disease'. And The British Dietetic Association also specifically recommends the MedDiet for people with coronary vascular disease or who have had a heart attack [45].

Although endorsements in relation to cancer prevention are less explicit, the MedDiet is in line with general dietary recommendations, such as high fruit and vegetable consumption and low consumption of saturated fat and red meat.

1.4 The MedDiet, past, present and future

1.4.1 Current trends

Since the early 1960s, the period when the MedDiet was first delineated by the epidemiologist Ancel Keys, there have been significant changes in eating habits in Mediterranean countries. The diet in Mediterranean countries has progressively become much more similar to that of North European countries in terms of meat and dairy produce consumption, although on average there is still a higher consumption of fruit, vegetables and cereals (Table 1.6).

The progressive departure from a traditional MedDiet is particularly evident in children and young adults. This is of significant public health concern since it is thought that moving away from a MedDiet is contributing to the large rise in the incidence of obesity in the young in many Mediterranean countries [47].

A number of different scoring systems have been developed in order to assess adherence to the MedDiet (see Chapter 8). One of these is the Mediterranean Adequacy Index (MAI) which measures the ratio of energy obtained from foodstuffs

Table 1.6 Mean availability (g per capita per day) of selected food groups in Mediterranean countries and the rest of the 15-country EU in the early 1960s and early 1990s [46]. With permission from Cambridge University Press.

	Fruits	Vegetables	Legumes	Cereals	Meat	Dairy produce	Vegetable oils: animal fats	Alcoholic beverages
1960s								
Mediterranean	264	416	19	435	105	376	6.3	274
Rest of EU	217	215	6	288	189	583	0.1	332
1990s								
Mediterranean	341	500	16	372	248	599	4.4	245
Rest of EU	279	257	7	272	236	682	0.2	360

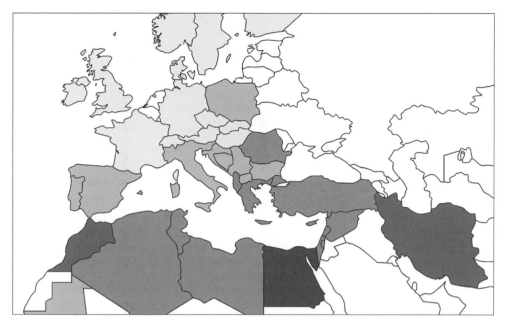

Figure 1.7   MAI in European and North African countries 2000–2003 [48]. ▨ 00–0.99; ▨ 1.00–1.99; ▨ 2.00–2.99; ▨ 3.00–3.99; ▨ 4.00–4.99. With permission from Cambridge University Press.

associated with the MedDiet divided by energy obtained from animal foodstuffs and processed foods. Hence a high value indicates better adherence to the MedDiet:

$$MAI = \frac{\% \text{ of energy (bread + cereals + legumes dry and fresh + potatoes* + vegetables + fresh fruit + nuts + fish + wine + vegetables oils)}}{\% \text{ of energy (milk + dairy products + meat + eggs + animal fats and margarines + sweet beverages + cakes, pies, and cookies + sugar)}}$$

The MAI has been used to assess adherence of the MedDiet in various countries of the world (Figure 1.7) [48].

In addition, the MAI has been used to monitor changing trends. Most Mediterranean countries showed a decrease in their MAI scores between the period 1961–1965 and the period 200–2003 (Figure 1.8). By contrast, some countries, such as Iran, the UK, Sweden, Denmark and Norway, showed an increase in their MAI, although their overall pattern is still a long way from a true MedDiet pattern as can be seen by their absolute MAI values (Figure 1.7). Egypt had highest MAI in 2005. So does this mean that Egyptians are particularly free of chronic degenerative disorders? Unfortunately, the answer is no. The average life expectancies for men and women in Egypt are only 66 and 70 years respectively (WHO, 2006 figures), and the major killer is CVD,

---

* Potatoes are not included in most estimates of the MedDiet.

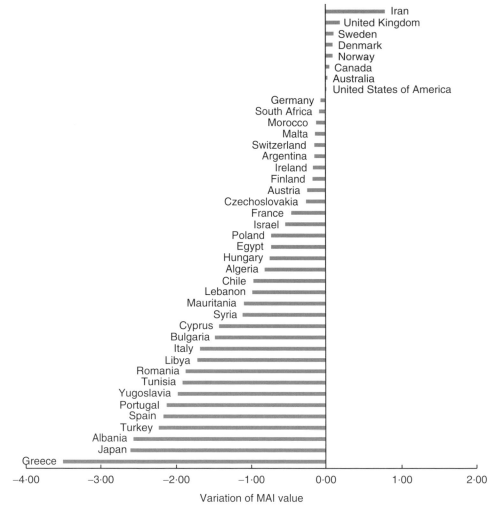

Figure 1.8 Changes to Mediterranean Adequacy Index 1961–1965 and 2000–2003 [48]. With permission from Cambridge University Press.

accounting for 34% of all deaths (WHO, 2006 figures). These figures may appear contradictory since the MedDiet is quintessentially associated with protection against CVD. There are important lessons from these figures as they highlight the limitations of the MAI[2]. Egypt is a low income country compared to Europe and the US, and the diet emphasises vegetables, pulses and has a relatively low meat consumption, and this eating pattern is reflected in the high MAI. However, consumption of two other key components of the MedDiet, namely olive oil and fish, is low, whereas by contrast saturated fat consumption is high due to the popularity of cooking with clarified butter (known as *samna* in Egypt). These figures are an argument in favour of emphasising the importance of the *whole* dietary pattern in reducing the risk of CVD, although other factors, such as smoking and health care access, could also be important.

---

[2] Similar reservations may also apply to other scoring systems for adherence to a MedDiet.

Many factors have been suggested that could contribute to changes in eating patterns in Mediterranean countries, and these include:

- Increased costs of some traditional Mediterranean foods (e.g. fish, olive oil). Depletion of fish from the Mediterranean sea has reduced consumption in Greece and Italy. However, fish consumption in Spain is still high – mostly due to using alternative supplies of fish from the Atlantic ocean and fish farming.
- Aspects of modernity [49]:
  - Changes in working patterns. This often results in fewer opportunities for a traditional lunch-time meal. Also, many modern jobs require far less physical activity than was the case in traditional Mediterranean society. Women working was associated with a decrease in consumption of pulses.
  - Increased availability of cheap industrialised foods.
  - New household appliances, which change food preservation and cooking techniques.
  - Migration
  - Tourism

Some of these changes particularly impact on poorer socio-economic groups whereas, by contrast, some are associated with increased purchasing power.

1.4.2 The Greek experience

Greece had the highest MAI in 1960–1965 (5.54) but this had decreased by 3.5 points by 2000–2005. This represents the largest reduction in adherence to the MedDiet over the last 40 years of any country (see Figure 1.8). Greece is also currently experiencing a dramatic rises in obesity rates, and it is estimated that one in five men and one in six women in Greece are now obese, and that approximately half the men and one-third of the women in Greece are overweight [50]. The situation is now serious in Greek children [51], and even Greek medical students have high rates of obesity [52]. Overall, Greece now has one of the highest rates of obesity in the developed world (Table 1.7).

Table 1.7   Obese population aged 15 and above. Data based on OECD (2010), 'Obesity', in OECD, *OECD Factbook 2010: Economic, Environmental and Social Statistics*, OECD Publishing, http://dx.doi.org/10.1787/factbook-2010-87-en

Country	Females	Males
France	10.4	10.5
Germany	12.8	14.4
Greece	18.3	14.3
Italy	9.2	10.6
Japan	3.3	3.4
Netherlands	12.2	10.2
Spain	14.7	15.1
Turkey	14.5	9.7
United Kingdom	24.4	23.6
United States	35.3	33.3

Limitations of comparing international obesity statistics

Comparisons of health statistics between countries is often fraught with difficulties due to differences in the way data are collected. In the case of obesity, data may be collected by experts or from self-reported surveys. However, self-reporting frequently underestimates the true situation. In addition, there is the consideration of whether or not to compensate for non-responders to self-reporting surveys: some countries do this but not others. Other differences between data from countries can include the age ranges that have been surveyed, and the year in which the data was collected. Hence national obesity figures only give a general indication of comparative obesity rates.

Several studies have been undertaken to examine whether the rise in obesity in Greece is linked to changing dietary patterns. Although the traditional Greek diet is often considered to represent the quintessential MedDiet, there have been major changes in eating patterns within the last generation. There is some evidence that reduced adherence to the MedDiet is linked to the rise in obesity in Greece [53], although the rise in obesity is also linked to reduced levels of physical activity and changes in socio-economic factors. The overall Greek population showed an increase in average calorie intake from 2900 kcal/per person/per day in the mid 1960s to 3700 kcal/per person/ per day by the 21st century, much of which can be attributed to increased consumption of animal fats [54]. There has also been a significant decline in physical activity. Socio-economic factors may also play a part in the large rise in obesity in Greek children: children are subject to high exposure of advertising for fast foods, and fat babies are still often seen as more desirable than thin children, possibly a legacy of deprivations during the Second World War. However, consumption of some traditional components of the MedDiet in Greece, such as olive oil and fruits and vegetables, is still high.

The rise of obesity in Cretans farmers is particularly poignant. Cretan farmers living in the 1960s were highlighted in the Seven Countries Study by Ancel Keys as representing a gold standard of healthy living, and this was attributed to a combination of their diet and relatively high levels of physical activity. In the 1960s their mean BMI was $22.9 kg/m^2$ (average weight 63 kg) for the 40–59 age group, but this had increased to a mean BMI of $29.8 kg/m^2$ (average weight 83 kg) by 2005 [55]. Energy intake cannot explain these changes since this *decreased* from 2820 kcal in the 1960s to 2412 kcal in 2005. Rather, the large reduction in physical activity from the 1960s to the 1990s is thought to be a contributory factor coupled with the low awareness on matters of health and diet of this socieconomic group [55].

1.4.3   Not all bad news

Although many Mediterranean countries are seeing a decrease in adherence to the MedDiet, other parts of the world have seen an increase in consumption of foods associated with the MedDiet. For example, much of the expansion in world consumption of olive oil over the last few years has been in non-Mediterranean countries such as the US, Northern Europe, Japan, Australia and Brazil. The availability of many foods associated with the MedDiet, such as olive oil, fruit and cereals, increased in non-Mediterranean northern Europe between the periods 1961–1965 and 2000–2004 [56].

1.4.4 Future prospects

The MedDiet is well placed to benefit from current consumer concerns related to eating and health due to the high consumption of fruits and vegetables, moderate consumption of dairy products and low consumption of red meat. In addition, its environmental impact is relatively low: Many Mediterranean foods can be grown locally (less 'air-miles'), and Mediterranean agriculture is associated with a lower production of greenhouse gases due to the low use of cattle raised under intensive conditions [57]. Indeed, even traditional Mediterranean foods such as Italian cheeses and hams are now being produced in the UK! [58]

References

1. Grigg, D. Food consumption in the Mediterranean region. *Tijdschrift voor Economische en Sociale Geografie*, 1999. **90**:391–409.
2. Janick, J. The origin of fruits, fruit growing, and fruit breeding. *Plant Breeding Rev*, 2005. **25**:255–320.
3. Salas-Salvado, J. et al. Diet and dietetics in al-Andalus. *Br J Nutr*, 2006. **96** Suppl 1:S100–4.
4. Nestle, M. Mediterranean diets: historical and research overview. *Am J Clin Nutr*, 1995. **61**:1313S–20S.
5. Trichopoulou, A. et al. Minutes of the Meeting on the Definition of the Traditional Mediterranean Diet. 2004.
6. Trichopoulou, A. et al. Traditional foods: why and how to sustain them. *Trends in Food Science & Technology*, 2006. **7**:498–504.
7. Keys, A. Mediterranean diet and public health: personal reflections. *Am J Clin Nutr*, 1995. **61**:1321S–3S.
8. German, J.B., Dillard, C.J. Saturated fats: what dietary intake? *Am J Clin Nutr*, 2004. **80**:550–559.
9. Pineo, C.E., Anderson, J.J.B. Cardiovascular benefits of the Mediterranean Diet. *Nutrition Today*, 2008. **43**:114–120.
10. Bach-Faig, A. et al. Evaluating associations between Mediterranean diet adherence indexes and biomarkers of diet and disease. *Public Health Nutr*, 2006. **9**:1110–1117.
11. Research. WCRFAIfC. Food, nutrition, physical activity, and the prevention of cancer: a global perspective. Washington DC: AICR, 2007.
12. Mason, J.B. et al. A temporal association between folic acid fortification and an increase in colorectal cancer rates may be illuminating important biological principles: a hypothesis. *Cancer Epidemiol Biomarkers Prev*, 2007. **16**:1325–1329.
13. Reguant-Aleix, J. et al. Mediterranean heritage: an intangible cultural heritage. *Public Health Nutr*, 2009. **12**:1591–1594.
14. Trichopoulou, A. et al. Modified Mediterranean diet and survival: EPIC-elderly prospective cohort study. *BMJ*, 2005. **330**:991.
15. Rivera, D. et al. Gathered Mediterranean food plants – ethnobotanical investigations and historical development. *Forum Nutr*, 2006. **59**:18–74.
16. Oldways. http://wwwoldwaysptorg/med_pyramidhtml 2009.
17. Simopoulos, A.P. The Mediterranean Food Guide. Greek column rather than an Egyptian pyramid. *Nutr Today*, 1996. **30**:54–61.
18. Fidanza, F., Alberti, A. The Healthy Italian Mediterranean Diet Temple Food Guide. *Nutrition Today*, 2005. **40**:71–8.
19. Gerber, M. Santé et alimentation Méditerranéenne au quotidien. Aix-en-Provence: Édisud, 2004.
20. Toobert, D.J. et al. Long-term effects of the Mediterranean lifestyle program: a randomized clinical trial for postmenopausal women with type 2 diabetes. *Int J Behav Nutr Phys Act*, 2007. **4**:1.
21. Iestra, J. et al. Lifestyle, Mediterranean diet and survival in European post-myocardial infarction patients. *Eur J Cardiovasc Prev Rehabil*, 2006. **13**:894–900.
22. Knoops, K.T. et al. Mediterranean diet, lifestyle factors, and 10-year mortality in elderly European men and women: the HALE project. *Jama*, 2004. **292**:1433–1439.

23   Padilla, M., Aubaille-Sallenave, F., Oberti B. *Eating behaviour and culinary practice*. John Libby Eurotext, 2001.

24. Bellisle, F. Infrequently asked questions about the Mediterranean diet. *Public Health Nutr*, 2009. **12**:1644–1647.

25. Pettinger, C., Holdsworth, M., Gerber, M. Meal patterns and cooking practices in Southern France and Central England. *Public Health Nutr*, 2006. **9**:1020–1026.

26. Esmarck, B. et al. Timing of postexercise protein intake is important for muscle hypertrophy with resistance training in elderly humans. *J Physiol*, 2001. **535**:301–311.

27. Kafatos, A. et al. Mediterranean diet of Crete: foods and nutrient content. *J Am Diet Assoc*, 2000. **100**:1487–1493.

28. Naska, A. et al. Siesta in healthy adults and coronary mortality in the general population. *Arch Intern Med*, 2007. **167**:296–301.

29. WCRF/AICR. World Cancer Research Fund/American Institute for Cancer Research. Food, Nutrition, Physical Activity, and the Prevention of Cancer: a Global Perspective. Washington DC: AICR, 2007.

30. Castillo-Garzon, M.J., Ruiz, J.R., Ortega, F.B, Gutierrez-Sainz, A. A Mediterranean diet is not enough for health: physical fitness is an important additional contributor to health for the adults of tomorrow. *World Rev Nutr Diet*, 2007. **97**:114–38.

31. Wong, A. Incident solar radiation and coronary heart disease mortality rates in Europe. *Eur J Epidemiol*, 2008. **23**:609–614.

32. Sofi, F., Cesari, F., Abbate, R., Gensini, G.F., Casini, A. Adherence to Mediterranean diet and health status: meta-analysis. *BMJ*, 2008. **337**:a1344.

33. Babio, N. et al. Adherence to the Mediterranean diet and risk of metabolic syndrome and its components. *Nutr Metab Cardiovasc Dis*, 2009. **19**:563–70.

34. Jacobs, D.R., Jr., Gross, M.D., Tapsell, L.C. Food synergy: an operational concept for understanding nutrition. *Am J Clin Nutr*, 2009. **89**:1543S–1548S.

35. Jacobs, D.R., Jr., Tapsell, L.C. Food, not nutrients, is the fundamental unit in nutrition. *Nutr Rev*, 2007. **65**:439–450.

36. Benetou, V. et al. Conformity to traditional Mediterranean diet and cancer incidence: the Greek EPIC cohort. *British Journal of Cancer*, 2008. **99**:191–195.

37. Rivellese, A.A. Diet and cardiovascular disease: beyond cholesterol. *Nutr Metab Cardiovasc Dis*, 2005. **15**:395–8.

38. Martinez-Gonzalez, M.A. et al. Mediterranean food pattern and the primary prevention of chronic disease: recent developments. *Nutr Rev*, 2009. **67** Suppl 1:S111–116.

39. Naska, A. et al. Dietary patterns and their socio-demographic determinants in 10 European countries: data from the DAFNE databank. *Eur J Clin Nutr*, 2006. **60**:181–90.

40. de Lorgeril, M., Salen, P. Modified Cretan Mediterranean diet in the prevention of coronary heart disease and cancer: an update. *World Rev Nutr Diet*, 2007. **97**:1–32.

41. Paolini, M., Nestle, M. Pitfalls of enzyme-based molecular anticancer dietary manipulations: food for thought. *Mutat Res*, 2003. **543**:181–189.

42. Liu, R.H. Health benefits of fruit and vegetables are from additive and synergistic combinations of phytochemicals. *Am J Clin Nutr*, 2003. **78**:517S–520S.

43. Pezzuto, J.M. Grapes and human health: a perspective. *J Agric Food Chem*, 2008. **56**:6777–6784.

44. Kris-Etherton, P., Eckel, R.H., Howard, B.V., St Jeor, S., Bazzarre, T.L. AHA Science Advisory: Lyon Diet Heart Study. Benefits of a Mediterranean-style, National Cholesterol Education Program/American Heart Association Step I Dietary Pattern on Cardiovascular Disease. *Circulation*, 2001. **103**:1823–5.

45. Mead, A. et al. Dietetic guidelines on food and nutrition in the secondary prevention of cardiovascular disease – evidence from systematic reviews of randomized controlled trials (second update, January 2006). *J Hum Nutr Diet*, 2006. **19**:401–419.

46. Trichopoulos, D., Lagiou, P. Mediterranean diet and overall mortality differences in the European Union. *Public Health Nutr*, 2004. **7**:949–951.

47. Baldini, M., Pasqui, F., Bordoni, A., Maranesi, M. Is the Mediterranean lifestyle still a reality? Evaluation of food consumption and energy expenditure in Italian and Spanish university students. *Public Health Nutr*, 2009. **12**:148–155.

48. da Silva, R. et al. Worldwide variation of adherence to the Mediterranean diet, in 1961–1965 and 2000–2003. *Public Health Nutr*, 2009. **12**:1676–1684.

49. Tessier, S., Gerber, M. Factors determining the nutrition transition in two Mediterranean islands: Sardinia and Malta. *Public Health Nutr*, 2005. 8:1286–1292.
50. Codrington, C., Sarri, K., Kafatos, A. Stakeholder appraisal of policy options for tackling obesity in Greece. *Obes Rev*, 2007. 8 Suppl 2:63–73.
51. Kosti, R.I. et al. Dietary habits, physical activity and prevalence of overweight/obesity among adolescents in Greece: the Vyronas study. *Med Sci Monit*, 2007. 13:CR437–444.
52. Bertsias, G., Mammas, I., Linardakis, M., Kafatos, A. Overweight and obesity in relation to cardiovascular disease risk factors among medical students in Crete, Greece. *BMC Public Health*, 2003. 3:3.
53. Panagiotakos, D.B., Chrysohoou, C., Pitsavos, C., Stefanadis, C. Association between the prevalence of obesity and adherence to the Mediterranean diet: the ATTICA study. *Nutrition*, 2006. 22:449–456.
54. Alexandratos, N. The Mediterranean diet in a world context. *Public Health Nutr*, 2006. 9:111–117.
55. Vardavas, C.I., Linardakis, M.K., Hatzis, C.M., Saris, W.H., Kafatos, A.G. Prevalence of obesity and physical inactivity among farmers from Crete (Greece), four decades after the Seven Countries Study. *Nutr Metab Cardiovasc Dis*, 2009. 19:156–62.
56. Vareiro, D. et al. Availability of Mediterranean and non-Mediterranean foods during the last four decades: comparison of several geographical areas. *Public Health Nutr*, 2009. 12:1667–1675.
57. Steinfeld, H., Gerber, P., Wassenaar, T., Castel, V., Rosales, M., de Haan, C. Livestock's long shadow. *FAO*, 2006.
58. Hargreaves, C. A Slice of Italy. *The Independent*, 7 January 2010, pp. 8–9.

Section 1
CONSTITUENTS

2 Constituents and Physiological Effects of Mediterranean Plant Foods

Summary

- Mediterranean plant foods are major sources of many essential nutrients including dietary fibre, essential fatty acids, various minerals including potassium, calcium and selenium, a wide range of vitamins (B vitamins, folate, vitamin C, provitamin A) and phytochemicals.
- The diverse types of plant foods and relatively high amounts (compared to a western diet) that are consumed as part of a MedDiet are important contributors to the health benefits of the MedDiet.
- There are quite high levels of dietary fibre and foods with a low glycaemic index in the MedDiet, and these will reduce the glycaemic load of a Mediterranean meal.
- Important sources of fats include nuts, seeds, pulses and green vegetables (both cultivated and collected from the wild).
- The MedDiet is a good source of B vitamins, and a particularly good source of folates due to the high consumption of vegetables.
- Most vitamin D is derived from sun exposure, and so people in sunny Mediterranean countries may particularly benefit from the possible health benefits of vitamin D against chronic degenerative disorders.
- The MedDiet is a rich source of phytochemicals including phenolics, terpenes, and sulphur-containing compounds.
- There are diverse sources and types of phenolics in the MedDiet, compared to the more limited range in a typical western diet.
- Dietary sources of terpenes include herbs (monoterpenes), olives (triterpenes), pulses, nuts and seeds (phytosterols), and red, orange and yellow fruits and vegetables (carotenoids).
- Carotenoids with provitamin A activity are an important source of vitamin A due to the low intake of meat.
- Sulphur-containing compounds are found in alliums and cruciferous vegetables, and the bioactive forms are generated when the plant cells are damaged.

2.1 Introduction

This chapter discusses significant aspects of the nutrient composition of the MedDiet. It particularly emphasises how some of these nutrients differ quantitatively or qualitatively from other diets and how these constituents have been linked to biochemical and physiological changes in experimental systems and in the body. Extending these observations to possible health benefits in humans requires an appreciation of interpreting epidemiological studies and so these discussions are deferred until later.

2.2   Carbohydrates

The MedDiet is characterised by the consumption of a diverse range of carbohydrates, and the major groups of carbohydrates and typical sources in the MedDiet are shown in Table 2.1. One carbohydrate that is consumed in relatively low amounts by many Mediterranean people is the sugar lactose. This is because the preference in the MedDiet is for cheese and yogurt rather than fresh milk. Cheese and yogurt are usually low in lactose because this sugar is removed in the whey during cheese making, and fermentation by lactobacilli – especially during yogurt making – converts some of the lactose to lactic acid[1]. Indeed, there is a high prevalence of lactose intolerance amongst Mediterranean people (which reaches 71% in Sicily and Turkey and is even higher in North African populations [1]), so fresh milk consumption is not advisable for these individuals. For the infant, however, lactose and other milk oligosaccharides from breast milk are thought to be very important for health since they help establish a population of bifidobacteria in the infant gut.

2.2.1   Glycaemic index

The carbohydrate profiles of diets are of particular interest because of their effects on postprandial glucose levels and potential effects on insulin resistance and diabetes. Carbohydrates that result in a postprandial rise in blood glucose are referred to as 'glycaemic', and the ability of a carbohydrate to raise blood glucose levels is quantified by its 'glycaemic index' (GI). Foods with a high GI produce a higher peak in postprandial blood glucose and a greater overall blood glucose response (which is calculated during the first 2 h after consumption) than do foods with a low GI. The primary factor determining the GI of a food is the content of readily-available glucose residues of the carbohydrates present in the food.

Many Mediterranean plant foods, such as unprocessed grains, legumes, non-starchy fruits and vegetables, have a low GI, although honey and bread – typical foods in the MedDiet – do have higher GI values (Table 2.2). However, the overall GI of the MedDiet is generally considered to be quite low [2].

Food preparation can have a significant impact on the GI of a foodstuff, and this is an important consideration when assessing the overall GI of a Mediterranean meal. For example, juicing a fruit raises the GI by releasing sugars (extrinsic sugars) that in an intact fruit are present inside cells (intrinsic sugars), and are associated with other cellular constituents which slow their rate of absorption. Ripe fruit generally has a lower GI than unripe fruit since starch (high GI) is converted to sugars (including fructose with a low GI) as the fruit ripens [4]. An Italian study found that potato dumplings, which are prepared by mixing cooked, mashed potato with wheat flour and boiling a second time, had a significantly lower GI than equivalent mashed potatoes [2]. Although mashing potatoes increases their GI, the authors of this study observed by

---

[1] However, lactose may be added to start the fermentation process in the commercial production of yogurt, and residual lactose levels can be high.

Table 2.1 Main carbohydrates in the MedDiet.

Carbohydrate (dp)	Sub-group	Examples	Sources in MedDiet
sugars (1–2)	monosaccharides	glucose, fructose	fruits, berries, honey
	disaccharides	sucrose	fruits, berries, vegetables
	sugar alcohols	sorbitol, mannitol, xylitol	some fruits
oligosaccharides (3–9)		raffinose, stachyose, verbascose inulin[1], fructo-oligosaccharides	pulses, some vegetables onions, leeks, asparagus
polysaccharides (≥10)	starch (α-glucans)	amylose, amylopectin, modified starchs	cereals, root vegetables, legumes
	non-starch polysaccharides (NSPs)	cellulose, hemicellulose, pectin, arabinoxylans, β-glucan, glucomannans, plant gums and mucilages	diverse plant foods

dp, degree of polymerization.
[1]Usually present as a mixture of dp's which can vary from 2 to 90.

Table 2.2 GI values of some foods in the MedDiet (adapted from [3]). With permission from John Wiley & Sons.

Food	Low GI	Medium GI	High GI
Bread	breads containing grains	pitta bread	white, brown, wholemeal
Pastas	pasta (hard wheat)	couscous	
Rice		white, brown	
Beans and pulses	peas, lentils, nuts		broad beans
Potatoes	new potatoes in their skins	boiled old potatoes	mashed potatoes
Fruit	most fresh fruit	dried fruit, apricots, peaches	fruit juices, water melons
Vegetables	all green and salad vegetables, carrots	beetroot, sweetcorn, sweet potato	pumpkin
Dairy produce	plain yogurt		
Sugars	fructose	sucrose, honey	glucose

scanning electron microscopy that 'the potato dumplings had a compact structure similar to that observed in other low-GI starchy foods. This is consistent with a reduction of the rate of starch accessibility owing to a combination of compact form and need for protein digestion to free trapped starch granules' (so-called resistant starch).

A number of other factors may influence GI values, as shown in Table 2.3. One of these factors is the type of starch present in a foodstuff. Starch exists as a mixture of amylose, a linear chain of glucose units linked by α 1, 4 bonds, and amylopectin, which in addition to α 1,4 linked glucose also has branches linked via α 1,6 linkages. Amylopectin is more easily hydrolysed by α-amylase in the gut than amylose, so foods with a higher proportion of amylopectin have a higher GI. Cooking also increases the GI by causing the starch grains to swell. Processing starch-rich foods can affect granule size and hence influence the GI. The acidity of a meal is one factor that

Table 2.3 Factors that affect the GI of a food [5]. With permission from Springer Science + Business Media (Springer).

Factor	Example
Type of monosaccharide	glucose
	fructose
	galactose
Type of starch	amylose
	amylopectin
	starch-nutrient interactions
	resistant starch
Cooking or food processing	degree of gelatinisation of starch
	particle size
	food form
	cellular structure
Food components	fat and protein
	dietary fibre
	anti-nutrients
	organic acids

may lower its overall GI, and a number of sources of acidity have been demonstrated to lower the GI of a Mediterranean meal including sourdough breads (common in Mediterranean countries such as Sardinia, Israel, and Lebanon) and vinegar [4]. Soluble fibre also tends to lower GI values [2], and the high level of soluble fibre in the MedDiet is thought to contribute to the reduced incidence of diabetes despite a high carbohydrate intake [5]. A regular meal pattern (and not consuming high GI foods between meals) is likely to be another important feature of the MedDiet that reduces the glycaemic response to a meal [6].

2.2.2 Honey

Honey is the traditional sweetener in the MedDiet and is used in place of sugar (sucrose). Honey is frequently found in combination with almonds and other nuts in sweet desserts such as Greek *baklava*, Southern French nougat and its Spanish equivalent known as *turron*. The aromas of honeys vary widely depending on the flower source, and some honeys are much sought after; the honeys produced from rosemary around Narbonne in the Languedoc region of France have been well-known since the time of the Romans.

The main sugars in honey are fructose and glucose – present in approximately equal amounts, together with smaller amounts of disaccharides and oligosaccharides (Table 2.4). The other noteworthy components in honey are various polyphenols (56–500 mg/kg). The overall compositions of honeys from different regions can vary widely.

In one study, the GI values of honeys were found to vary between 32 and 87 with an average GI of 55 [7]; honeys with a higher fructose content will have a lower GI. This compares with a GI of 68 for sucrose, the main sweetener also likely to be used in cooking. A high fructose intake, mainly from the use of high fructose corn syrup, is linked with obesity in the western diet, but feeding honey to rats did not produce a comparable increase in triglycerides (see [7]). It has also been

Table 2.4 Approximate composition of honey (from [7]). With permission from American College of Nutrition.

Component	Amount (g/100 g)
Water	16.8
Total sugars	80.1
Fructose	35
Glucose	28.7
Disaccharides	2.6
Oligosaccharides	13.8
Minerals	0.6
Amino acids, proteins	0.5
Acids	0.8

Table 2.5 Physiological properties of dietary carbohydrates [11]. Reprinted with permission from Macmillan Publishers Ltd, copyright 2007 Nature.

	Glycaemic	Cholesterol-lowering	Increase calcium absorption	Source of SCFA[1]	Promote healthy gut microflora	Increase stool output	Immuno-modulatory
monosaccharides	✓						
disaccharides	✓		✓				
sugar alcohols				✓		✓	
oligosaccharides			✓	✓	✓		✓
starch	✓			✓[2]		✓	
NSP		✓		✓		✓[3]	

NSP, non-starch polysaccharides.
[1]Short chain fatty acids.
[2]Resistant starch only.
[3]Some forms of NSP only.

hypothesised that fructose consumption may result in an increase in plasma urate, which increases the antioxidant capacity of plasma.

2.2.3 Physiological effects of carbohydrates

Carbohydrates have a variety of influences on human physiology and some of these are shown in Table 2.5. These physiological changes may have important implications for human health. For example, complex carbohydrates that help prevent rapid increases in blood sugar, or those that act as dietary fibre, are linked with a reduced incidence of some cancers and with a reduced risk of CVD [8]. The importance of these observations in relation to the MedDiet is considered in Chapters 11 and 12. Adherence to a MedDiet has also been found to reduce post-prandial glucose increases in diabetic patients [9] and this is associated with an improvement in insulin sensitivity [10] (see Chapter 10).

Table 2.6 Sources of dietary fibre in the MedDiet.

Fibre	Examples	Food sources	Role
Insoluble dietary fibre	cellulose, some hemi-celluloses, lignin	wheat bran, edible skins of seeds of fruits and vegetables, pulses	increase stool weight and decrease transit time
Soluble dietary fibre	β-glucans, pectins, mucilages, some hemicelluloses	fruits, oats, barley, pulses	reduce lipid and glucose absorption, some are fermentable
Resistant starch	RS1 – physically enclosed starch, RS3 retrograded starch	RS1 – milled grains or seeds; RS3 – cooked and cooled potato, bread, rice	fermentable to SCFA
Prebiotics	inulin, oligofructose, lactulose, oligosaccharides	onion, garlic, leek, pulses	stimulate beneficial bacteria in colon
Animal-derived fibre	chitin	shells of crustaceans	cholesterol lowering

2.2.4 Fibre

Composition

Some carbohydrates, including sugar alcohols, many oligosaccharides and non-starch polysaccharides, escape digestion in the small intestine and reach the large intestine intact. These carbohydrates constitute a major part of 'dietary fibre' (Table 2.6). Most of the non-starch polysaccharides are obtained in the diet from plants, where they are present as components of plant cell walls or as storage carbohydrates. The so-called primary plant cell wall consists of a mesh of cellulose (a polymer of glucose), together with pectin and various forms of hemicellulose. Hemicelluloses are a diverse family that includes various polymeric sugars (known as glycans) composed of mixtures of glucose, galactose, arabinose, rhamnose and xylose. In some plants a secondary cell wall develops which contains lignin. Lignin is not a carbohydrate, but rather a complex polyphenolic substance. Lignin is found in woody tissues and in seeds, wheat bran and apples and is highly resistant to degradation. Cellulose, some hemicelluloses and lignin make up the bulk of insoluble dietary fibre.

Some MedDiets are associated with the consumption of significant quantities of a non-plant-derived insoluble dietary fibre, namely chitin. This is the major constituent of the shells of crustaceans and is consumed on a regular basis in some Mediterranean countries in fish soups and stews since these often include the finely ground shells of prawns and other crustaceans. There is some limited evidence that specific derivatives of chitin may help prevent colon cancer, but it is not established whether or not chitin from the diet has similar health benefits.

Soluble fibres include pectin, β-glucans, inulin and some hemicelluloses. Pectin is present in the cell walls of some fruits and is partially broken down during fruit ripening. Pectin is well known for its gelling properties (*pektikos* is the Greek for 'congealing'). B-glucans are found in oats, barley and rye, whereas the major sources of inulin in the MedDiet are onions and grain products. Inulin is the second most common storage carbohydrate produced by plants after starch and acts as an energy reserve. Onions build up reserves of inulin during their first year of growth and they would then use this if they were allowed to commence a second year of growth. Inulin is also found in leeks, garlic, asparagus, Jerusalem artichokes and the roots of chicory and dandelions. Inulin is a polymer of fructose (i.e. a fructan) and the chain length can vary depending on the food source. Fructose polymers with degrees of polymer-isation of <10 are sometimes referred to as oligo-fructose or fructo-oligosaccharides. Although inulin is quite heat stable, prolonged cooking breaks it down into fructose, which gives slow-cooked onions their sweetness. Inulin is an example of a fermentable soluble fibre. Gums are forms of dietary fibre added to various processed foods, but these will not constitute part of a traditional MedDiet.

  Pulses are important sources of both insoluble and soluble dietary fibre in many Mediterranean countries. Chickpeas and lentils are especially widely consumed in Provence (France), Spain and North African Mediterranean countries. Hemicelluloses (arabinans) and cellulose were identified as the main forms of insoluble dietary fibre in chickpeas [12]. In addition to these insoluble fibres, some pulses also contain high levels of galactose-containing oligosaccharides (α-galactosides) such as raffinose, stachyose and verbascose. Another α-galactoside called ciceritol has been identified as the major type in chickpeas [12]. These α-galactosides pass undigested into the large intestine where they are fermented by bacteria, leading to flatulence. Soaking and cooking techniques can significantly reduce the levels of these sugars prior to consumption and thus flatulence whilst still retaining the desirable dietary fibre components. These galactosides may also have beneficial effects since studies have shown that they also increase the levels of beneficial bifidobacteria in the colon.

Physiological effects

The physiological effects of fibre include reducing cholesterol absorption and regulating gut transit time. Some types of soluble fibre, including inulin, other oligosaccharides, pectin, β-glucan, lactulose and resistant starch, are fermentable by gut bacteria and are referred to as 'prebiotics' – that is, a food source that stimulates the growth of beneficial gut bacteria, particularly lactobacilli and bifidobacteria (see box below). Dietary prebiotics are particularly high in some fruits, vegetables, legumes and pulses (see Table 2.6) and hence are consumed in significant quantities in the MedDiet. It has been suggested that in non-Mediterranean European countries, there is a higher proportion of insoluble fibre, mainly from grains. Hence, although total intake of dietary fibre in Mediterranean and non-Mediterranean countries may be similar quantitatively (one estimate is 20 g per day [13]), there are significant qualitative differences. The estimated intake of fibre required to perform a prebiotic function is about 2–10 g per day. One study of the contemporary Spanish diet found intake to be only about 1.5 g per day [14] although levels may well be higher for a more traditional MedDiet. Evidence that a high intake of dietary fibre is associated with a reduced risk of CVD, diabetes, obesity, some gastrointestinal diseases including acid reflux and duodenal ulcers and some forms of cancer is discussed in later chapters [15, 16].

Gut bacteria

The adult human gut is thought to contain about 100 trillion (10^{14}) micro-organisms – which is ten times more than the total number of human cells in the body. These are mainly strict anaerobes such as *Bacteroides* and *Bifidobacterium*, with smaller numbers of facultative anaerobes which include *Lactobacillus* spp.

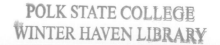

and *Enterobacteriaceae*. Some bacteria such as *Streptococcus bovis*, *Bacteriodes*, Clostridia and *Helicobacter pylori* are implicated in the pathogenesis of gastro-intestinal cancers, whereas there is evidence that other bacteria such as *Lactobacillus acidophilus* and *Bifidobacterium longum* inhibit colon tumour development.

The MedDiet is characterised by a high intake of fermented dairy products, such as live yogurt and goat's cheese, and these are good sources of beneficial bacteria such as Bifidobacteria and *Lactobacillus* spp. [17]. Beneficial bacteria consumed from food sources are referred to as probiotics. It is thought that there is a high attrition rate as probiotic bacteria transit through the stomach and upper gut. Once in the colon, dietary prebiotics will help the remaining probiotic bacteria to thrive, and hence a diet combining probiotics and prebiotics is optimal. (Manufacturers of probiotics are now mimicking natural dietary interactions by developing so-called synbiotic products that combine probiotic bacteria-rich yogurts together with a prebiotic food source.)

Colonic bacteria produce a wide variety of fermentation products, both harmful and beneficial, from dietary substances. Some fermentation products have potential cancer-preventative properties and these include butyrate (a fermentation product from fibre), conjugated linoleic acid (from linoleic acid), enterolactone (from the lignan secoisolariciresinol found in flaxseed and sesame seed) and urolithins A and B (from ellagic acid found in strawberries, walnuts and pomegranates) [18]. These fermentation products may variously help protect against colon cancer by controlling colon cell proliferation, preventing the overgrowth of pathogenic micro-organisms and by stimulating intestinal immunity. Interestingly, there is wide variation between individuals in their ability to generate these beneficial metabolites, and there is now good evidence that this is due to variations in the colonic microflora between individuals [19]. Other colonic bacteria, without glucuronidase activity, induce a decrease in the recirculation of oestrogens and facilitate oestrogen excretion, thus decreasing exposure to the potential tumour-promoting activity of oestrogens [20].

2.3 Fats

Plant foods are an important source of fats in the MedDiet. Olive oil is the major source of monounsaturated fatty acids (MUFAs) (see Chapter 6), although some types of nuts are an additional source (Table 2.7).

There are several plant sources of polyunsaturated fatty acids (PUFAs) in the MedDiet. The *n*-6 (omega-6) fatty acid linoleic acid (18:2 *n*-6) (LA) is found in nuts, and it is the predominant fatty acid in many seeds such as sunflower seeds and corn, and hence in oils made from these seeds. Due to their lower cost, corn oil and sunflower oil are increasingly replacing olive oil for cooking in some Mediterranean countries. Sunflower and pumpkin seeds are eaten with an aperitif in some Mediterranean countries. It is noteworthy that, unlike seed oils, seeds retain their anti-oxidants and this may help reduce the increased oxidant stress in the body resulting from consuming PUFAs.

Many Mediterranean plant foods are rich sources of the *n*-3 fatty acid α-linolenic acid (ALA) (18:3 *n*-3), and a balanced MedDiet readily achieves an intake of 1–2 g per day which satisfies the recommended intake of ALA of ≥ 0.5% total energy intake. Walnuts are one of the best sources, four walnuts providing about 1.2 g of ALA [22]. Other types of nuts contain far lower levels of ALA. Some vegetables, such as spinach and pulses, and herbs are also good sources of ALA (Table 2.8).

Table 2.7   Sources of MUFA in the MedDiet (based on [21]).

Food	MUFA (g/100 g oil)
Olive oil	76
Almonds	32
Hazelnuts	46
Pine nuts	19
Pistachios	23
Walnuts	9

Table 2.8   ALA content of various plant foods (based on [22, 25]).

Food	ALA per portion (g)	Portion size (g)
white beans	0.29	135
chickpeas	0.15	135
red lentils	0.14	135
green lentils	0.11	135
peas	0.06	135
purslane	0.32	80
spinach	0.22–0.48	250
lettuce	0.06	80
walnuts	1.2	4 walnuts

The richest known plant source of ALA is purslane, a leafy plant resembling lamb's lettuce. Purslane is a common ingredient in many Mediterranean countries such as Greece and is generally collected from the wild. Purslane has been reported to have quite high levels of oxalic acid and so is not recommended for people with a predisposition to kidney stones. Many other wild plants are also rich in ALA [23] and this could contribute to their health benefits [24].

ALA is the metabolic precursor for the long chain n-3 PUFAs eicosapentaenoic acid (EPA) (20:5 *n*-3) and docosahexaenoic acid (DHA) (22:6 *n*-3). Humans can accumulate some EPA from plant sources of ALA since we have a limited ability to convert ALA into EPA. For example, eating about four walnuts every day, a rich source of ALA, was found to significantly boost levels of EPA in volunteers [22]. However, further conversion to DHA in humans is thought to be very low and, correspondingly, DHA levels did not alter after eating walnuts [22]. Terrestrial plants do not themselves convert ALA into EPA and DHA and hence are not a source of these longer chain fatty acids. By contrast, phytoplankton do readily convert ALA into EPA and DHA, and this provides a ready source of these fatty acids for fish, and subsequently for humans.

2.4   Organic acids

Organic acids give fruits and vegetables their tartness. Commonly-occurring organic acids in plants include malic acid, citric acid, oxalic acid and ascorbic acid (ascorbic acid is considered in the Section 2.6). The proportion of sugar to acid often increases as fruits ripen and this changes a previously unpalatable fruit into one that is readily eaten. Oxalic acid is a common constituent of green leafy vegetables, parsley, beetroot, carrots and tea. High levels (up to 1–2 g/100 g wet weight) are present in spinach and purslane [26], two popular ingredients in Mediterranean cuisine. Oxalic acid is a well-known inhibitor of calcium absorption, due to the formation of insoluble complexes, but studies indicate that it does not significantly influence iron absorption [27].

2.5 Minerals

Calcium is necessary for bone development. Levels build up during adolescence and start to decrease from adulthood, sometimes to such an extent that osteoporosis may develop. Milk from cows and dairy products is the main source of calcium for many populations in northern Europe and the US, but yogurt and cottage from goat and sheep milk will be more important in the MedDiet. Some Mediterranean plant foods are also good sources of calcium, such as almonds (250 mg/100 g), oranges (40 mg/100 g) and cruciferous vegetables (25–30 mg/100 g). Consumption of 15–20 almonds, two oranges and a dish of cruciferous vegetables provides the same amount of calcium as 30 g of hard cheese, and without the saturated fat [28]. Potassium helps prevent hypertension and contributes to calcium metabolism. It is widely distributed in fruits and vegetables (100–300 mg/100 g).

Major sources of selenium in the MedDiet are cereal products, garlic, fish and sesame seeds. Uptake of selenium from the soil into plants is highly variable depending on the levels present in the soil, and levels in animal products are related to their feed. Selenium is involved in antioxidant defences. Selenium is essential for the synthesis of glutathione peroxidase, an enzyme that inactivates hydrogen peroxide by using glutathione as a reducing agent (see Chapter 9). Selenium is incorporated into glutathione peroxidase (and other selenium-containing proteins) as part of the amino acid selenocysteine. This selenocysteine residue is critical for the functioning of selenium-containing proteins. Like other non-essential amino acids, selenocysteine can be synthesised by the body. It uses the codon UGA that can also function as a stop codon in protein synthesis, and selenocysteine is now considered as the 21st naturally-occurring amino acid in the body. Selenium can replace sulphur in some sulphur-containing phytochemicals such as allicin (which is found in garlic), and this will tend to occur in soils that are rich in selenium. Some Se-containing phytochemicals have superior health benefits, such as anti-cancer activity, at least in experimental systems, compared to their S-containing counterparts [29].

2.6 Vitamins

2.6.1 Water soluble vitamins

B vitamins

Although animal products[2] are a major source of B vitamins, cereals also make a significant contribution. B group vitamins are precursors for cofactors for many enzymes involved in metabolic reactions. For example, riboflavin (Vitamin B_2) is the precursor for FAD. FAD, and its reduced form $FADH_2$, are involved in oxidation-reduction reactions. $FADH_2$ reduces NADP to NADPH, and NAPDH in turn can reduce glutathione (GSSG) to reduced glutathione (GSH). GSH is one of the main

---

[2] For example, the tradition in some Mediterranean countries of preserving pork liver provides a source of vitamins B_9 and B_{12}.

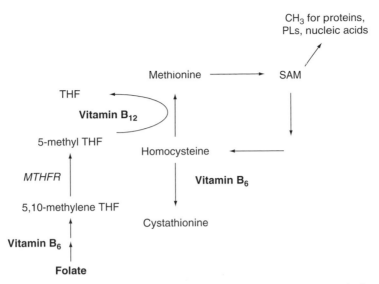

Figure 2.1   Roles of folate, vitamin B_6 and vitamin B_{12} in homocysteine metabolism. MTHFR: methylene tetrahydrofolate reductase; THF: tetrahydrofolate; SAM: S-adenosyl methionine; PLs: phospholipids.

reductants in the cell and it helps protect against many chronic degenerative disorders associated with oxidative stress (see Chapter 9).

Folates (also called vitamin B_9) are present in liver and leafy vegetables and other dietary sources mainly as 5-methyl tetrahydrofolate (THF) and 10-formyl THF. Folate intake in a traditional MedDiet is high, probably because of the high intake of fruits and vegetables, and plasma folate levels were found to be a good biomarker for adherence to a MedDiet [30]. Cancer prevention by a diet rich in folate is thought to be linked to the role of folate as a cofactor for nucleotide synthesis and DNA methylation, processes that affect carcinogenesis (see Chapter 12). Folate, together with vitamins B_6 and B_{12}, is also linked to a reduced risk of CVD. Together, these vitamins reduce the level of homocysteine, a risk factor for CVD, by converting it to methionine (Figure 2.1).

Vitamin C

Vitamin C is a water soluble antioxidant and also regenerates vitamin E from the radical formed during redox reactions. Severe vitamin C deficiency causes scurvy, but a mild deficiency may be associated with immune deficiency. Vitamin C is found mainly in citrus fruits which are widely eaten in Mediterranean countries, and orange juice is the primary source of vitamin C for many people. Other sources are tomatoes, sweet peppers, strawberries and cruciferous vegetables [28]. Fruits and vegetables should be eaten raw since vitamin C is not heat stable.

2.6.2   Fat soluble vitamins

Pro-vitamin A and vitamin A

Vitamin A is a lipid soluble vitamin that is important for vision and vitamin A deficiency (xerophthalmia) can lead to blindness. Animal products are the only sources of preformed vitamin A, but these are not significant in the MedDiet. Instead, most vitamin A is obtained from pro-vitamin A carotenoids such as α-carotene, β-carotene and β-cryptoxanthin which are present in some yellow, orange and red fruits and vegetables (see Section 2.7.4). Vitamin A is important for controlling cellular differentiation, and deficiencies lead to skin alterations and are associated with some cancers.

Vitamin D

'It is estimated that one billion people worldwide are either vitamin D insufficient or deficient' [31].

For most people, more than 90% of their vitamin D requirement comes from exposure to the sun, and this is probably especially true for people living in the sunny Mediterranean. However, vitamin D will be considered in this chapter on plant foods. The most overt signs of severe vitamin D deficiency are rickets in children and osteomalacia and osteoporosis in adults, and this reflects the role of vitamin D in increasing calcium uptake and enhancing bone formation. In addition to these well-established roles for vitamin D, there is now increasing evidence that low vitamin D status increases the risk for a wide range of other conditions, including some types of cancer (such as colon, prostate, breast), diseases with an autoimmune component such as type 1 diabetes and multiple sclerosis, and asthma [32–34]. Part of this evidence comes from the observation that living at higher latitudes is associated with an increased risk of these disorders [35]. Since higher latitudes receive less overhead sunshine, this reduces vitamin D production. Based on these observations, it has been proposed that sunlight, and thus higher vitamin D status, could be a factor contributing to the lower levels of some chronic degenerative disorders in Mediterranean countries [36].

Vitamin D is synthesised from the precursor 7-dehydrocholesterol in the skin. 7-Dehydrocholesterol is converted into pre-vitamin D by sunlight (UVB, 290–315 nm), and this is then converted, first in the liver and then in the kidneys, into biologically active vitamin D (1,25-dihydroxy-vitamin D_3) (Figure 2.2). Hence vitamin D is not a true vitamin since it does not need to be supplied by the diet, but rather is often considered to be more analogous to a steroid hormone. If sun exposure is restricted, then vitamin D levels can be low. This is true even in sunny Mediterranean countries since elderly Greeks living in institutions and Muslim women wearing the veil are two groups that have been found to have low vitamin D levels [37].

Oily fish are one of the few good dietary sources of vitamin D, and levels ranging between about 100–1000 IUs per serving have been reported. The higher levels are present in the fat and red muscle of wild fish with the fat of herring and the red muscle of tuna being especially rich sources. Farmed fish are a good source as long as they have been fed a fish diet, since these receive feed naturally rich in vitamin D, whereas fish fed pelleted food receive far lower amounts of vitamin D [39]. There are various estimates of the optimal daily requirement of vitamin D required for humans, with some recent evaluations putting this as high as 2000 IUs per day [40]. This amount would be difficult to achieve from dietary sources. By contrast, sunbathing for 15–30 minutes can provide 10,000–20,000 IUs [34]. Since it is generally considered that dietary sources of vitamin D

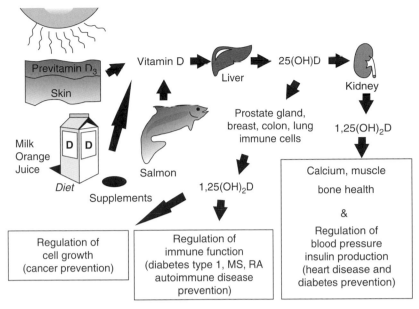

Figure 2.2 Production and physiology of vitamin D [38]. With permission from Elsevier.

are insufficient to compensate for lack of sunshine, foods (such as milk and orange juice) are supplemented with this vitamin in some countries.

Vitamin D acts via binding nuclear receptors, and this is congruent with thinking of vitamin D as a steroid hormone (most of which act via nuclear receptors) rather than as a vitamin. Many tissues express vitamin D receptors, and these are implicated in diverse physiological and pathological processes. Mice engineered not to express vitamin D receptors (so-called knockout mice) have increased numbers of chemically-induced tumours at some sites compared to normal mice treated with these chemicals [41]. Vitamin D receptors belong to a family of nuclear receptors which also includes receptors for vitamin A and for factors activated in response to xenobiotics, and these different receptors interact in complex and coordinated ways. These nuclear receptors provide a framework that helps explain the diverse processes in which vitamin D is implicated, including immunoregulation, cell growth and cell death, the production of insulin and renin [32] and in the intestinal detoxification of dietary toxins [31]. The vitamin D receptor may also play a role in triggering defences against viral and mycobacterial infections, and low winter sunshine/low vitamin D status has been even postulated to explain the higher rates of flu in the winter months [42].

The precise role of vitamin D in cancer and other diseases has not yet been fully established, and this is complicated by other dietary components such as folate which can modify the actions of vitamin D [43]. However, many nutritionists now feel that current concerns over sun exposure and skin cancer should be balanced with the need for moderate sunshine in order to allow the body to produce adequate vitamin D. Since the vitamin D status of most Mediterranean people is due to their exposure to sunlight, rather than to their diet, sun exposure is a possible confounding factor in epidemiological studies when considering Mediterranean people, their diet and their health.

Vitamin D and human evolution

Vitamin D has played an important role for animals and plants for millions of years. Since vitamin D absorbs radiation in the same wavelength band as proteins and DNA (290–320 nm), it has been suggested that it may have played a sun-protective role since the beginning of life on Earth [39]. Early humans evolved in Africa under the sun, and one of the traits that evolved was the ability to use sunlight to convert the vitamin D precursor 7-dehydrocholesterol in the skin into pre-vitamin D. As humans migrated out of Equatorial regions to more northerly latitudes with decreasing sunlight, so melanin pigmentation decreased, and it has been suggested that the main reason for this was to enable enough vitamin D to be made in the skin.

Vitamin E

The main sources of vitamin E are vegetable oils, especially sunflower oil (30–80 mg/100 ml) and safflower oil (30 mg/100 ml), whereas olive oil contains only a moderate amount (12–15 mg/100 ml). Nuts frequently consumed in the MedDiet are a good source of vitamin E (almonds 25 mg/100 g; pistachios 5 mg/100 g). Vitamin E deficiency is associated with neurological and neuromuscular disorders. Vitamin E is a lipid soluble antioxidant vitamin that blocks the lipid peroxide chain reaction. The radical that is formed is regenerated by vitamin C. Vitamin E also stabilises cell membranes, and decreases thromboxane synthesis. In experimental systems, vitamin E protects against oxidation of LDL, and atherosclerotic plaques from rupture. However, intervention studies with vitamin E against CVD have produced conflicting results (see Chapter 11).

2.7 Phytochemicals

A huge body of evidence now suggests that phytochemicals contribute to the health benefits of plant foods (see Chapters 10–13). Many synonyms for the term 'phytochemical' are used. To a plant biochemist, phytochemicals are often referred to as 'plant secondary metabolites' to reflect their metabolic origin. Nutritionists may refer to phytochemicals as 'bioactives' or, somewhat disparagingly, as 'non-nutrients'.

It is estimated that many plant genomes contain more than 40,000 genes whereas, by comparison, the human genome contains only about 20,000–25,000 genes [44]. One of the main reasons for the extraordinarily high numbers of genes in some plants is their investment in genes needed to produce phytochemicals: about 15–20% of plant genes are for enzymes that synthesise secondary metabolites. Secondary metabolites are essential for plants since they must perform diverse functions which help compensate for the fact that, unlike animals, plants cannot run away from prey or adverse conditions, but rather must cope with literally being rooted to the spot. Overall, many thousands of phytochemicals have now been isolated from plant foods.

The diverse roles of phytochemicals for plants include defence against various adversities and attraction for reproduction (Table 2.9). As might be anticipated from these roles, plants respond to environmental factors by regulating the amounts and types of phytochemicals that they produce. This has important implications regarding levels of phytochemicals in food plants since growing conditions will influence

Table 2.9   Functions of phytochemicals for plants.

Defence against herbivores, microbes, viruses, competing plants
Signal compounds to attract pollinating or seed-dispersing animals
Protection from uv radiation and oxidants

Table 2.10   Internet databases for phytochemical content of plant foods.

Database	Description	URL
euroFIR BASIS	All phytochemicals Composition data and health benefits	www.polytec.dk/eBasis/Default.asp
Phenol-Explorer	Polyphenols only Composition data	www.phenol-explorer.eu/
USDA	Wide range of nutrients Composition data	www.nal.usda.gov/fnic/foodcomp/search/

phyochemical levels and so possibly also affect the health benefits of plant foods. This is discussed in Chapter 3.

The increasing awareness of the importance of phytochemicals for human health has stimulated the development of various internet data bases with information on the phytochemical composition of food plants (Table 2.10).

The MedDiet is a particularly rich source of phytochemicals due to the high consumption of a diverse range of plant foods. Although experimental studies have identified specific mechanisms of action for many individual phytochemicals, it is far less clear how phytochemicals act and interact *in toto* as part of an overall diet. There is evidence that a low intake of phytochemicals is associated with many age-related disorders (Chapters 10–13). However, currently there is insufficient understanding of the health benefits of individual phytochemicals to be able to ascribe recommended daily allowances (RDAs). (Although inroads in this direction are now being made for polyphenols [45].) The picture is complicated because the effects of low intakes of phytochemicals are observed in disorders that may have multiple environmental and genetic causes and that develop over many years. Also, individual phytochemicals may not play a precise role. For example, many phytochemicals are functionally interchangeable as antioxidants. There are, however, a few phytochemicals that play a more clearly defined role in disease prevention. A good example is the specific requirement of the eye for lutein and zeaxanthin, and a low intake of these phytochemicals has been linked to an increased risk of age-related macular degeneration (Chapter 13).

Although it is certainly not the case that all phytochemicals are benign, plant breeding has produced cultivars with reduced levels of toxic phytochemicals compared to their wild predecessors. Most plants that contain toxic phytochemicals are not consumed by humans, but in some cases processing techniques can reduce levels of toxic phytochemicals. For example, olives are inedible in their raw state, and must be extensively treated to reduce levels of the bitter phytochemical oleuropein before they can be consumed (see Chapter 5).

Table 2.11 Major phytochemical classes.

Class	Sub-classes of nutritional interest	Typical physico-chemical properties
Phenolics	Flavonoids	water soluble*
	Non-flavonoids	
Terpenes	Monoterpenes	volatile
	Carotenoids	fat soluble
	Phytosterols	fat soluble
Sulphur-containing compounds	Glucosinolates	water soluble
	Allium compounds	
Acetylenes		
Nitrogen-containing compounds	Alkaloids	stable

*When present as glycosides.

2.7.1 Classes of phytochemicals

Phytochemicals can be categorised into five basic classes as shown in Table 2.11 [46]. The vast majority of dietary phytochemicals are phenolics, terpenes or sulphur-containing compounds. Although caffeine is a commonly-consumed dietary alkaloid, most alkaloids are too toxic to be of dietary significance. Many alkaloids are, however, important pharmaceutical agents.

Useful information about the properties of a phytochemical can often be gleaned simply by knowing the class, or sub-class, to which it belongs. Broadly speaking, phytochemicals within a particular class share common physico-chemical properties, such as lipophilicity, and these physico-chemical properties can in turn influence many important aspects of a phytochemical such as its stability during cooking, absorption by the body and mode of action in the body. For example, carotenoids are fat soluble, and they are also moderately heat stable and so remain active during cooking (Table 2.11).

2.7.2 Sensory properties of phytochemicals

A visit to a Mediterranean market with its vibrant colours and aromatic smells is a feast for the senses. Since it is various phytochemicals that confer colour and flavour to plant foods, those responsible can be described as 'Nature's food additives'. More-over, some phytochemicals also act as natural defences against attack, be it from micro-organisms, insects or larger animals, and hence this analogy with artificial food additives can be extended to say that some phytochemicals are Nature's preservatives.

Colours

Certain classes of phytochemicals are responsible for the colours of fruits and vegetables. The yellow colour of some vegetables is due to the presence of the sub-class of phenolics known as flavonoids (*flavus* = yellow). The colour spectrum from orange to reds is frequently due to carotenoids, whereas reds to purples are often due to anthocyanins (Table 2.12). There is some overlap between phytochemicals on the colour spectrum; for example some carotenoids, like flavonoids, are yellow. Green

Table 2.12 The colour spectrum of Mediterranean food plants.

Colour	Class	Typical source
red	capsanthin (carotcnoid)	red pepper
	lycopene (carotenoid)	tomato
orange	β-carotene (carotenoid)	carrot
	β-cryptoxanthin (carotenoid)	orange juice
yellow-orange	zeaxanthin (carotenoid)	corn
yellow	lutein (carotenoid)	leafy vegetables
	flavonoids	leafy vegetables
green	cholorophyll	all green vegetables
blue to violet	anthocyanins	many types of berries

colouration is due to the presence of chlorophyll and this may mask the presence of other pigments. These other colours may become apparent during plant development as the chlorophyll breaks down revealing other colours, such as occurs during the ripening of fruits.

Smell and taste

The human genome has more genes dedicated to the sense of smell than to any other function (about 1000, although only about one third of these are functional) [47]. Smell can be defined as the recognition of external odour molecules by the nose. The perception of 'flavour' is a more complex phenomenon, and is due to stimulation of both the taste receptors (sweet, salt sour, bitter and unami) on the tongue and to stimulation of olfactory receptors at the back of the nose (retronasal smell) by volatile molecules that are emitted by chewing food.

Smell versus flavour perception

Smell = perception of external odour molecules by the nose (orthonasal)
Flavour perception = perception of taste + internal volatile molecules (retronasal smell)

The psychological response to taste is thought to be 'hard-wired' from birth: sweet is pleasant whereas bitter is unpleasant. By contrast, response to odour is thought to be mostly learnt [47]. This could have important implications for acceptance of a Mediterranean dietary pattern by those individuals unfamiliar with Mediterranean foods, since strong-tasting unfamiliar Mediterranean foods such as garlic and anchovies may provoke a strongly adverse response.

Many different types of phytochemicals contribute to the aroma and taste of plant foods [48] (Table 2.13). Monoterpenes, a sub-class of terpenes, impart the pleasant aroma of many fruits and herbs. Isothiocyanates are responsible for many of the sulphurous smells that are generated when brassicas and alliums are chopped. Some

Table 2.13 Phytochemical classes that confer flavour.

Flavour property	Phytochemical class	Example	Typical food source
Aromatic	mono-terpenes	limonene	herbs, lemons
Bitter	glucosinolates alkaloids	sinigrin, progoitrin	cruciferous vegetables
	flavonoids	naringin	grapefruit
		tangeretin	orange
		quercetin	onion, endive, wine
		epigallocatechin gallate	green tea
Astringent		catechin polymers	red wine
Sulphurous	isothiocyanates	allyl isothiocyanate	cruciferous vegetables
	sulphur-containing compounds	allicin	garlic
Tart/acid	hydroxycinnamic acid derivatives organic	chlorogenic acid	quince, tomato
	acids	malic	apple

foodstuffs, such as tea and red wine, have another feature that contributes to their overall sensation, namely astringency. Astringency is the drying or puckering mouth-feel detectable throughout the oral cavity. It involves a complex reaction between high molecular-weight phenolics and proteins in the mouth and saliva.

Plants produce bitter-tasting toxins in order to deter predation. Although humans have evolved to dislike bitterness in order to avoid eating potentially toxic plants, moderate levels of bitterness add interest and complexity to Mediterranean cuisine. Cultural conditioning during childhood is an important influence on what is considered an enjoyable level of bitterness in foods, and this can be expressed in terms of an individual's 'bitterness acceptance threshold'. In addition, we have bitterness *detection* thresholds for phytochemicals. These thresholds have been determined for a wide range of phytochemicals since they are an important determinant of consumer acceptance for plant foods. For example, bitterness is not usually seen as a desirable taste in carrots, but the levels of bitter compounds (6-methoxymellein and falcarindiol) in carrots may increase during storage. This does not create a problem as long as the concentrations of bitter phytochemicals remain below the detection threshold, and so some desirable bitter compounds may be consumed without consumer resistance. Green tea is brewed in water at about 80°C in some cultures in the Far East, rather than with boiling water, in order to reduce the extraction of bitter compounds.

Many Mediterranean greens, both cultivated and collected from the wild, such as wild chicory, wild rocket and dandelion, are sought for their bitterness. These greens are eaten raw in salads, sometimes by complementing the bitterness with a sweet dressing. If the level of bitterness is too high, the greens can be lightly boiled as this leaches out some of the bitter compounds. Fruits that are too bitter to be eaten raw, such as quince and bitter (Seville) oranges, are cooked with sugar and made into preserves, making for an interesting overall taste.

The saying 'The dose makes the poison' (attributed to Paracelsus 'the father of toxicology') can be applied to bitter phytochemicals, since many phytochemicals that are toxic at high concentrations have very beneficial effects when consumed in moderation. This biphasic dose response, namely a beneficial effect at low doses but

Table 2.14 Phytochemicals as preservatives.

Rate of production	Mechanism of production	Examples
Preformed	–	Monoterpenes in herbs
Fast	Following decompartmentalisation between enzyme and substrate	Isothiocyanates in Brassicas; Sulphur-compounds in Alliums
Slow	Induction of a biosynthetic pathway	Resveratrol (grapes)

Table 2.15 Some possible health benefits of anti-microbial phytochemicals found in the MedDiet.

Phytochemical class	Example	Action in plant	Possible health benefits
Phenolic monoterpenes	Thymol	Anti-bacterial	Anti-bacterial
S-containing compounds	Allicin derivatives from garlic	Anti-viral, anti-bacterial, anti-fungal	Anti-bacterial action against *Helicobacter pylori* and hence possibly stomach cancer
Phytoalexins	Resveratrol	Anti-fungal	Experimental evidence for protection against many age-related diseases
	Falcarinol	Anti-fungal	Experimental evidence for protection against cancer

toxicity at higher doses is currently a very active area of nutrition research (see Chapter 9). However, consumer preference has led to the development of many varieties of vegetables with very low levels of bitter phytochemicals, and this may also result in reduced health benefits [48].

Preservatives

Many phytochemicals can be thought of as preservatives since they act as anti-spoiling agents due to their anti-microbial properties. Some anti-microbial phytochemicals are constantly present in the plant. Herbs are low-lying plants that are very susceptible to attack and many herbs constantly produce phenolic monoterpenes to prevent infection (for example, thymol in thyme). Other phytochemicals are only produced by plants as and when they are required. The rate at which these phytochemicals are produced is associated with how quickly they are needed for defence duties, since it is a waste of metabolic energy for a plant to produce a phytochemical that it does not require (Table 2.14). Inducible phytochemicals are called 'phytoalexins' (from the Greek *phyton* meaning plant and *alexin* meaning to ward off). The best-known phytoalexin in relation to the MedDiet is resveratrol, which is produced by grapes infected with the fungus *Botrytis cinerea*. Resveratrol subsequently finds its way into wine. Although it is normal viticulture practice to keep fungal infection in grapes to a minimum (apart from grapes destined for Sauterne-type wines), interest in the potential health benefits of resveratrol is leading to wines being produced with enhanced levels of this phytochemical (see Chapter 7).

Anti-microbial phytochemicals are thought to be responsible for a number of the health benefits attributed to food plants and to plant products such as wine (Table 2.15). Many of these phytochemicals are cytotoxic to human cells, and this

Table 2.16 Phenolics in some Mediterranean food plants (adapted from [49]).

Phenolic	Division	Examples	Food sources
Flavonoids	flavonols	quercetin	onion, apple, cos lettuce, broccoli, berries, red wine, olives, capers, coriander leaves
		kaempferol	endive, leek, black tea, capers
		myricetin	grapes, red wine
	flavones	apigenin, luteolin	celery, parsley, oregano
	flavanones	hesperetin, naringenin	citrus fruits
	flavan-3-ols	epicatechin, epicatechin gallate, epigallocatechin, epigallocatechin gallate	green tea
		catechin	red wine
	proanthocyanidins (polymeric flavan-3-ols)		chocolate, cinnamon, kidney beans, hazlenuts
	anthocyanidins	cyanidin, delphinidin	berries, red wine, aubergine
	isoflavones	genistein, daidzein	chickpeas, lentils, beans
Non-flavonoids	phenolic acids	gallic acid	wine, cereals, coffee, fruits and vegetables
	cinnamic acid derivatives	p-coumaric acid, caffeic acid, ferulic acid	fruits and vegetables
		chlorogenic acid	coffee
	stilbenes	resveratrol	grapes, red wine, peanuts
	lignans	secoisolariciresinol, matairesinol	linseeds (flax seeds), sesame seed, strawberries, carrots

is not surprising in view of their inherent requirement to kill microbial cells. Fortunately, some appear to be more potent at killing tumour cells than normal cells, and this may contribute to the cancer-preventing properties of consuming plant foods rich in these phytochemicals (see Chapter 12). The inherent toxic nature of many of these phytochemicals also causes the body to induce a battery of defence enzymes to neutralise them, and this may coincidentally make cells more resistant to pathological changes associated with various diseases such as cancers and CVDs (see Chapter 9).

2.7.3   Phenolics

Over 8000 plant phenolics have been identified. Phenolics are all based on the phenol structure, namely a benzene ring with a hydroxyl group (-OH) attached. Monophenols have a single benzene ring; structurally-speaking this group also includes tocopherols such as vitamin E, but these are generally classified with vitamins rather than with phenolics. The majority of phenolics have more than two benzene rings and these are referred to as polyphenols. Phenolics can be divided into two groups, namely flavonoids and non-flavonoids (see Table 2.16). The basic structures are shown in Figure 2.3.

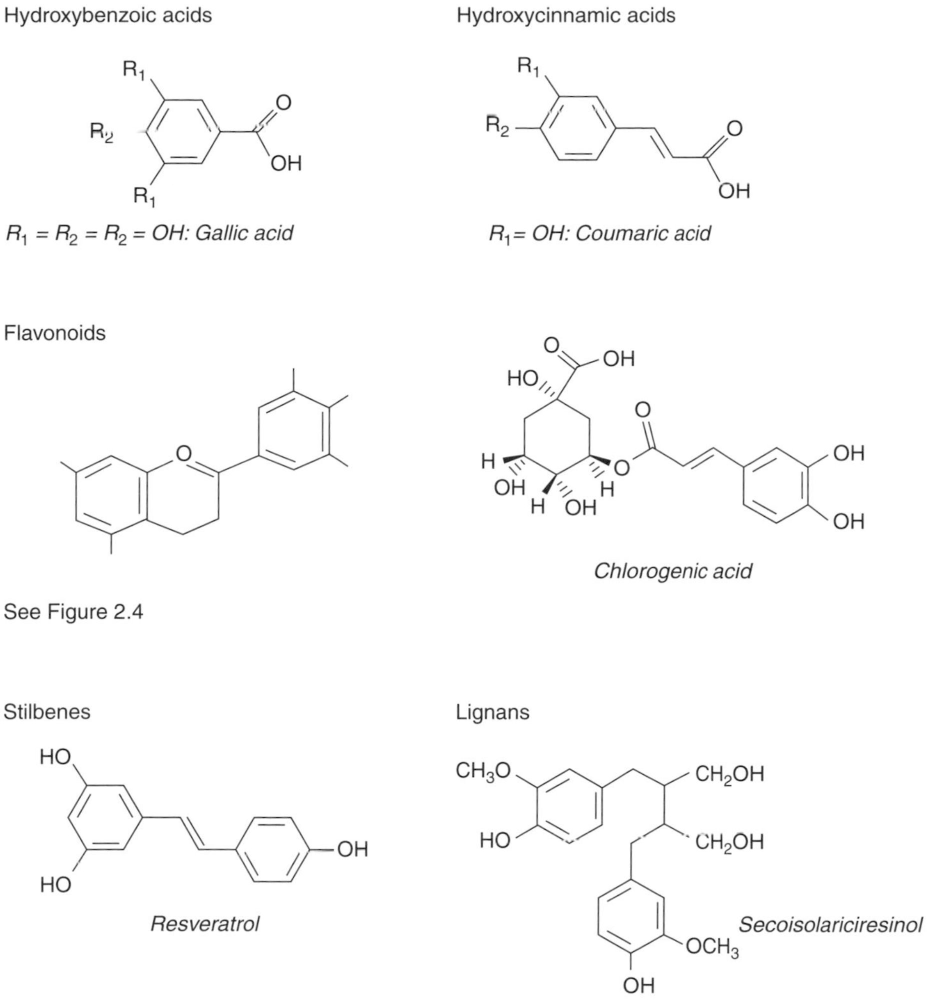

Hydroxybenzoic acids

Hydroxycinnamic acids

$R_1 = R_2 = R_2 = OH$: Gallic acid

$R_1 = OH$: Coumaric acid

Flavonoids

Chlorogenic acid

See Figure 2.4

Stilbenes

Lignans

Resveratrol

Secoisolariciresinol

Figure 2.3   Chemical structures of some phenolics [50].

Flavonoids

Over 5000 flavonoids have been identified and they are consumed in many different beverages, fruits and vegetables (see Table 2.16). Flavonoids are mainly present in the outer epidermal layers of leaves and in the skin of fruits, where they help protect the plant against UV damage. They also confer disease resistance for fruits and vegetables and contribute to their yellow colour.

Flavonoids are polyphenolic compounds (two or more phenol-based rings), and are divided into sub-classes according to their chemical structures. The main types found in the MedDiet are flavonols, flavones, flavanones, flavan-3-ols (flavanols), and anthocyanidins (Figure 2.4). Most types of flavonoids are present in plants conjugated to sugars (the exception being flavan-3-ols). This affects how they are absorbed from the gut, since the sugar moiety must usually be cleaved off before they can be absorbed (see Chapter 4). Many flavonoids have interesting actions in experimental systems, such as antioxidant activity and pro-apoptotic effects on cancer cells. However,

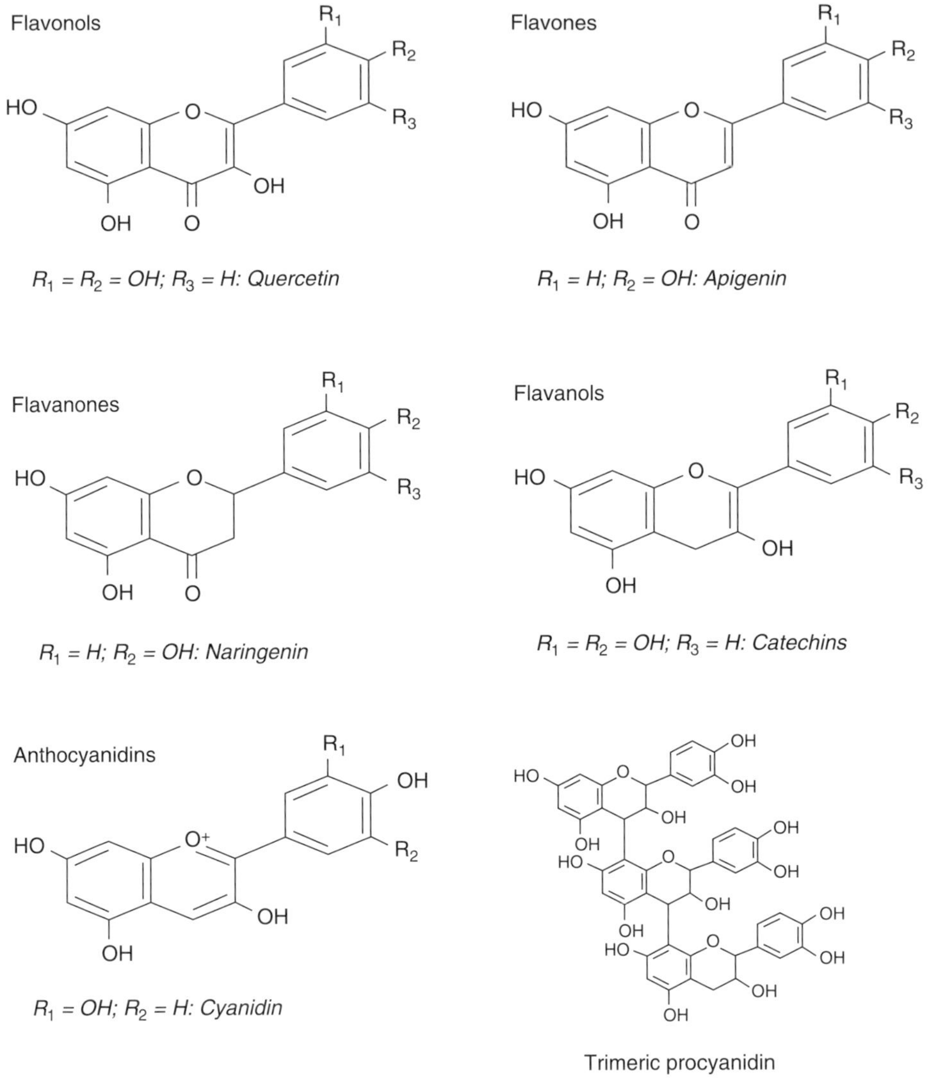

Flavonols

$R_1 = R_2 = OH; R_3 = H$: Quercetin

Flavones

$R_1 = H; R_2 = OH$: Apigenin

Flavanones

$R_1 = H; R_2 = OH$: Naringenin

Flavanols

$R_1 = R_2 = OH; R_3 = H$: Catechins

Anthocyanidins

$R_1 = OH; R_2 = H$: Cyanidin

Trimeric procyanidin

Figure 2.4   Chemical structures of some flavonoids [50].

although there is increasing epidemiological evidence that flavonoids may help prevent age-related diseases such as cancer, their precise mechanisms of action in humans are still controversial.

A few studies have looked at the total flavonoid content in a Mediterranean diet. It was estimated that consumption of flavonoids (flavones, flavonols and flavanols) in a traditional Greek Mediterranean diet is about twice that of a typical N. European or N. American diet [51]. The flavonoids in the Greek diet were also found to come from more varied sources, with a significant contribution from herbs. The major sources of flavones and flavonols in the Greek diet were apples (20%), herbs such as parsley (19%) and dill (6%), onions (16%), olives (7%), spring onions (7%), red wine (6%) and spinach (5%), while apples (44%) and red wine (44%) were equal contributors to the total flavanol (catechin) intake [52]. By contrast, tea was the

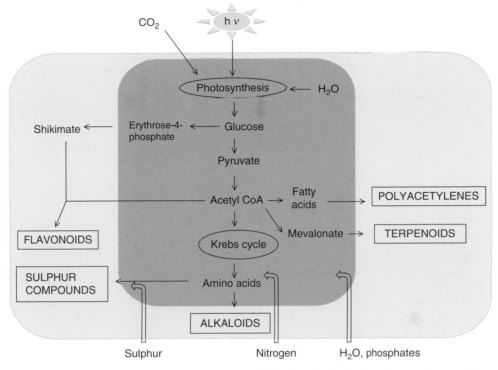

Figure 3.2 Relationship between primary metabolism (dark shading) and secondary metabolism (light shading) in plants and sources of nutrients from the soil (↰).

plants can radically modify their size, so too their production of phytochemicals is very sensitive to environmental conditions.

In order to understand factors that influence the phytochemical composition of plants, it is necessary to understand the underlying metabolic processes that regulate their production. There are two principle metabolic processes in plants, referred to as primary metabolism and secondary metabolism (Figure 3.2). Primary metabolism involves the production of carbohydrates, amino acids and fatty acids that are required for growth and other vital functions such as respiration and photosynthesis. Carbohydrates arise from the 'fixing' of the carbon in CO_2 into sugars during photosynthesis. Amino acids require the uptake of nitrogen from the soil. Primary metabolic pathways are basically similar in all plants. Secondary metabolic pathways, by contrast, can vary widely between different taxonomic groups. These pathways generate the diverse range of phytochemicals, i.e. secondary metabolites, found in plants. Secondary metabolites do not participate directly in growth but they serve diverse roles such as protecting plants against predation by herbivores and micro-organisms, and as attractants for pollinators or seed dispersers. In general, the products of secondary metabolism are far more responsive to growth conditions than the products of primary metabolism.

Primary metabolism for plant growth requires adequate levels of soil nutrients such as nitrogen (N) and phosphates, adequate water, and sunlight to produce sugars during photosynthesis. Sugars are also the starting point for the production of phytochemicals by secondary metabolic pathways.

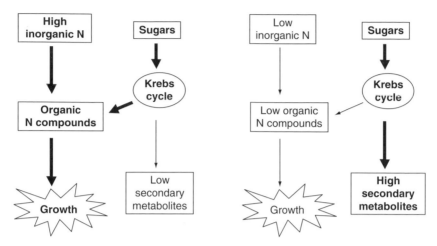

Figure 3.3 Influence of soil N on production of secondary metabolites in plants. Left: High levels of soil N favour growth (represented by thick arrows). Right: Low soil N results in more carbon fixed during photosynthesis into sugars being channelled into secondary metabolite production (thick arrows).

3.2.2   Soil

Secondary metabolite production in plants is often inversely related to the rate of primary metabolism. A soil rich in N favours primary metabolism and less secondary metabolism, whereas an N poor soil may lead to increased levels of phytochemicals (Figure 3.3). This has been shown to occur with brocolli which produces far higher levels of glucosinolates in N poor soil than in N rich soil [1]. One possible explanation for this is that plants cannot excrete the carbon that is converted into sugars during photosynthesis, so if there are insufficient levels of N to be used with carbon for protein synthesis, then more of the carbon fixed into sugars during photosynthesis is channelled into producing secondary metabolites (see Figure 3.3). In this way, phytochemicals can act as a 'store' of carbon fixed during photosynthesis.

N availability in organically cultivated soil is generally lower than inorganic N supplied by chemical fertilisers. This is thought to be one of the reasons why organically-grown plants tend to have a higher level of some secondary metabolites than the same plants grown in soils supplemented with inorganic fertilisers [3]. For example, one study found that organically-grown tomatoes had far higher levels of flavonoids compared with their non-organic counterparts [4]. However, limiting N is not always associated with an increase in phytochemical levels: increasing the amount of N-fertiliser supplied to carrots raised, rather than lowered, their carotene content [5].

Other elements in the soil may also affect the composition of plants. Brassicas require sulphur from the soil in order to produce sulphur-containing glucosinolates. It is thought that brassicas use a similar uptake mechanism for selenium. Hence, there is competition between sulphur and selenium for uptake, and it has been found that soils rich in selenium can under some circumstances reduce the uptake of sulphur and result in decreased levels of glucosinolates [1]. Not only do selenium and sulphur compete for uptake, but there is some evidence that selenium can substitute for sulphur in phytochemicals in onions and garlic, although the health significance of the resulting seleno-phytochemicals needs further elucidation [6]. Although selenium has wide-ranging health effects, many food plants incorporate selenium from the soil in non-edible parts and hence there will be no health benefit. For example, most of the selenium taken up by tomatoes is in the leaves rather than the fruit [7].

3.2.3 Sun

Mediterranean cuisine has been dubbed the 'cuisine of the sun'[1]. Whereas Mediterranean vegetables are traditionally grown outside and directly exposed to sunlight, many Mediterranean vegetables grown for the north European market are grown under glass. Hence it is of interest to examine if these different growing conditions could affect the potential health benefits of the vegetable. A number of studies have examined the effects of UV-B (280–315 nm) exposure on the micronutrient composition of plant foods since most glasshouses do not absorb UV-B light from the sun and so plants grown in glasshouses are not exposed to UV-B. Some studies have found that vegetables exposed to UV-B produce more carotenoids, vitamin C, glucosinolates or flavonoids compared to plants not exposed to UV-B, although the effects seem to be species-specific [8]. For example, the carotenoid content of some green-leaved lettuces was approximately doubled by UV-B exposure, whereas there was a decrease in carotenoid content in red-leaved varieties [9]. There were increases in flavonoids and carotenoids in some, but not all, cultivars of tomatoes following exposure to UV-B [9, 10]. Hence, the nutrient content of some food plants could be adversely affected by growing them in greenhouses. It is thought that plants stimulate phytochemical production when exposed to UV light in order to protect themselves against potential damage by photo-oxidation: flavonoids and carotenoids act as 'sunscreens', and vitamin C can neutralise free radicals.

3.2.4 Water

It has been shown that vegetables such as tomatoes and brassicas grown with a decreased water supply produce increased levels of phytochemicals [11]. Controlled reduction in water supply, known as 'regulated deficit irrigation', is increasingly being used to control vegetative growth in fruits (where this is economically favourable) whilst at the same time encouraging phytochemical production, for example to increase anthocyanin production in grapes during veraison (the stage when grapes turn colour). There is the added benefit of reducing water need.

Grafting is also used to increase drought resistance in traditional Mediterranean agriculture, for example the practice of grafting peach on to almond root stock. Grafting has been shown to favourably modify phytochemical content [11].

3.2.5 Other environmental factors

Another important trigger for phytochemical production is attack by predators such as bacteria, fungi, insects or larger herbivorous animals. Since plants cannot run away from their predators, they defend themselves with chemical deterrents. There are many ways they do this, such as simply discouraging eating due to a disagreeable

---

[1] The title of a book by Roger Vergé on the cooking of the South of France (Papermac, 1981).

scent, by interfering with the feeding and digestive system of the predator, or by poisoning the predator. For example, levels of glucosinolates, which deter predation, increased 3-fold in broccoli following insect attack [12]. Many herbs store monoterpenes in specialised structures in their leaves. If these leaves are damaged, the aroma of the terpenes is released which can act as an anti-feedant signal.

Although it is often useful for the plant to have its defences ready prepared, the speed of infection by fungi is slow enough to allow time for the plant to produce defence phytochemicals only when required. These sophisticated defence phyto-chemicals are known as phytoalexins. The phytoalexin resveratrol is produced by grapes infected by the fungus *Botrytis cinerea* and this phytochemical is of interest for its possible role in wine for protecting against CVD and cancer (see Chapter 7). Resveratrol levels are also influenced by exposure of the grape vines to sunlight (UV irradiation), and this environmental factor may be a more significant determinant of resveratrol levels than fungal infection [13]. Other phytochemicals traditionally thought of as phytoalexins, i.e. only produced following infection, are now known to be present in apparently healthy tissue. For example 'healthy' carrots can contain polyacetylene-type phytoalexins. These probably accumulate during storage and are of health interest as they have been found to inhibit the growth of cancer cells in culture.

Although the debate continues regarding the health benefits of organic versus non-organic produce [14], environmental factors associated with organic food production often favour increased production of defence phytochemicals [15]. However, exceptions have been reported, and one study found that non-organic grapes had higher levels of the purple pigments anthocyanins than grapes grown organically. This was attributed to a combination of the very hot summer and spraying with pesticides, which, the authors of the study suggested, acted together as more important stressors for phytochemical production than growing the vines organically [16].

Variations in nutrient content are not restricted to cultivated plants. Geographical location influences the growing conditions of wild plants, and the same edible wild plants originating from different geographical locations can have substantially different levels of polyphenols [17].

Flavonoids are particularly responsive to various environmental stresses such as diseases, insects, climate and ultraviolet radiation, and these exposures can also be seasonally influenced. It has been suggested that seasonal factors such as sunlight and water availability contribute to the large variations in the flavonoid content reported for some leafy vegetables (e.g. lettuce 1.9–30 mg/kg quercetin; endive 15–95 mg/kg kaempferol; leek 11–56 mg/kg kaempferol) [18].

In summary, many different growth conditions can influence the nutrient content of plants, and the extent of this is likely to vary with the plant and with the nutrient under consideration. There is a strong emphasis in the traditional MedDiet on the use of seasonal, outdoor-grown produce, and this can result in food plants that not only have enhanced levels of beneficial phytochemicals but are also tastier.

3.3   Plant cultivar

Varieties of food plants available to consumers in Mediterranean countries may differ from those available to their counterparts in more northerly countries. Breeding programmes have produced a huge range of cultivated varieties i.e. 'cultivars' that are selected for yield, taste, disease resistance and 'performance' – a term that includes

Table 3.1 Variations between cultivars in phytochemical content.

Plant	Phytochemical	Fold variation between cultivar*	Ref
Sweet red peppers	β-cryptoxanthin	7	[5]
Tomatoes	lycopene	2965	[5]
Oranges	β-cryptoxanthin	100	[5]
Lettuce	total flavonoid	763	[20]
Endive	total flavonoid	6	[20]

* These analyses may not always be considering like with like since other factors that can affect the levels of phytochemicals such as part of the plant analysed, age and growing conditions may not have been taken into consideration.

factors such as shelf life and uniformity of production. Different cultivars are commercially more appropriate in different circumstances. Hence the type of sweet pepper or tomato grown and supplied to a North European market may be different to that grown and supplied in the Mediterranean.

Retailers may consider fruits and vegetables with uniform size and appearance and with good shelf life to be more commercial than fruits and vegetables containing high levels of phytochemicals. However, phytochemical levels can vary widely between cultivars of the same food plant (Table 3.1). Indeed, it is has been claimed that choice of cultivar is a more important determinant of polyphenol and glucosinolate levels than other influences such as storage and growth conditions [1, 19].

The organoleptic (sensory) properties of food plants can sometimes give an indication of the relative phytochemical content. For example, it is not surprising that deep red tomato varieties have far higher levels of the red pigment lycopene than yellow varieties. Grape variety guides the selection of wine by many consumers, although the wine drinker may be less aware that grape variety also influences the composition of phenolics in the wine. Some glucosinolate breakdown products found in brassicas contribute to taste and there has been a trend towards producing varieties with milder tastes [1]. One glucosinolate present in some brassicas that contributes little to flavour is glucoraphanin, found at high levels in broccoli, and this lack of flavour impact has enabled breeders to increase levels of this putative cancer-preventative agent without detracting from the taste.

Familiarity is an important factor that influences consumer choice and this may impact on phytochemical consumption. This can be illustrated by considering lettuce cultivars, since these vary widely in flavonoid content (Table 3.1). Iceberg lettuce is a popular choice in northern countries but not in southern countries, and this cultivar has a very low flavonoid content compared to the traditional Italian variety Lollo Rosso, which as its name implies is a red variety and has a high content of red anthocyanins. Cos – the cultivar of choice in many Mediterranean countries – has intermediate levels of flavonoids.

Traditional Mediterranean agricultural practices favoured cultivars with good disease resistance and good keeping qualities, which were particularly important factors prior to the introduction of pesticides. Many phytochemicals, including flavonoids and glucosinolates, contribute to disease resistance and hence disease-resistant varieties of fruit and vegetables may contain higher levels of these phytochemicals. Disease-resistant varieties tend to be favoured by organic farmers, and this is one of the reasons why organic produce often contains higher levels of phytochemicals. Root vegetables and fruits are often stored for extended periods prior to consumption. Hence cultivars with good storage properties were important in the Mediterranean, at least until the introduction of post-harvest pesticides and refrigeration. Some phytochemicals can increase storage time. For example, the polyacteylene compounds in carrots confer resistance to storage rot by the fungus *Botrytis cinerea*.

There is a burgeoning industry of selective breeding programmes and genetic engineering (GM foods) to boost the levels of phytochemicals. Although some of these 'functional foods' have increased phytochemical content, there is currently considerable consumer resistance to buying GM plant foods.

3.4   Food retailers and food processing

Locally produced and fresh fruits and vegetables are very important to many Mediterranean consumers, whereas this may not be of such importance in other societies. These considerations can have significant effects on the type of produce supplied by retailers. Root vegetables that are consumed within a short time after harvest may be supplied with earth still clinging to them. This is a positive feature for some consumers, but others may favour washed produce, which may also be sprayed to increase shelf life, for example sprout suppressants on potatoes.

Some parts of plants that are routinely discarded by retailers in some countries, such as the 'tops' (leaves) of beetroots and turnips, are still used in traditional Mediterranean cuisine. Removing the outer leaves of vegetables for 'ready-to-eat' produce may improve shelf appeal, but it can also affect nutritional quality. For example, the outer leaves of Savoy cabbage contain up to 150-fold more lutein and 200-fold more β-carotene than the inner leaves [5]. These outer leaves may be used in stuffed cabbage recipes, popular in both Mediterranean countries and elsewhere. The phytochemical-rich outer layers of some vegetables are too tough to be acceptable for consumption due to high levels of indigestible lignans. But the frugality of peasant-based cuisines, such as the MedDiet, is more likely to result in these phytochemical-rich outer layers being used for making a tasty stock than being thrown away. By contrast, modern-day western consumers are more likely to prefer off-the-shelf ready-prepared 'baby' vegetables.

3.4.1   Anatomical distribution of nutrients

Many phytochemicals are not evenly distributed in plants. The skins of onions and garlic contain far higher levels of phenolic antioxidant compounds than the flesh [21]. Although normally discarded, whole garlic cloves with their skins intact are often roasted in meat dishes (such as 'chicken with 40 cloves of garlic'), although it is not known if any of the phenolics leach into the flesh of the garlic during cooking. Many nutritionally-desirable phytochemicals also accumulate in the skins of fruits, vegetables and nuts since this is where they are best able to protect the plant against photo-oxidation or predation. A very visible example is the accumulation of anthocyanins in the skins of purple varieties of aubergine, whereas the flesh is totally devoid of these pigments. In nuts, removing the skin (known as the pellicle) results in a dramatic decrease in their overall total antioxidant capacity (see Chapter 5).

Table 3.2 Classification of fruits [24]. With permission from Taylor & Francis Group.

Climacteric fruits (ripen once picked)	Non-climacteric fruits (stop ripening once picked)
Apple	Cherry
Apricot	Cucumber
Banana	Grape
Guava	Grapefruit
Kiwifruit	Lemon
Mango	Lime
Papaya	Lychee
Passion fruit	Mandarin
Peach	Melon
Pear	Orange
Persimmon	Pineapple
Plum	Pomegranate
Sapodilla	Raspberry
Tomato	Strawberry

On the other hand, processing some types of fruits for juice may actually increase the phytochemical content by mechanically extracting phytochemicals from the skin. For example, pomegranate juice is made by pressing the whole fruit and contains high levels of the hydrolysable tannin punicalagin which is present in the peel and would not be eaten in the fresh fruit [22].

Grains are another good example where there is an uneven distribution of phytochemicals. Grain consists of an outer layer of bran, a middle layer called the endosperm, and an inner germ layer. The outer bran and inner germ are the main sources of lignans, phytosterols and fibre, whereas the endosperm is rich in carbohydrate. Refining removes most of the bran and germ layers and thus many of the nutritionally important phytochemicals (see Chapter 5).

3.4.2 Freshness

Local fruit and vegetable markets remain very popular in Mediterranean countries. The food is generally less expensive and fresher than in supermarkets. Freshness as perceived by the consumer and the retailer is mostly based on appearance. However, not-so-obvious post-harvest deterioration in phytochemicals can be significant. This can be the result of enzymatic effects, microbial spoilage or temperature-induced changes. For example, post-harvest storage has been found to substantially reduce levels of glucosinolates [23] and carotenoids [5] found in brassicas.

Fruits sold in the Mediterranean are usually sold after they have ripened on the tree. However, some Mediterranean fruits grown for export can be picked unripe since they will ripen after picking (so-called climacteric fruits) (Table 3.2). This reduces damage in transit and increases storage time. Fruit ripening involves a wide range of changes such as chlorophyll degradation, increased biosynthesis of carotenoids, anthocyanins and monoterpenes, and increased degradation of pectin-containing plant cell walls [24]. Fruits that ripen during storage are often perceived by the consumer as developing less taste than tree-ripened fruit, but whether or not this has any effect on the health benefits is not known.

References

1. Verkerk, R. et al. Glucosinolates in Brassica vegetables: The influence of the food supply chain on intake, bioavailability and human health. *Mol Nutr Food Res*, 2008. 53:S219–S265.
2. Ingrouille, M., Eddie, B. *Plants: diversity and evolution*. Cambridge: Cambridge University Press, 2006, p. xiv.
3. Zhao, X. et al. Does organic production enhance phytochemical content of fruit and vegetables? Current knowledge and prospects for research. *Horttechnology*, 2006. 16(3):449–456.
4. Mitchell, A.E. et al. Ten-year comparison of the influence of organic and conventional crop management practices on the content of flavonoids in tomatoes. *J Agric Food Chem*, 2007. 55(15):6154–6159.
5. van den Berg, H. et al. The potential for the improvement of carotenoid levels in foods and the likely systemic effects. *Journal of the Science of Food and Agriculture*, 2000. 80:880–912.
6. Arnault, I., Auger, J. Seleno-compounds in garlic and onion. *J Chromatogr A*, 2006. 1112(1–2):23–30.
7. Carvalho, K.M. et al. Effects of selenium supplementation on four agricultural crops. *J Agric Food Chem*, 2003. 51(3):704–709.
8. Jansen, M. et al. Plant stress and human health: Do human consumers benefit from UV-B acclimated crops? *Plant Science*, 2008. 175:449–458.
9. Caldwell, C., Britz, S. Effect of supplemental ultraviolet radiation on the carotenoid and chlorophyll composition of green house-grown leaf lettuce (Lactuca sativa L.) cultivars. *Journal of Food Composition and Analysis*, 2006. 19:637–644.
10. Giuntini, D. et al. Changes in carotenoid and ascorbic acid contents in fruits of different tomato genotypes related to the depletion of UV-B radiation. *J Agric Food Chem*, 2005. 53(8):3174–3181.
11. Martınez-Ballesta, M. et al. Agricultural practices for enhanced human health. *Phytochem Rev*, 2008. 7:251–260.
12. Kuhlmann, F., Muller, C. Independent responses to ultraviolet radiation and herbivore attack in broccoli. *J Exp Bot*, 2009. 60(12):3467–3475.
13. Schmidlin, L. et al. A stress-inducible resveratrol O-methyltransferase involved in the biosynthesis of pterostilbene in grapevine. *Plant Physiol*, 2008. 148(3):1630–1609.
14. Dangour, A.D. et al. Nutrition-related health effects of organic foods: a systematic review. *Am J Clin Nutr*, 2010. 92(1):203–210.
15. Afssa, *Évaluation nutritionnelle et sanitaire des aliments issus de l'agriculture biologique*. Rapport Afssa, 2003.
16. Vian, M.A. et al. Comparison of the anthocyanin composition during ripening of Syrah grapes grown using organic or conventional agricultural practices. *J Agric Food Chem*, 2006. 54(15):5230–5235.
17. Schaffer, S. et al. Antioxidant properties of Mediterranean food plant extracts: geographical differences. *J Physiol Pharmacol*, 2005. 56 Suppl 1:115–124.
18. Hertog, M., Hollman, P., Katan, M. Content of potentially anticarcinogenic flavonoids of 28 vegetables and 9 fruits commonly consumed in the Netherlands. *J Agric Food Chem*, 1992. 40:2379–2383.
19. Amarowicz, R. et al. Influence of postharvest processing and storage on the content of phenolic acids and flavonoids in foods. *Mol Nutr Food Res*, 2009. 53 Suppl 2:S151–83.
20. DuPont, M.S. et al. Effect of variety, processing, and storage on the flavonoid glycoside content and composition of lettuce and endive. *J Agric Food Chem*, 2000. 48(9):3957–3964.
21. Ichikawa, M. et al. Identification of six phenylpropanoids from garlic skin as major antioxidants. *J Agric Food Chem*, 2003. 51(25):7313–7317.
22. Seeram, N.P., Schulman, R.N., Heber, D. *Pomegranates: ancient roots to modern medicine. Medicinal and aromatic plants – industrial profiles*; v. 43. 2006, Boca Raton: CRC/Taylor & Francis.
23. Rungapamestry, V. et al. Effect of cooking brassica vegetables on the subsequent hydrolysis and metabolic fate of glucosinolates. *Proc Nutr Soc*, 2007. 66(1):69–81.
24. Prasanna, V., Prabha, T.N., Tharanathan, R.N. Fruit ripening phenomena – an overview. *Crit Rev Food Sci Nutr*, 2007. 47(1):1–19.

4 Influences of Food Preparation and Bioavailability on Nutritional Value

Summary

- Food preparation techniques can significantly influence phytochemical levels in plant foods. For example, chopping and pureeing generate bioactive compounds in garlic and also liberate lycopene in tomatoes.
- Virgin olive oil (VOO) is an important cooking ingredient in the MedDiet. Although frying with VOO reduces its phenolic content, there is relatively low peroxidation of lipids in the oil. VOO can favourably influence the composition of fried fish. Marinating with VOO or other sources of antioxidants such as herbs and red wine can reduce the formation of harmful carcinogens during frying.
- Glucosinolates, carotenoids and flavonoids are relatively heat stable compared to many vitamins.
- Factors that affect the way phytochemicals are liberated from the food matrix, absorbed across the gut, distributed around the body, and are metabolised and excreted, are very important for understanding the potential health benefits of these compounds. These influences are expressed in terms of the bioavailability of a phytochemical.
- Dietary fibre can influence the composition of gut bacteria and possibly of bacterial metabolism of phenolics in the gut.
- Individuals can be classified as 'responders' or 'non-responders' in terms of their abilities to metabolise certain phytochemicals, and this may in turn influence the health benefits of these compounds.
- Genetic variations between individuals influence the metabolism of some phytochemicals to bioactive forms.

4.1 Introduction

The way foods are prepared can have a major impact on their nutritional value. Chopping, cooking and other ways of preparing foods are all influential, although there is currently only limited epidemiological evidence linking food preparation techniques with effects on health. Once consumed, metabolic processes in the body influence the levels of nutrients that reach target tissues, and some of these processes are genetically determined. The concentration of a nutrient that reaches its target tissue can be evaluated by determining the 'bioavailability' of the compound. Although bioavailability was originally used to describe how pharmaceutical agents behave in the body, this term is now increasingly being applied in relation to nutrition.

The Mediterranean Diet: Health and Science, First Edition. Richard Hoffman and Mariette Gerber.
© 2012 Richard Hoffman and Mariette Gerber. Published 2012 by Blackwell Publishing Ltd.

Bioavailability of a nutrient has been defined as 'the fraction of an ingested nutrient that becomes available to the body for utilisation in physiological functions or for storage' [1].

4.2 Food preparation

4.2.1 Chopping

Many water soluble nutrients, such as some phytochemicals and vitamins, are stored in the plant cell vacuole (Figure 4.1). Breaching the outer wall of a plant cell by chopping or other physical action is usually sufficient to liberate these nutrients. There may be significant losses of water soluble nutrients, such as folates and flavonoids, if the chopped vegetables are then washed in water. However, as this may also significantly reduce taste compounds, it is more normal to wash intact fruit or vegetable prior to chopping.

Chopping and other forms of mechanical processing can also help liberate phytochemicals that are normally tightly bound inside the plant cells. For example, carotenoids are not generally found in the aqueous environment of plant cells, but rather they are bound to proteins in the chloroplasts in green leafy vegetables or as semi-crystalline bodies in fruits and roots. The carotenoid lycopene is present in tomatoes in a semi-crystalline form in specialised storage organelles called chromoplasts (a specialised form of an organelle called a plastid). Extensive processing of tomatoes during the manufacture of purees involves both mechanical homogenization and heat treatment, and this greatly facilitates the release of lycopene. It has been found that processed tomato products have superior health

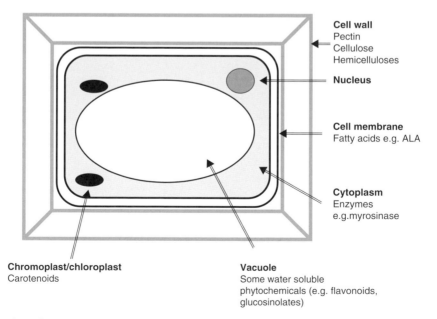

Figure 4.1   Sub-cellular locations of some plant constituents. (ALA: alpha linolenic acid.)

benefits compared to raw tomatoes, and this may be due to the increased bioavailability of lycopene. In very ripe fruits, carotenoids are often dissolved in oil droplets and this presumably makes them more easily absorbed by the body. Chopping can also have detrimental effects on carotenoids since this procedure increases the exposure of carotenoids in cells to light and oxygen, and these are known to be factors that increase the breakdown of some carotenoids. For example, one study found that commercially shredded carrots retained only 59% of total carotenes three hours later [2].

Another consequence of chopping can be to increase the production of beneficial phytochemicals by activating enzyme-substrate systems. The best known of these are the alliinase-alliin system in alliums and the myrosinase-glucosinolate system in brassicas. Both of these generate a range of bioactive metabolites due to decompart-mentalisation of the enzyme, which is thought to be located in the cytoplasm in the intact cell, and its substrate, which in the intact cell is located in the cell vacuole (Figure 4.1). There may be considerable variability in the extent to which these two enzyme systems are activated during food preparation. Preparation of alliums usually involves a significant degree of chopping or crushing, and this will facilitate the generation of bioactive compounds. Allowing time for the bioactive products to be generated after causing cell damage may have health implications; one study found that waiting 10 minutes after crushing garlic before cooking with it greatly increased anti-platelet activity [3]. By contrast, there may be minimal activation of myrosinase during the preparation of brassicas such as cauliflower and broccoli since these are usually only cut to separate the florets. A few brassicas, such as cabbages, may be chopped to a greater extent and so result in greater activation of myrosinase. Other factors such as vitamin C and pH also affect the activity of myrosinase and, overall, it has been suggested that food preparation is a significant factor affecting the overall levels of bioactive compounds in brassicas [2].

It is not only nutrients in vegetables that can be influenced by cutting. There was found to be an increased rate of PUFA oxidation in filleted fish compared to the rate of oxidation that occurred in intact fish. Some oxidation has been found to occur even in frozen fish. However, this should be balanced by the likelihood that frozen fillets will usually be eaten soon after thawing, whereas PUFAs in whole fish kept in the fridge for several days before consumption will also be subject to oxidation.

4.2.2 Cooking

Eating plant foods raw is very popular in Mediterranean cuisine, and the accompanying olive oil-based dressing for a salad or oil-based dip enhances the bioavailability of fat-soluble phytochemicals. Vegetables are also cooked in a myriad of ways: roasted in the oven, stuffed (e.g. peppers or tomatoes), fried, marinated, and as ingredients in soups, pies, tarts or in a casserole of mixed vegetable such as a French *ratatouille* or a Greek *briami*. The UK preference for boiling vegetables in water is far less common.

Frying and grilling

The main oil used for frying in traditional Mediterranean cuisine is olive oil. A significant proportion of the antioxidant phenolics in virgin olive oil (VOO) is destroyed by frying. Levels of hydroxytyrosol and its derivatives, major antioxidants in VOO, were found to decrease by 40–50% following heating to 180C for 10 minutes [4]. These antioxidants are linked to some of the health benefits of consuming VOO, and hence raw VOO and VOO used for frying may not have the same health benefits.

Although frying and grilling develops many desirable flavour compounds in foods, these processes can also generate carcinogenic heterocyclic aromatic amines (HAs), especially in meat. Both the flavour compounds and the HAs are products of the so-called Maillard reaction, a reaction between reducing groups on sugars and amines, mostly on proteins.

The Maillard reaction

The Maillard reaction is responsible for changes in the colour, flavour and nutritive value of food. The reaction was first demonstrated by Louis-Camille Maillard in 1912 when he addressed the French Academy and described some of his experiments. He had made the very simple observation that when sugars and amino acids in water are gently heated together, a yellow-brown colour develops. This may not seem of great significance, but Maillard was shrewd enough to realise that since biology is teeming with sugars and amino acids, this reaction would have far-reaching implications. It is now known that this apparently simple reaction can lead to a huge variety of further products. Some of these are potentially harmful such as carcinogenic heterocyclic amines and acrylamide in foods, and pathological products produced in the body such as advanced glycation end products.

Marinating meat and fish in olive oil was originally a technique widely used in Mediterranean countries for tenderising tough meat from animals raised in poor conditions. Serendipitously, there is now good evidence that marinating with VOO helps prevent carcinogens from forming during frying and grilling. Free radicals are involved in HA formation, and the inhibition of HA formation by marinating is probably linked to the high content of anti-oxidant phenolics in VOO since refined olive oil was found to be less effective [6]. Marinades that contain onion and garlic, herbs or red wine also have a high antioxidant capacity, and these marinades have also been found to inhibit HA formation [7, 8].

Pan-frying is the most popular way of preparing many Mediterranean fish, and another benefit of fish fried in VOO is that they absorb significant quantities of antioxidant phenolics, terpenic acids and vitamin E from the oil (Table 4.1). These absorbed antioxidants may be a useful source of daily requirements. In one study, it was calculated that one serving of fried fish could provide 17–26% of the daily vitamin E requirement and 23–77% of the total daily antioxidant intake when this is compared to the normal daily intake in the Netherlands [9].

Besides absorbing antioxidants, pan-frying fish also results in an exchange of fatty acids between those present in the fish and those in the oil. This has the potential to adversely affect the fatty acid composition of the fish depending on the type of frying oil used. One study found that the n-6 fatty acid content of sardines rose 19.9-fold when they were fried in sunflower oil and the n-3 fatty acid content fell 3.3-fold [2].

Table 4.1 Antioxidants in fish fried in virgin olive oil (from [9]). With permission from Elsevier.

Fish[1]	α-tocopherol (mg/100g)	Olive oil polyphenols[2] (mg/100g)	Terpenic acids[3] (mg/100g)	Total antioxidants (mg/130g serving)
raw	ND–0.08	ND	ND	–
fried	2.29–2.92	0.72–2.14	2.9–12.6	7.8–21.7

ND, not detected.
[1]Average of 8 fin fish (sand smelt, picarel, anchovy, striped mullet, bogue, scad, hake, sardines).
[2]Average of 9 polyphenols (predominantly tyrosol and hydroxytyrosol).
[3]Average of 3 terpenic acids (predominantly oleanolic acid).

Frying in olive oil had less adverse effects: *n*-6 fatty acid content rose 4-fold and *n*-3 fatty acid content fell 2.2-fold.

Frying vegetables in olive oil increases the bioavailability of some fat soluble phytochemicals. During cooking, olive oil not only helps liberate fat soluble phytochemicals from the food matrix, but the phytochemicals then dissolve in the oil, and so are far more readily absorbed by the body than if no oil is present. This is particularly significant for the ability of the body to absorb highly fat soluble carotenoids such as lycopene in tomatoes.

Boiling

Water soluble nutrients from vegetables boiled in water may leach out and be lost. A very visible example of this is the appearance of purple betalains in the water from boiled beetroots. The loss in health benefits from leaching may be substantial. For example, it has been shown that up to 90% of glucosinolates in brassicas can end up in the cooking water [10]. Similarly, there can be substantial leaching into the cooking water of water soluble vitamins, including folates and other B vitamins and vitamin C [11]. Several techniques used in Mediterranean cooking ensure that nutrients leached from cooked vegetables are not lost to the consumer. Making a sauce using the cooking liquid from cooked brassicas ensures no loss of the beneficial glucosinolates and vitamins. Soups are very popular in many traditional Mediterranean cuisines, and since the liquid is consumed, there will be no loss of water soluble phytochemicals. Another technique is to cook vegetables in a small amount of water with added olive oil. The olive oil will dissolve some of the phytochemicals left in the saucepan that may otherwise be lost.

Cooking can have beneficial as well as detrimental effects on food quality. Cooking breaks down plant cell walls and hence facilitates the liberation of nutrients from plant cells. It was found that 65% of β-carotene was absorbed from cooked carrot puree, whereas only 40% was absorbed from raw carrot [5]. On the other hand, frying and grilling can have detrimental effects.

Heat stability

Many vitamins and some phytochemicals, such as alliin-derived products from garlic, are not heat stable. However, a number of phytochemicals, including

Table 4.2   Heat stability of phytochemicals.

Relatively stable to heating	Not stable to heating
glucosinolates	allicin
carotenoids	vitamin A
flavonoids	vitamin B1 (thiamine)
	folate
	vitamin C

glucosinolates, carotenoids and flavonoids are surprisingly stable to moderate levels of cooking – although prolonged cooking at high temperature will ultimately result in their breakdown (Table 4.2). Frying onions for a short period of time resulted in only a slight loss of flavonoids [12]. The food matrix can have a major influence on the relative heat stability of phytochemicals. Fat content and antioxidants influence the heat stability of carotenoids, and this helps explain why carotenoids may be more heat stable in one food source compared to another [2]. Heating also has the interesting effect of dissociating the carotenoid astaxanthin from a protein complex present in the carapace of lobsters, thus changing their colour from blue-green to a pinkish-red.

4.3   Nutrient bioavailability

4.3.1   Pharmacokinetics of phytochemicals

The bioavailability of the major nutrients such as proteins, carbohydrates, fats, vitamins and minerals are, on the whole, very high. Active transport mechanisms ensure good uptake of these nutrients from the gut and anabolic pathways incorporate them into components in the body or catabolic pathways generate energy. Information on these processes are readily available in nutrition textbooks and hence they will not be further considered here.

The bioavailability of phytochemicals is far more variable. This is because phytochemicals in the body are treated as foreign chemicals or 'xenobiotics', and so, in this respect, phytochemicals behave like pharmaceutical agents. The bioavailability of drugs is studied using pharmacokinetic analysis. Pharmacokinetics describes how a drug is absorbed, how it distributes around the body, how it is metabolised and how it is excreted. Hence these processes are collectively given the acronym ADME. Many nutrients must first be liberated from the food matrix. Hence the overall acronym of LADME forms a useful framework in order to understand the bioavailability of phytochemicals, an area that could be dubbed 'nutrikinetics' (Figure 4.2). Many drugs fail to make it to the market, not because they lack efficacy in experimental systems *in vitro* or even in animal studies, but rather because of their poor pharmacokinetics. Similarly, many phytochemicals that have beneficial effects in laboratory experiments may have no health benefits in humans (besides possibly in the gut itself) if their pharmacokinetic properties are poor.

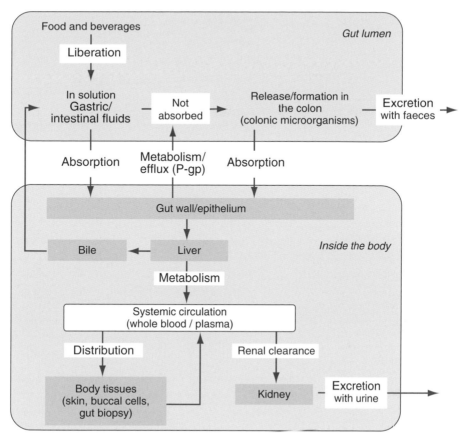

Figure 4.2   Nutrikinetics of phytochemicals [13]. Reproduced with permission from Elsevier.

4.3.2   Liberation

Although some phytochemicals are only loosely associated with the food matrix, others must be liberated from plant cell walls or other components of the food matrix before they can be absorbed in the gut. Food preparation techniques such as chopping, and chewing (mastication) break down plant cell walls and release phytochemicals locked inside. The mechanical process of liberating fat soluble phytochemicals is significantly facilitated by olive oil or fats present in meat or cheese.

4.3.3   Absorption

Many phytochemicals are absorbed by enterocytes lining the small intestine, whereas others are absorbed in the colon.

Absorption of phenolics

Flavonoid glycosides
Most flavonoids (flavanols being the main exception) exist in plants as glycosides, i.e. with one or more sugar residues attached. Current evidence indicates that flavonoid glycosides must be deglycoslyated at some stage by glycosidases (enzymes

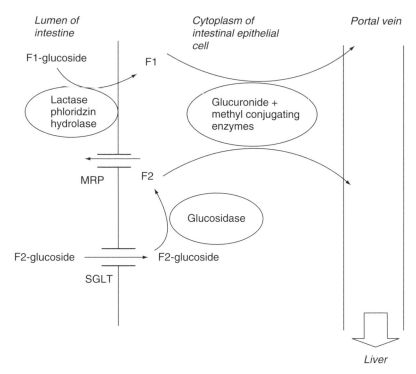

Figure 4.3 Update and metabolism of flavonoid-glucosides at enterocytes. SGLT: sodium-dependent glucose transporter; MRP: multidrug resistance protein (efflux pump); F: flavonoid.

that cleave off sugars) before they can be absorbed [14]. There are two ways by which this has been demonstrated to occur: (1) a glucosidase (i.e. a glycosidase that specifically cleaves off glucose) called lactase phloridzin hydrolase present on the surface of the brush border of epithelial cells of the small intestine (enterocytes) cleaves some flavonoid glucosides enabling the free flavonoid to then be absorbed by diffusion (Figure 4.3). (2) Some glucosides are taken up by active transport by a glucose transporter (SGLT1) into epithelial cells and then hydrolysed by a glucosidase in the cytoplasm of the epithelial cell (Figure 4.3). Interestingly, it has been suggested that some flavonoid glucosides may compete with dietary glucose for uptake by SGLT1 expressed on enterocytes and hence a meal rich in certain flavonoid glucosides may reduce glucose absorption and hence the overall glycaemic load of a meal [15].

An efflux pump, known as multidrug resistance protein, expressed on the cell membranes of enterocytes has been identified that pumps flavonoid aglycones out from the enterocytes and back into the gut (Figure 4.3). There is evidence that efflux pumps can be induced by dietary flavonoids and they can have a significant effect on the net absorption across the gut.

The type of sugar attached to a flavonoid influences where in the gut it will be absorbed. This is because different glycosidases are expressed in different regions of the gut. Quercetin can be attached to a range of sugars and hence different quercetin glycosides can be absorbed in different parts of the gut. In onions, quercetin is attached to glucose, and glucosidases on or in enterocytes can cleave the glucose

---

Lactase phloridzin hydrolase

Lactase phloridzin hydrolase (LPH) is better known simply as 'lactase', the enzyme that breaks down the milk sugar lactose into glucose and galactose. Many adult Mediterranean people have lost the ability to produce LPH (a phenomenon known as 'lack of persistence'). Loss of the enzyme results in lactose intolerance, and this is associated with bloating and flatulence due to the fermentation of undigested lactose to CO_2 and methane by colonic bacteria.

---

enabling the free quercetin to be absorbed in the small intestine. In tomatoes, quercetin is attached to rhamnose and glucose. Quercetin-rhamnoglucoside is not a substrate for glucosidases in the small intestine and so passes unabsorbed into the colon. Bacteria in the colon produce rhamnosidases (along with a wide range of other glycosidases), and hence quercetin from tomatoes is absorbed in the colon – albeit less efficiently – rather than in the small intestine [5].

Non-glycosylated phenolics

Some phenolics occur naturally in non-glycosylated forms including flavanols and many phenolic acids such as chlorogenic acid (a major phenolic in coffee) and gallic acid (present in berries, red wine and nuts). Phenolic acids, and monomeric forms of flavanols such as catechin and epicatechin, are well absorbed. However, it is currently uncertain whether polymeric forms of flavanols, such as red wine proanthocyanidins, are broken down in the gut to their monomeric components (i.e. flavanols such as catechin) or to smaller components before they are be absorbed [5, 16]. Failure to absorb proanthocyanidins would limit any therapeutic effects of the intact molecules to the gut itself.

Attaching sugars to flavonoids increases aqueous solubility. (Plants do this to enable them to store flavonoids in the aqueous cell cytoplasm.) During wine making, some quercetin glycosides from grapes are converted into the less soluble aglycones. Fortunately, ethanol in wine acts as a solubilising agent for the flavonoids, and this may explain why there is better absorption of some flavonoids from wine compared with grape juice [14].

Absorption of carotenoids

Carotenoids are fat soluble and their uptake is strongly influenced by the presence of lipids in the gut. During cooking or chewing, carotenoids partition into fat: this can be observed by the way that carotenoid-rich foods such as tomatoes or chorizo sausage colour cooking fat. It has been estimated that about 5 g of dietary fat is associated with the optimal absorption of carotenoids from a meal; higher amounts of fat do not lead to higher levels of carotenoid absorption [17]. Cooking tomatoes in olive oil greatly increases the absorption of lycopene compared to tomatoes not cooked in olive oil [18]. In the intestine, carotenoids transfer to mixed micelles (i.e. spheres containing more than one type of lipid). The lipids and carotenoids in the mixed micelles are believed to then transfer to the brush border of enterocytes [5].

In the enterocytes, triglycerides and carotenoids are packaged into chylomicrons and released into lymph and transported into tissues.

Absorption of sulphur compounds

There are a few reports from gut models indicating that glucosinolates may be absorbed intact, although the relevance of this to humans is not clear [19]. There is stronger evidence that glucosinolate breakdown products (GBPs), such as isothiocyanates, are readily absorbed. If these are generated during food preparation or chewing, they can be absorbed in the small intestine. Otherwise, GBPs can be generated from glucosinolates by bacteria in the colon, enabling absorption to occur there.

Dietary effects on absorption

Many phytochemicals are not absorbed in the small intestine because they are bound to fibre. These fibre-bound phytochemicals pass through the upper gut and into the colon. Here, the actions of colonic bacterial enzymes can release phytochemicals, enabling them to be absorbed across the colon wall [20, 21]. Thus, whereas soluble phenolics are absorbed relatively quickly in the small intestine (peak plasma levels 1–2 hours after consumption), fibre-bound phenolics are absorbed more slowly (peak plasma levels may be eight hours) since they are absorbed in the colon [22]. Fruits contain high levels of hydrolysable tannins that are tightly bound to fibre and proteins [23]. It is thought that these pass through the gut to the colon where they can be fermented by bacteria, releasing various metabolites that may have physiological effects either in the colon itself or after absorption.

Dietary fibre can also influence absorption of phytochemicals in the gut in other ways. Firstly, fibre modifies the activity of colonic bacteria which may in turn influence the metabolism and absorption of flavonoids in the colon. Secondly, soluble fibre in the form of pectin was found to increase the absorption of quercetin, and this might be attributed to an alteration of the absorptive capacity of the small intestine through an improvement of its morphological and physiological properties [24].

4.3.4   Distribution

Distribution involves the movement of nutrients around the circulation and to the target tissue. The behavior of a nutrient in blood plasma can be described using standard pharmacokinetic terminology. Plotting plasma concentration versus time enables a number of useful parameters to be determined (Figure 4.4). The peak plasma concentration is known as C_{max}, and the time to reach C_{max} is T_{max}. The terminal plasma half-life ($t_{1/2}$) can be calculated from the terminal exponential part of the curve. The total amount of nutrient in the plasma is calculated from the area under the curve (AUC). The AUC gives an indication of the bioavailability of a nutrient. Figure 4.4 shows the plasma concentration-time curves for a nutrient from two sources, source A (black line) and source B (grey line). It can be seen that the AUC for the nutrient from source A (black line) is twice that of the AUC for the nutrient from source B (grey line). Hence, the nutrient from source A has twice the bioavailability compared with its bioavailability from source B.

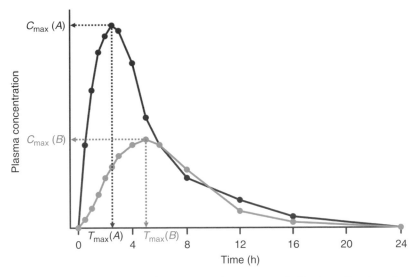

Figure 4.4 Plasma concentration-time curves of a compound after ingestion from two different dietary sources A (black line) and B (grey line) [25]. With permission from Wiley-VCH Verlag GmbH & Co. KGaA.

The peak plasma concentration (C_{max}) of a phytochemical is often compared to the concentration exerting a biological effect in cell culture models. It is often argued that only if these two values are similar is there the likelihood that a compound can exert a beneficial effect *in vivo*. However, this correlation may not always be straightforward since some phytochemicals selectively accumulate in tissues. For example, the carotenoids lutein and zeaxanthin selectively accumulate in the macula in the eye at far higher concentrations than are found in the plasma (probably due to a specific uptake mechanism). There is also a limited amount of evidence that some phenolics accumulate in tissues to concentrations that are greater than those present in the plasma [26]. Cell culture studies have demonstrated that isothiocyanates such as sulphoraphane can accumulate in cells to concentrations that are several hundred-fold higher than outside the cell, reaching millimolar concentrations [27].

4.3.5 Metabolism

The main aim of metabolising a xenobiotic, be it a phytochemical or a drug, is to convert it into a form that can be more readily excreted. There are two stages, and these are referred to as phase 1 metabolism and phase 2 metabolism (Table 4.3).

Phase 1 metabolism introduces functional groups, especially hydroxyl groups, into hydrophobic molecules to increase their polarity and this usually also increases their water solubility. The major group of enzymes involved in phase 1 metabolism is the cytochrome P450 mixed function oxygenases (cytochrome P450s or CYPs), mostly present in the liver. There are many isoforms of CYPs and different isoforms metabolise different xenobiotics.

Phase 2 metabolism conjugates phase 1 metabolites with various water soluble groups. Phase 2 metabolism takes place in both the small and large intestine and in the liver. Further metabolism can also occur in the target tissue (Figure 4.5). The main groups that are added to phase 1 metabolites are glutathione, glucuronate, and

Table 4.3 Main groups of xenobiotic metabolising enzymes.

Enzyme	Representative isoforms	Typical reaction
Phase 1 cnzymes		oxidation, reduction, hydrolysis
cytochrome P450s	CYP1A	oxidation
Phase 2 enzymes		conjugation
Glutathione S-Transferases (GSTs)	GSTM1, GSTT1, GSTP1, GSTA1	addition of glutathione
UDP-glucuronosyltransferases (UGTs)		addition of glucuronate
sulphotransferases (SULTs)		addition of sulphate
N-acetyltransferases (NATs)		addition of acetate

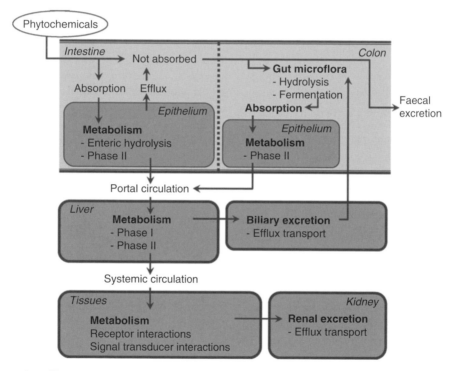

Figure 4.5 The main sites of metabolism [28]. With permission from Elsevier.

sulphate groups. These conjugations are catalysed by glutathione S-transferases (GSTs), UDP-glucuronosyltransferases (UGTs) and sulphotransferases (SULTs) respectively. As for CYPs, phase 2 enzymes exist in many different isoforms (see Table 4.3).

Although most reaction products of phase 1 enzymes are inert, reactive electrophiles are sometimes generated. These can damage macromolecules such as DNA and increase the risk of cancer. For example, heterocyclic amines (HAs) generated in meat cooked at high temperatures undergo metabolic activation to genotoxic compounds. Studies have shown that cytochrome P450s are key enzymes involved in the metabolic activation of one of the most abundant heterocyclic amines known as 2-amino-1-methyl-6-phenylimidazo [4,5-b]pyridine (PhIP) [29]. HAs are not genotoxic prior to activation, demonstrating that inhibition of phase 1 metabolism can prevent the carcinogenic activity of these compounds. This has important implications for cancer prevention by phytochemicals and is discussed further in Chapter 12.

Phase 2 enzymes usually catalyse reactions that inactivate, ie detoxify, a xenobiotic and facilitate excretion. Hence, whereas most phase 1 enzymes can be thought of as 'activating' enzymes, phase 2 enzymes are 'detoxifying' enzymes. This has led to the concept that selective induction of expression of genes encoding phase 2 enzymes may have the potential to protect against chemical carcinogenesis.

Metabolism of phenolics

Unlike some phytochemicals, phenolics do not need to undergo phase I metabolism since they already possess the necessary hydroxyl groups to which phase 2 enzymes can attach chemical groups. Many types of phenolics, including flavonoids, chlorogenic acid and gallic acid are rapidly conjugated by phase 2 enzymes in the intestinal enterocytes, principally by UGTs that add glucuronate groups. The conjugates travel from the enterocytes via the hepatic portal vein to the liver, where they may be taken up by hepatocytes (although how these polar metabolites are taken up is unclear). They may then be further conjugated with glucuronate, methyl or sulphate groups. Phenolics that are not absorbed in the small intestine pass to the colon where they may be metabolised by colonic bacteria.

Due to rapid conjugation, few flavonoids are found in plasma in the forms that were present in the foods from which they originate. For example, quercetin is found in the plasma entirely in conjugated forms. Micromolar concentrations of conjugated forms can be achieved following consumption of flavonoid-rich foods. There is now a great deal of interest in determining the biological properties of flavonoid metabolites. Most studies so far suggest that conjugated flavonoids are less active than the unconjugated forms. Antioxidant activity can be greatly reduced, and this is not surprising since conjugation occurs on free hydroxyl groups, and it is these groups that are responsible for the antioxidant activity of polyphenols. Hence, it is questionable if polyphenols are acting in the body as direct antioxidants (see Chapter 9). It has also been speculated that deconjugation can occur inside cells and that conjugates may act as storage 'pools' that can provide active polyphenols. However, it is not clear if cells can take up conjugated phenolics. Alternatively, it is possible that deconjugation may occur outside the cell.

Flavonoid metabolites and inflammatory diseases

A wide range of chronic degenerative disorders including cancer and CVD are associated with an inflammatory response (see Chapter 9). This involves an influx of neutrophils and macrophages to sites of inflammation. When activated, these cells can produce glucuronidases, and there is increasing evidence that these glucuronidases can cleave flavonoid glucuronides liberating the free flavonoid [30, 31]. In this respect, the flavonoid glucuronides can be considered as transporter molecules in the blood, and the active parent (non-conjugated) flavonoid can be regenerated specifically at a site of inflammation such as an atherosclerotic plaque (see also Section 11.3.2). Hence, this mechanism provides a possible explanation for biological activity of dietary flavonoids despite the fact that circulating flavonoid glucuronides may not themselves be biologically active.

Metabolism of carotenoids

In contrast to phenolics, carotenoids are not substrates for phase 2 conjugating enzymes. Provitamin A carotenoids are cleaved to retinol, the main precursor of vitamin A. The metabolism of non-provitamin A carotenoids is less clear, although limited evidence suggests that they undergo oxidation, cleavage and chain shortening in a manner somewhat analogous to the β-oxidation of fatty acids. It is presently unclear whether carotenoid metabolites are more or less active than the parent molecule, although some cell culture studies suggest that lycopene metabolites have the potential to act as tumour preventative molecules [32].

Metabolism of sulphur compounds

Conjugation with glutathione is the major route of metabolism for isothiocyanates and occurs in both the small intestine and in the liver.

4.3.6   Excretion

There is wide variability between the levels of phytochemicals that are excreted intact in the urine. For most flavonoids it is thought that bile is the major route of excretion [5]. The amount of urinary excretion of isothiocyanates is influenced by cooking and chewing.

4.3.7   Inter-individual variations in phytochemical pharmacokinetics

The metabolism of phytochemicals can vary significantly between individuals, and these variations can influence how much of an ingested phytochemical reaches body tissues. Two important reasons for inter-individual variations in phytochemical metabolism are:

- dietary variations between individuals
- genetic variations

Variation in diet

Diet can modify the bacterial population in the gut, as demonstrated by the effects of prebiotics such as inulin (found in onions) and probiotic bacteria (from yogurt) on the composition of bacteria in the colon. Variations in gut flora are thought to be a reason for differences between people in their metabolism of dietary phenolics. This has led to the concept of individuals being classified as either metabolite 'producers' or metabolite 'non-producers'. For example, the conversion by colonic bacteria of ellagitannins, such as punicalagin in pomegranates, to urolithins shows wide inter-individual variability. This may influence the health benefit to be gained from consuming pomegranates since urolithins have been shown to inhibit the growth of cultured cancer cells. There is also wide inter-individual variation in the metabolism of plant lignans. Many types of plant lignans are metabolised by intestinal bacteria to the mammalian lignans enterodiol and enterolactone and these are of interest as possible cancer-preventative agents. Studies have shown that the efficiency of conversion of plant lignan precursors to mammalian lignans varies greatly between individuals, ranging from 0 to 100%. Another well-known example, although not directly related to the MedDiet, is the conversion of the isoflavone daidzein, found in soya, to equol. Epidemiological studies have shown that the health effects of soya are better understood by recognising that a population can be divided into equol producers and equol non-producers [33]. Gut bacteria can also hydrolyse phytochemical conjugates such as glycosides, glucuronides and sulphates – which may be biologically inactive – into biologically active de-conjugated phytochemicals. Thus it can be concluded that variations in diet can influence the composition of colonic bacteria and hence the production of some biologically active phytochemicals.

Dietary phenolics can induce phase 2 enzymes such as UGTs in the intestine and liver. Phase 2 enzymes are major detoxifying enzymes in the body and help remove toxic compounds. By increasing the expression of UGTs in the intestinal cells, phenolics may help create a barrier to the absorption of harmful carcinogens and this may represent an important defence shield in the body [34]. Further protection may be afforded by the induction of efflux pumps, which pump toxins from the enterocytes back into the lumen of the intestine, and by the increased expression of phase 2 enzymes that occurs in the liver.

Carotenoids are not substrates for phase 2 enzymes. However, there are well-described variations in plasma concentrations in individuals given similar doses of carotenoids, and this has led to the concept that there are 'good' and 'bad' responders to carotenoids. These differences are thought to reflect both differences in absorption and in clearance.

Genetic variation

There are many isoforms of phase 2 enzymes such as GSTs, UGTs and SULTs. Isoforms of an enzyme (also known as isoenzymes) all catalyse essentially the same reaction, but are regulated in different ways and may be localised in different organs in the body. Some genes for isoforms of phase 2 enzymes are polymorphic, i.e. the gene exists in two or more forms in different individuals in a population. Epidemiological and experimental studies indicate that some genetic polymorphisms may influence the health benefits from consuming certain vegetables. This has been particularly well studied in relation to the consumption of brassicas.

Different isoforms of GSTs have different capacities to metabolise sulphoraphane. One isoform of GST, known as GSTM1, is expressed at high levels in the liver and seems particularly important for conjugating sulphoraphane with glutathione. The gene for GSTM1 is polymorphic, and some people have a polymorphism in the GSTM1 gene that prevents the production of any functional GSTM1 enzyme. Such individuals are said to have a 'null' genotype for GSTM1. It has been speculated that individuals who do not express GSTM1 will have greater protection against cancer since sulphoraphane would be expected to be less metabolised and so would be present longer in the body where it is able to exert a therapeutic effect (such as by inducing other forms of GSTs which may conjugate carcinogens). However, epidemiological studies have produced confusing results. In some populations (particularly Asians), GSTM1 null individuals do indeed appear to have greater protection from cancer if they consume brassicas. However, in US populations, GSTM1 positive individuals appear to gain the greater cancer protection from consuming broccoli or other cruciferous vegetables [35]. It is estimated that approximately 50% of the population do not express GSTM1, and hence understanding the role of this polymorphism in relation to the health benefits of brassicas is of great interest.

UGTs are also highly polymorphic. Glucuronidation is an important route for the metabolism of many flavonoids, but the significance of polymorphisms in UGT has not been established.

References

1. Fraser, P.D., Bramley, P.M. The biosynthesis and nutritional uses of carotenoids. *Prog Lipid Res*, 2004. **43**(3):228–265.
2. Ruiz-Rodriguez, A. et al. Effect of domestic processing on bioactive compounds. *Phytochem Rev*, 2008. **7**:345–384.
3. Cavagnaro, P.F. et al. Effect of cooking on garlic (Allium sativum L.) antiplatelet activity and thiosulfinates content. *J Agric Food Chem*, 2007. **55**(4):1280–1288.
4. Gomez-Alonso, S. et al. Changes in phenolic composition and antioxidant activity of virgin olive oil during frying. *J Agric Food Chem*, 2003. **51**(3):667–72.
5. Donovan, J.L. et al. Absorption and metabolism of dietary secondary metabolites. In *Plant secondary metabolites: occurrence, structure and role in the human diet*, ed. A. Crozier, M.N. Clifford and H. Ashihara. 2006, Oxford: Blackwell. xii.
6. Persson, E. et al. Influence of antioxidants in virgin olive oil on the formation of heterocyclic amines in fried beefburgers. *Food Chem Toxicol*, 2003. **41**(11):1587–1597.
7. Gibis, M. Effect of oil marinades with garlic, onion, and lemon juice on the formation of heterocyclic aromatic amines in fried beef patties. *J Agric Food Chem*, 2007. **55**(25): 10240–10247.
8. Busquets, R. et al. Effect of red wine marinades on the formation of heterocyclic amines in fried chicken breast. *J Agric Food Chem*, 2006. **54**(21):8376–8384.
9. Kalogeropoulos, N. et al. Recovery and distribution of natural antioxidants (a-tocopherol, polyphenols and terpenic acids) after pan-frying of Mediterranean finfish in virgin olive oil. *Food Chemistry*, 2007. **100**:509–517.
10. Song, L., Thornalley, P.J. Effect of storage, processing and cooking on glucosinolate content of Brassica vegetables. *Food Chem Toxicol*, 2007. **45**(2):216–224.
11. Leskova, E. et al. Vitamin losses: retention during heat treatment and continual changes expressed by mathematical models. *Journal of Food Composition and Analysis*, 2006. **19**:252–276.
12. Le Marchand, L. Cancer preventive effects of flavonoids – a review. *Biomed Pharmacother*, 2002. **56**(6):296–301.
13. Holst, B., Williamson, G. Nutrients and phytochemicals: from bioavailability to bioefficacy beyond antioxidants. *Curr Opin Biotechnol*, 2008. **19**(2):73–82.
14. Scholz, S., Williamson, G. Interactions affecting the bioavailability of dietary polyphenols in vivo. *Int J Vitam Nutr Res*, 2007. **77**(3):224–235.
15. Clifford, M., Brown, J.E. Dietary flavonoids and health – broadening the perspective. In *Flavonoids: chemistry, biochemistry, and applications*, Ø.M. Andersen and K.R. Markham, Editors. 2006, CRC: Boca Raton, Fla.; London.
16. Yang, C.S. et al. Bioavailability issues in studying the health effects of plant polyphenolic compounds. *Mol Nutr Food Res*, 2008. **52 Suppl 1**:S139–151.
17. van Het Hof, K.H. et al. Dietary factors that affect the bioavailability of carotenoids. *J Nutr*, 2000. **130**(3):503–506.

18. Fielding, J.M. et al. Increases in plasma lycopene concentration after consumption of tomatoes cooked with olive oil. *Asia Pac J Clin Nutr*, 2005. **14**(2):131–136.
19. Verkerk, R. et al. Glucosinolates in brassica vegetables: the influence of the food supply chain on intake, bioavailability and human health. *Mol Nutr Food Res*, 2008. **53 Suppl 2**:S219–S265.
20. Goni, I., Serrano, J., Saura-Calixto, F. Bioaccessibility of beta-carotene, lutein, and lycopene from fruits and vegetables. *J Agric Food Chem*, 2006. **54**(15):5382–5387.
21. Saura-Calixto, F., Serrano, J., Goni, I. Intake and bioaccessibility of total polyphenols in a whole diet. *Food Chemistry*, 2007. **101**:492–501.
22. Perez-Jimenez, J. et al. Bioavailability of phenolic antioxidants associated with dietary fiber: plasma antioxidant capacity after acute and long-term intake in humans. *Plant Foods Hum Nutr*, 2009. **64**(2):102–107.
23. Arranz, S. et al. High contents of nonextractable polyphenols in fruits suggest that polyphenol contents of plant foods have been underestimated. *J Agric Food Chem*, 2009. **57**(16): 7298–303.
24. Nishijima, T. et al. Chronic ingestion of apple pectin can enhance the absorption of quercetin. *J Agric Food Chem*, 2009. **57**(6):2583–2587.
25. Cermak, R. et al. The influence of postharvest processing and storage of foodstuffs on the bioavailability of flavonoids and phenolic acids. *Mol Nutr Food Res*, 2008. **53 Suppl 2**:S184–93.
26. Manach, C. et al. Polyphenols: food sources and bioavailability. *Am J Clin Nutr*, 2004. **79**(5):727–747.
27. Zhang, Y. Role of glutathione in the accumulation of anticarcinogenic isothiocyanates and their glutathione conjugates by murine hepatoma cells. *Carcinogenesis*, 2000. **21**(6):1175–1182.
28. Lampe, J.W., Chang, J.L. Interindividual differences in phytochemical metabolism and disposition. *Semin Cancer Biol*, 2007. **17**(5):347–353.
29. Pool-Zobel, B., Veeriah, S., Bohmer, F.D. Modulation of xenobiotic metabolising enzymes by anticarcinogens – focus on glutathione S-transferases and their role as targets of dietary chemoprevention in colorectal carcinogenesis. *Mutat Res*, 2005. **591**(1–2):74–92.
30. Shimoi, K., Nakayama, T. Glucuronidase deconjugation in inflammation. *Methods Enzymol*, 2005. **400**:263–272.
31. Shimoi, K. et al. Deglucuronidation of a flavonoid, luteolin monoglucuronide, during inflammation. *Drug Metab Dispos*, 2001. **29**(12):1521–1524.
32. Mein, J.R., Lian, F., Wang, X.D. Biological activity of lycopene metabolites: implications for cancer prevention. *Nutr Rev*, 2008. **66**(12):667–683.
33. Hall, M.C., O'Brien, B., McCormack, T. Equol producer status, salivary estradiol profile and urinary excretion of isoflavones in Irish Caucasian women, following ingestion of soymilk. *Steroids*, 2007. **72**(1):64–70.
34. Sergent, T. et al. Molecular and cellular effects of food contaminants and secondary plant components and their plausible interactions at the intestinal level. *Food Chem Toxicol*, 2008. **46**(3):813–841.
35. Traka, M., Mithen, R. Glucosinolates, isothiocyanates and human health. *Phytochem Rev*, 2009. **8**:269–282.

5 Guide to the Composition of Mediterranean Plant Foods

Summary

- Consumption of a diverse range of fruits, vegetables, pulses, grain products, herbs and spices, and nuts and seeds is a defining feature of the MedDiet.
- Consumption of fruits and vegetables is higher in European Mediterranean countries than in some North African countries.
- Green leafy vegetables include not only various crucifers, salad vegetables and others widely consumed in Northern Europe, but also vine leaves and wild greens. The latter are a particularly rich source of physiologically active constituents (phytochemicals and n-3 fatty acids).
- Alliums, especially onions and garlic, are consumed in high amounts, and preparation and cooking methods influence the levels of bioactive ingredients.
- Fruits are usually eaten fresh and seasonally. Citrus fruits are an important source of vitamin C, figs and dates are rich in fibre and some fruits are particularly rich in certain phytochemicals (e.g. β-carotene in apricots, punicalagin in pomegranates, monoterpenes in Citrus).
- Black olives contain lower levels of bitter-tasting oleuopein than green olives and so need less processing. Processing methods can have a major effect on levels of putative bioactive compounds.
- Pulses are very important in Mediterranean cuisine especially when incomes are low. Mashed fava (broad) beans is the national dish of Egypt and chickpeas are particularly popular in Turkey and Spain. Pulses are a good source of fibre, phytosterols and lignans.
- Whole grain wheat products are consumed in a traditional MedDiet, but refining significantly reduces levels of the complex mixture of bioactive constituents.
- Herbs and spices help define the different Mediterranean cuisines, and are often consumed in far higher levels than in Northern cuisines.
- Nuts and seeds are used in both sweet and savoury dishes and are rich in protein, fats (mostly unsaturated) fibre, vitamins, minerals and phytochemicals, with some nuts being particularly rich in certain nutrients (e.g. walnuts: α-linolenic acid; pistachio: β-sitosterol; almonds: α-tocopherol).

The Mediterranean Diet: Health and Science, First Edition. Richard Hoffman and Mariette Gerber.
© 2012 Richard Hoffman and Mariette Gerber. Published 2012 by Blackwell Publishing Ltd.

5.1   Types of plant foods consumed as part of a MedDiet

5.1.1   Consumption

Many everyday meals in Mediterranean countries are based on vegetables, and the vast range of imaginative and tasty main-course vegetable dishes reflects the skills of Mediterranean cooks. Fruit is often eaten instead of a sweet dessert after a meal. By contrast, vegetables in a typical meal in Northern Europe are consigned to be the side dish that accompanies the meat. Hence it is not surprising that consumption of vegetables in many Mediterranean countries is higher than in many North European countries such as the UK (Table 5.1). It is worth noting, however, that there is wide variation in eating patterns even between Mediterranean countries, with consumption of fruits and vegetables in North African Mediterranean countries tending to be much lower than in European Mediterranean countries and Turkey [1].

As well as fruits and vegetables, a traditional MedDiet includes many other plant foods such as wild greens and an abundance of aromatic herbs and spices. Pulses are widely used in soups and stews, often to enhance and extend small amounts of meat, most commonly from poultry. Cereal products, such as bread or pasta, accompany all main meals and are usually made from only partially refined cereals. Many plant foods, particularly when minimally refined, are an important source of dietary fibre. For more information on the botany and usage of vegetables, *Mediterranean Vegetables* by Clifford A. Wright (which discusses 200 different varieties) is recommended [2].

5.1.2   Diversity of consumption

The consumption of a wide variety of fruits and vegetables is one of the defining features of a traditional MedDiet and encompasses not only cultivated plants but also includes plants collected from the wild, a practice still common in some parts of the Mediterranean. The wide diversity of consumption of fruits and vegetables in

Table 5.1   Fruit and vegetable consumption in Mediterranean countries and the UK (FAOSTAT 2003).

	Consumption (g/per capita/per day)	
	Fruit	Vegetables
Egypt	244	490
France[1]	260	389
Greece	402	753
Italy	356	488
Morocco	170	332
Spain	307	392
Tunisia	233	545
Turkey	293	630
United Kingdom	315	249

[1]Includes both Mediterranean and non-Mediterranean regions.

the MedDiet will greatly increase the number of possible beneficial interactions between constituents in the different foods as well as between their metabolic products. Although this chapter discusses individual plant foods and their constituents and physiological effects that have been described for them, it is quite likely that *diversity* of consumption is very important for the overall health benefits of the MedDiet.

Diversity of consumption and cancer risk

Diet diversity scores have been used to assess variety of fruit and vegetable consumption. A number of these studies have shown an inverse association between diversity of fruit and vegetable consumption and cancer risk. For example, increasing variety in consumption of vegetables was inversely associated with lung cancer risk amongst current smokers in the EPIC cohort, an effect over and above the inverse association with quantity [3].

5.2 Vegetables

5.2.1 Green leafy vegetables

Cruciferous vegetables

Cruciferous vegetables (crucifers) have been consumed in Mediterranean countries since before Roman times [2]. Crucifer means 'cross bearer', and refers to the four petals of the flowers which are in the shape of a cross. Many of the best-known crucifers are members of the single genus *Brassica* and these include cabbage, broccoli, cauliflower, kale, kohlrabi, mustard, swede (rutabaga), turnips and Spring greens (American: collard greens). Other cruciferous vegetables that are not members of the genus *Brassica* include rocket (American: arugula), horseradish, radish and watercress. Although popular in the UK, brussel sprouts are not widely consumed in Mediterranean countries.

Crucifers are well-known for their sulphur-containing glucosinolates and the glucosinolate content of some crucifers is shown in Table 5.2. Glucosinolates are water-soluble glycosides which are stored in the plant. The glucosinolates are normally spatially separated in plants cells from the enzyme myrosinase, but when plant cells are damaged, myrosinase comes into contact with glucosinolates and can hydrolyse them, forming pungent glucosinolates breakdown products (GBPs). GBPs act as anti-feedants for the plant and deter predation. These same products are generated during chopping and chewing and, depending on the starting substrate, include various isothiocyanates and indoles. Glucosinolates, or more commonly their hydrolysis products, are responsible for the characteristic flavour of some crucifers. For example, glucosativin and its hydrolysis product sativin, give the distinct pungent flavour of rocket [4].

The absorption of glucosinolates in humans is not clear, but may be quite low since these molecules are relatively polar and charged at neutral pH. By contrast,

Table 5.2 Glucosinolate content of crucifers (from [5]).

Crucifer	Glucosinolate content (mg/100 g FW)	Major glucosinolates
Brassica oleracea		
○ Savoy cabbage	61.4–72.2	GIB, SIN, GBS
○ Kale	65.4–151.1	GIB, SIN, GBS
○ Green broccoli	23.0–64.6	PRO, GRA, GNA, GBS
○ White cauliflower	19.5–42.6	GIB, PRO, SIN, GBS
Brassica rapa		
○ Turnip*	50.4–81.7	PRO, GNA, GBN, GST
Eruca sativa		
○ Rocket (mg/g DW)	8.7–12.8	GSA, GRA, GER

GIB: glucoiberin; PRO: progoitrin; SIN: sinigrin; GRA: glucoraphanin; GNA: gluconapin; GBN: glucobrassicanapin; GBS: glucobrassicin; NGBS: neo-glucobrassicin; GST: gluconasturtiin; GER: glucoerucin; GSA: glucosativin. *Turnip greens contain GNA and GBN [6].

isothiocyanates and other bioactive GBPs have low molecular weights and low polarity and as a consequence they are efficiently absorbed across the gut [5]. Mild cooking does not inactivate myrosinase, and so active GBPs can be produced during chewing and subsequently absorbed in the small intestine. However, moderate levels of cooking inactivate the plant myrosinase and under these circumstances the inactive glucosinolates pass intact into the colon. Once in the colon, microbial metabolism of glucosinolates can make a major contribution to the production of active GBPs which can then be absorbed by the body.

Sulforaphane and other GBPs are recognised by the body as xenobiotics (foreign chemicals) and they induce both phase 1 and phase 2 metabolising enzymes, particularly glutathione-S-transferases (GSTs) [5]. GSTs rapidly conjugate GBPs with glutathione in the small intestine and liver, and the conjugated GBPs are ultimately excreted. The ability of GBPs to potently induce GSTs also increases the overall defence capability of cells against assault from other xenobiotics, including carcinogens. This is thought to be an important mechanisms for reducing cancer risk, and a number of epidemiological studies have shown a relationship between above average intake of Brassicas and a reduction in cancer [7].

Crucifers are also a good source of carotenoids. Spinach, kale and turnip greens have high levels of lutein, a carotenoid required for the correct functioning of the eye. The outer leaves of savoy cabbage contain substantially higher levels of carotenoids than the inner leaves (150 times the level of lutein and 200 times the level of β-carotene) [8]. These high levels of antioxidant carotenoids protect the outer leaves from photo-oxidation caused by sunlight. Higher levels of carotenoids are also found in the outer sun-exposed leaves of other green leafy vegetables.

Lettuces

Lettuce-based salads are widely consumed throughout the Mediterranean. The 'romaine' type lettuce, also known as Cos (possibly named after the Greek island), is more heat tolerant and is favoured over iceberg or looseleaf varieties. Exposure of the leaves of Cos lettuce to light causes them to produce antioxidants, particularly carotenoids, to protect against photo-oxidation. Cos lettuce contains up to ten times more carotenoids (β-carotene, lutein, zeaxanthin) than iceberg lettuce. Red lettuces (Lollo Rosso) are a source of anthocyanins. Dressing salad leaves with olive oil may enhance the bioavailability of fat-soluble phytochemicals, especially carotenoids.

Chicory

Early varieties of lettuce contained the bitter principle lactucin, but this has now mostly been bred out. However, moderate levels of this compound and related substances are still present in chicory, giving chicory its desired bitterness. Wild chicory is one of the most commonly-collected wild greens in Mediterranean countries. The roots of chicory are rich in inulin, and this used to be dried and used like coffee.

Spinach and related plants

Spinach is grown throughout the Mediterranean and it is a common side dish in Mediterranean cuisine. It also crops up in 'green' pies (such as Greek *spanokopita* and Tuscan *scarpazza*) where it is sometimes used interchangeably with Swiss chard or other greens. Spinach is an excellent source of folate and carotenoids, and it also contains methoxylated flavonol derivatives that are reported to have anti-mutagenic properties [9]. Spinach contains high levels of oxalic acid and this reduces calcium absorption due to the formation of insoluble calcium oxalate. However, iron absorption was reported to not be affected following consumption of spinach, presumably because the iron oxalate that is formed is soluble [10].

Smaller leafed relatives of spinach such as amaranth and orache are still eaten in some Mediterranean countries but must be boiled to reduce their oxalate content. Swiss chard, a close relative to spinach, is exceptionally rich in lutein and also has a very high flavonoid content (2700 mg/kg compared with 1000 mg/kg in spinach).

Vine leaves

A common dish in Eastern Mediterranean countries is rice and/or minced meat wrapped in vine leaves. Perhaps the best known of these dishes is Greek *dolmades*. It is usual to use vine leaves that have been preserved in brine, and hence these dishes can provide a source of green leaves throughout the year. Brined vine leaves were found to contain a variety of flavonoids and hydroxycinnamates, and extracts of the leaves demonstrated anti-inflammatory and anti-oxidant activities in *in vitro* assays and in animal models [11].

Vine leaves as a source of resveratrol?

There is much interest in increasing the levels of resveratrol in wine due to its purported health benefits [12]. Besides grapes, vine leaves also produce resveratrol and resveratrol derivatives, and levels increase significantly in vines exposed to UV light, reaching concentrations up to 750 µg/g FW [13]. If these levels were found in brined vine leaves used for consumption, this could translate into a significantly higher intake of resveratrol compounds than would be obtained from a couple of glasses of red wine, and without the dangers associated with alcohol consumption.

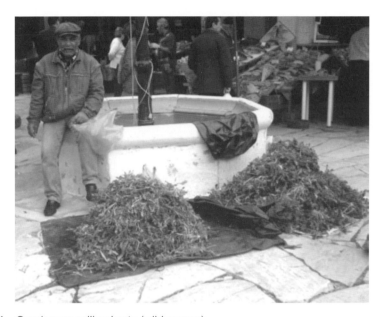

Figure 5.1   Greek man selling horta (wild greens).

Wild greens

Stalls piled high with wild greens, such as dandelions and wild chicory, are still a common site in some Mediterranean countries (Figure 5.1). It has been estimated that there are more than 150 edible wild greens in Mediterranean regions. Some that are widely consumed in Mediterranean countries include the leaves of purslane, wild fennel, smooth sow thistle, watercress, hawthorn, common golden thistle, common Mallow and borage, the stems of wild asparagus and wild leek, and the fruit of the strawberry tree [14]. Some examples are illustrated in Figure 5.2. In Greece, a huge variety of wild greens is consumed as part of a traditional MedDiet, and daily consumption was estimated at 20 g per day, which represents 10% of the total daily vegetable intake [15]. In the traditional Graecanic (Greek) area in Southern Calabria, Italy, more than 40 species (referred to as *ta chòrta*) were found to be regularly consumed [16]. By contrast, consumption in nearby Ragusa, Sicily was mainly restricted to six species [17]. This study suggests that the decision regarding which species to eat is not necessarily based on availability but may be strongly embedded

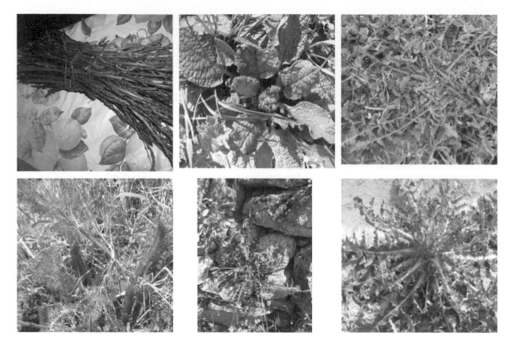

Figure 5.2   Examples of wild greens [18]. Clockwise from top left: wild asparagus shoots; borage; wild chicory; dandelion; French scorzanera; wild fennel.

in the local culture [14]. This may possibly help explain why most consumers in countries such as the UK do not collect wild greens although most of those shown in Figure 5.2 do in fact grow in the UK. (An excellent reference source on wild greens in the UK is *Food for Free* by Richard Mabey.)

Consumption of many wild greens is seasonal: Spring is the most popular time since the young leaves are usually less bitter. To avoid collecting greens at times of the year when the level of bitter compounds could be dangerous, precise timing for collection is often embedded in religious dates. Thus Easter is a traditional time in several Mediterranean countries for collecting wild asparagus, and this is then made into an omelette to be eaten by the community.

Many wild greens are eaten in salads. For example, *salada campanela* from Provence in France includes wild chicory, perennial lettuce, rampion, buck's horn plantain and corn salad, and Spanish *ensalada del campo* includes sow thistles, poppy, wild chicory, hawksbeard and prickly goldenfleece dressed with vinegar and extra virgin olive oil [14]. Wild greens may be boiled in water prior to use in order to remove water-soluble bitter compounds. Cooked wild greens are also used in a range of traditional soups and pies. Although some culinary practices such as boiling or the use of sweeteners are sometimes used to reduce excessive bitterness, a certain degree of bitterness is desirable for some Mediterranean people, and indeed is perceived as healthy [16]. One study found that consumption of wild greens was greater in Southern Italy compared with Northern Italy, and this was attributed to both a greater retention of traditional knowledge about these plants and to the greater appreciation in the South for bitter tastes [18].

Bitterness in wild greens is a double-edged sword: a certain level may have health benefits whereas excessive levels can be toxic. Many bitter compounds in wild greens

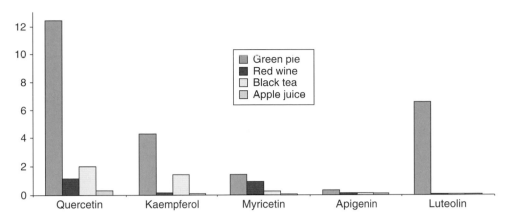

Figure 5.3 Flavonoid content of green pies (mg/100 g) and selected beverages (mg/100 ml) [22]. With permission from Elsevier.

act as plant defences against predation and are often present at far higher levels than in their cultivated counterparts. Wild greens, like berries, were probably an important part of the diet of our hunter-gatherer forebears. Humans can tolerate a certain level of toxic dietary compounds due to the presence of an efflux pump known as p-glycoprotein which is expressed on gut cells and pumps out toxins that accumulate in cells[1].

Wild greens have significant nutritional value, and even today they constitute an important source of nutrition for some people in the Mediterranean. For example, villagers in a rural area of Crete who consumed a lot of wild greens were found to have far better indicators of cardiovascular health than otherwise similar villagers who ate few wild greens [19]. The potential importance of wild greens for health has been recognised by major funding from the European Union, and some of the fruits of this research have been collated in a book [20].

At present, the compositional analysis of wild greens is mainly limited to those collected in Greece, Spain and Italy. Data from these studies have demonstrated that wild greens are particularly good sources of antioxidants and n-3 fatty acids. Wild greens collected in Crete were found to contain the antioxidant vitamins C and E, polyphenols and the carotenoids lutein and β-carotene, with generally higher levels than their cultivated counterparts [21]. One detailed study examined the flavonoid content of wild greens in Crete and pies made from these wild greens [15]. The wild greens were found to be excellent sources of flavonols, with one wild green (broad leaf dock) containing twice as much quercetin as onions – which is generally considered to be one of the richest sources of this flavonol. Pies are made from these greens in Crete from finely chopped greens that are cooked in a small amount of water with a lot of olive oil. (Using only a small amount of water will also minimise loss of water soluble phytochemicals.) It was calculated that two pieces of the pie (100 g) would make a significant contribution to the dietary flavonoid content – equivalent to 12 times more quercetin than a glass of red wine and three times more quercetin than a cup of black tea (Figure 5.3) [22].

---

[1] This pump is also exploited by cancer cells to pump out anti-cancer drugs that are derived from natural products.

The study of Ragusa, Sicily also found that wild greens from this commune, especially wild chicory, had remarkably high levels of antioxidants [17]. High levels were retained even after cooking the greens in a small amount of water, which was the traditional preparation method. Total levels of phenolics in the various wild greens ranged between 25 and 292 mg/100 g, and wild asparagus had 124 mg/100 g of quercetin which is far higher than that found in onions (34 mg/100 g). The most abundant carotenoids were β-carotene and lutein.

Another antioxidant that has recently been identified in plants is melatonin [23]. Although better known as a sleep regulator produced by the pineal gland, some studies suggest that melatonin may have diverse health benefits, such as protection against neurodegenerative disorders [24]. Purslane, which is commonly collected from the wild, is a particularly rich source of plant melatonin [25]. Purslane has small succulent leaves that have a delicious fresh pea taste; it has been grown in the UK in the past, but is not now readily available. However, it is easily grown from seed.

Many wild greens are good sources of the *n*-3 fatty acid alpha linolenic acid (ALA), and these plants also have relatively low ratios of *n*-6 fatty acids: *n*-3 fatty acids. Levels of *n*-3 fatty acids of up to 182 mg/100 g were reported in one study of wild greens that are still collected in Crete [26]. Purslane has the highest known levels of ALA in the plant kingdom, with concentrations reaching 400 mg/100 g [27].

Despite their potential health significance, wild greens are not yet represented on most depictions of the MedDiet such as the Oldways pyramid. In addition, culinary guidance on wild greens for people living outside areas of traditional knowledge is still somewhat limited. There are very few recipes in most Mediterranean cookery books, although *Mediterranean Vegetables* by Clifford A. Wright [2] and the Plants for a Future website (http://www.pfaf.org/index.php) are useful sources of further information.

5.2.2   Other green vegetables

Celery

Celery was first used medicinally and only later cultivated as a vegetable, and it crops up in many Mediterranean dishes, usually as a flavouring agent. Celery is a good source of the flavone apigenin (19 mg/100 g [28]). Apigenin administered in its pure form in experimental systems has a wide range of anti-proliferative and anti-tumour effects, although like most flavonoids it is subject to extensive metabolism, and its contribution to health as part of a normal diet is not known [29].

Parsley

Parsley is eaten in some Mediterranean countries in quantities that are comparable to vegetables. For example, parsley is a main ingredient in the Lebanese salad *tabbouleh* which is based on bulgur wheat. Parsley is a good source of vitamin C and of lutein and zeaxanthin, carotenoids found in the retina. Parsley is exceptionally rich in apigenin with levels of 630 mg/100 g FW being reported, and parsley was found to be the main source of this flavone in the traditional Greek MedDiet [30].

Asparagus

Both cultivated asparagus (*Asparagus officinalis*) and wild asparagus (*Asparagus acutifolius*) are consumed in Mediterranean countries, although most published information comes from studies on the cultivated variety. Asparagus is a good source of folate and of the carotenoids lutein, β-carotene and – unusually – capsanthin (which is only found elsewhere in any significant quantities in red peppers) [31]. Asparagus is also a very good source of flavonoids (principally rutin) [32], and of phytoestrogens (most of which is the lignan secoisolariciresinol) [33]. Some people excrete a sulphurous smelling urine after consuming asparagus, and this is believed to be due to methanthiol and other sulphur-containing compounds which are produced from asparagusic acid in those individuals who are able to absorb this compound across the gut (a good illustration of inter-individual variation in phytochemical bioavailability) [34].

Globe artichoke

Globe artichokes are consumed in many Mediterranean countries, and Spain and Italy are the top producers. Artichokes were originally used medicinally, particularly for liver complaints since they are thought to act as cholagogues (i.e. they increase the flow of bile into the duodenum). They are a rich source of phenolics including cynarin, chlorogenic acid and narirutin [35]. The therapeutic benefits of artichokes have in the past mostly been ascribed to cynarin, although it is now thought that these benefits are probably due to additive and synergistic interactions between several compounds, including various phenolics [36]. Artichokes also contain inulin, fibre, minerals and plant sterols, and they were estimated to be one of the richest vegetable sources of plant sterols in the Spanish diet [37]. Large green varieties are boiled, but small violet ones can be eaten raw, both being accompanied with a 'vinaigrette' made of wine vinegar and olive oil. They are also consumed as part of various dishes *à la provençale*, tagines, etc.

Courgettes, squashes

These vegetables are all members of the genus Cucurbita, and wild members are bitter due to the presence of cucurbitans. Yellow squashes contain various carotenoids, especially β-carotene.

5.2.3 Root vegetables

Root crops consumed in Mediterranean countries include carrots, turnips and beetroot. The leaves of turnips and beetroot are also eaten in some countries such as Portugal and Italy, although carrot leaves – which are edible – are rarely consumed. Carrots are well known for their α-carotene and β-carotene content (up to 65 mg/100 g), and they also contain phytosterols, chlorogenic acids and the polyacetylene falcarinol that has anti-tumour effects in experimental systems. The red pigmentation of beetroot is due to a group of phytochemicals called betalains. As with most Mediterranean vegetables, root vegetables are often married with olive oil. Goat's cheese and yogurt are popular partners for beetroot. These fats may enhance the bioavailability of fat-soluble phytochemicals.

Table 5.3 Consumption of onions in Mediterranean countries and the UK (FAOSTAT 2003).

	Consumption (g/per capita/per day)
Egypt	8
France	14
Greece	52
Italy	24
Morocco	58
Spain	44
Tunisia	27
Turkey	47
United Kingdom	25
EU 15	19

5.2.4 Alliums

The allium family includes several important culinary vegetables such as onions, shallots and leeks, and herbs such as garlic and chives. Onions have been used in Mediterranean cooking for thousands of years: onions were cultivated by the ancient Egyptians (*circa* 3200 BC), and onions and garlic were discovered at the Minoan royal palace at Knossos on Crete (2700–1450 BC) [2]. A wide range of beneficial effects are attributed to alliums, including protection against CVD and cancer. Many of these effects are attributed to various organo-sulphur compounds, most of which are generated from cysteine sulphoxides (which are modified sulphated amino acids) when the allium is cut or damaged.

Onions

Frying onions in olive oil is probably the most common first step in Mediterranean cuisine, and consumption of onions is high in many Mediterranean countries (Table 5.3). The frying time may be only a few minutes in the case of an Italian *soffrito*, or much longer if the aim is to develop the sweetness in the onions or to produce the dark brown base for a Catalan *sofregit* (which may take up to an hour or more). Catalans also hold hugely popular festivals in early Spring to eat – and celebrate – a type of onion called a *calçot*. Brown onions are the most popular choice for cooking, and milder red onions, Spanish onions and shallots are usually cooked for only short periods or are used raw in salads. Onions are also added to stews without any prior cooking.

Onions contain several quite distinct groups of constituents including flavonoids, inulin and cysteine sulphoxides. Yellow and red onions are major dietary sources of the flavonoid quercetin, but white onions contain very little. The quercetin is conjugated to various sugars, mainly glucose, and these glucosides are present at particularly high concentrations in the outer dry skin of onions where they protect the onion from soil microbes. But high levels do still remain after peeling. Quercetin is one of the most studied of all phytochemicals, and a wide range of potentially cancer-preventative actions have been identified in experimental systems [38]. Quercetin is moderately stable during cooking, and since onions are usually cooked

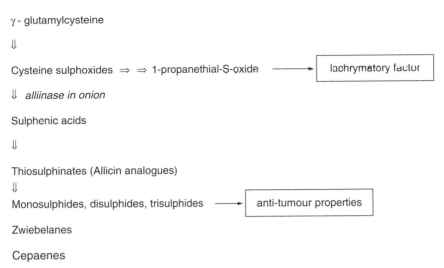

γ - glutamylcysteine

⇓

Cysteine sulphoxides   ⇒ ⇒ 1-propanethial-S-oxide ——————→ | lachrymatory factor |

⇓ *alliinase in onion*

Sulphenic acids

⇓

Thiosulphinates (Allicin analogues)
⇓
Monosulphides, disulphides, trisulphides ——————→ | anti-tumour properties |

Zwiebelanes

Cepaenes

Figure 5.4 Major organo-sulphur compounds produced during the processing of onions.

in dishes which are eaten in their entirety, this will minimise loss of this phytochemical. When onions are cooked in water, there is a significant transfer of quercetin glucosides to the cooking water, turning this liquid into a good source of these flavonoids [39]. Frying onions has beneficial effects by breaking down the onion cells to release the quercetin, and the frying oil increases the absorption of quercetin across the gut [39]. Drinking red wine with a meal rich in onions may also have unexpected benefits since the alcohol in red wine has been shown to increase the absorption of quercetin across the gut in animal models [40]. Apart from quercetin, onions also contain smaller quantities of the flavonoids isorhamnetin and kaempferol [41]. The flavonoid content of leeks consists almost entirely of kaempferol. Anthocyanins are responsible for the colour of red onions.

The sulphur compounds in onions become apparent to the cook during their preparation due to the generation of the lachrymatory (tear-inducing) factor cycloalliin (1-propanethial-S-oxide). This is generated from isoalliin, the major cysteine sulphoxide in onions, by the enzyme alliinase during cutting due to the decompartmentalisation of substrate and enzyme (Figure 5.4). Other sulphur-containing compounds are also generated when onions are cut, and some of these have anti-tumour properties, although some are inactivated during cooking [42].

Onions are also a major dietary source in the MedDiet of the fructose-containing polysaccharide inulin. Inulin is a prebiotic and may afford protection against colorectal cancer. Inulin is hydrolysed to fructose during cooking which gives onions that have been fried for prolonged periods their sweet taste. Onions are also a good source of the polysaccharide pectin, and pectin has been demonstrated to enhance quercetin absorption in animal models, although the relevance of this to human nutrition has not been established [43].

Garlic

The 19th century Irish-American Augustus Saint-Gaudens said of garlic 'What garlic is to food, insanity is to art.' Fortunately, the culinary and health properties of garlic

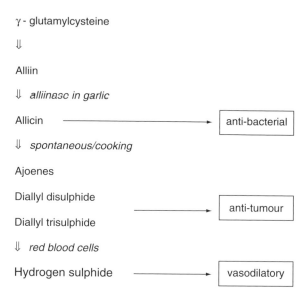

Figure 5.5 Formation of sulphur compounds from garlic and possible physiological effects.

are now more widely appreciated in the US and North European countries. In Mediterranean cuisine, the appreciation of garlic, both as a food and as medicine, goes back to the time of the ancient Egyptians. Garlic is eaten raw in various salad dressings and sauces. Catalan *allioli* is simply raw garlic mashed with salt and olive oil (all-i-oli means 'garlic and oil'). Less pungent variants are French *aiolli* (with the addition of egg yolks), and Greek *skordalia* which includes potatoes. Garlic is a basic ingredient in countless Mediterranean recipes, and it assumes centre stage in garlic soup or when the garlic is roasted whole.

Various studies have claimed that garlic has antifungal and antibacterial properties, protects against the early stages of stomach and colorectal cancer, reduces the likelihood of getting the common cold, lowers cholesterol, lowers blood pressure and reduces blood clotting. But these claims are not without controversy [44]. Inconsistent results may arise between human studies if different types of garlic preparations are consumed. These preparations include raw or cooked garlic, as well as various herbal garlic supplements such as garlic powder or 'aged' garlic preparations. In experimental studies, the amounts of garlic used may be far higher than would be consumed as part of a normal diet. The benefits of raw and cooked garlic are probably not the same due to the heat labile nature of some of the putative pharmacologically active organo-sulphur compounds. Garlic also contains minerals and oligosaccharides, although flavonoid levels are low compared to onions.

The major precursor organo-sulphur compound in garlic is alliin. Chopping or crushing garlic brings alliinase into contact with alliin to form allicin (Figure 5.5). Allicin is responsible for garlic's characteristic sulphurous odour. The effect of time on generating allicin is well known to the cook since foods containing garlic left overnight in the fridge will often taste more 'garlicky' the following day. Allicin is not heat stable and is rapidly converted into a range of sulphur-containing products including ajoene, diallyl disulphide and diallyl trisulphide (Figure 5.5).

Preparation and cooking procedures that maximise the production of allicin from alliin are important since many of the beneficial effects of garlic have been attributed to allicin and/or its breakdown products. This was nicely illustrated by a study that examined the activities of various garlic preparations using an *in vitro* anti platelet assay. An extract made from intact garlic that had previously been heated for ≥6 minutes at 200C had no anti-platelet activity, and this is probably because no allicin was present in the garlic due to heat inactivation of alliinase. By contrast, garlic that was crushed and left for up to 10 minutes was found to retain modest anti-platelet activity and allicin activity even when cooked for moderate times, indicating that if time is given for active compounds to be produced, then some activity may be retained even when heated [45].

Studies have established that allicin is also an important anti-bacterial compound in garlic [46], and allicin was found to be crucial for inhibition of the bacterium *H. pylori* in *in vitro* experiments [47]. The relative instability of allicin to heat suggests that consuming raw garlic would be optimal for it to be effective as an antibacterial. These studies on the anti-platelet and anti-bacterial properties of garlic point to the benefits of maximum contact between alliinase and its substrate alliin. This would be achieved in the kitchen by macerating garlic in salt and/or oil (a common procedure in Spanish cooking) rather than chopping or slicing it, and by leaving garlic before using it so as to allow time for allicin to be produced. Cooking will reduce the amount of allicin present since neither allicin nor alliinase are heat stable. Hence, the consumer may obtain quite different health benefits from the same amount of garlic depending on how the garlic has been prepared.

Various breakdown products of allicin including diallyl sulphide, diallyl disulphide, diallyl trisulphide and ajoene have chemopreventative properties in experimental systems [48]. Diallyl disulphide and diallyl trisulphide are also implicated in the cardioprotective properties of garlic since there is evidence that the vasodilatory actions of garlic in the body are due to the production of hydrogen sulphide from diallyl disulphide and diallyl trisulphide by red blood cells [49]. Hydrogen sulphide relaxes smooth muscle cells surrounding blood vessels, which results in vasodilation and thus a lowering of blood pressure.

The sulphur-containing phytochemicals in garlic are synthesised from sulphur obtained from the soil. If the soil is rich in selenium, then selenium can substitute for the sulphur and so produce a series of so-called seleno-compounds. In animal studies, these seleno-compounds have been found to be superior to their sulphur-containing counterparts [50]. However, their significance for human health has not been established. Other alliums that also obtain sulphur from the soil will also manufacture seleno-compounds if grown in selenium-rich soil.

5.2.5 Solanaceous vegetables

Tomato

Tomatoes are closely associated with Mediterranean cooking, although they were only introduced into Europe from S. America in the 16th century and it was another three centuries before they became widely accepted as a foodstuff. Tomatoes appear in a huge variety of Mediterranean dishes such as *gazpacho* – the cold tomato soup of Andalusia, as part of vegetable stews such as French *ratatouille*, as a sauce for pasta, stuffed and baked in the oven, and in an endless variety of salads.

Table 5.4 Nutrient composition of raw tomatoes (USDA; www.phenol-explorer.eu/).

	Nutrient	**Amount /100 g**
Minerals	potassium, mg	237
Vitamins	α-tocopherol, mg	0.54
	vitamin A, IU	833
	vitamin C, mg	12.7
	total folate, μg	15
Carotenoids	β-carotene, μg	449
	α-carotene, μg	101
	lycopene, μg	2573
	lutein + zeaxanthin, μg	123
	phytoene, μg	1860
	phytofluene, μg	820
Phenolics	naringenin-7-glucoside, μg	140
	rutin, μg	140
	chlorogenic acid, mg	1.84
	caffeic acid, mg	0.45
	ferulic acid, mg	0.27

Data from an EPIC study found that consumption of tomatoes and tomato products in Mediterranean countries was generally quite high compared to non-Mediterranean countries. Greece with 164±84 g/day had the highest consumption, and this compares with only 42±27 g/day in the UK and an average across all EPIC countries of 60±59 g/day [51].

Constituents

Tomatoes and tomato products are the main source of lycopene in the MedDiet (from the Latin name for tomato, *Lycopersicum esculentum*), and they are also an important source of other carotenoids, as well as vitamin C, chlorogenic acid, flavonoids, vitamin E, and trace elements such as copper, iron, and chromium (Table 5.4). A study on dietary sources in Spain found that tomatoes ranked first as a source of lycopene (71.6%); second as a source of vitamin C (12.0%), pro-vitamin A carotenoids (14.6%) and β-carotene (17.2%); and third as a source of vitamin E (6.0%) [52]. In one study, the major flavonoid was identified as chalconaringenin (which gets broken down to naringenin and comprised 35–71% of the total flavonoid content), with smaller quantities of rutin and other flavonoids [53]. Tomatoes also contain a wide range of other bioactive compounds including carbohydrates, free amino acids, fibre, minerals, vitamins, and – in green tomatoes – glycoalkaloids.

There are wide variations between tomatoes in their phytochemical content. Flavonoid content was found in one study to vary between 4 to 26 mg /100 g FW depending on the type of tomato [53]. The EuroFir database gives values of lycopene ranging from 0.8–63 mg/100 g FW, although most estimates are approximately 10 mg/100 g FW.

The accumulation of phytochemicals in tomatoes, and hence amounts consumed, is influenced by growth conditions. Lycopene synthesis is favoured at temperatures between 16 and 21 °C and inhibited at temperatures above 30 °C. There is no consistency between studies that have compared phytochemical levels in tomatoes grown organically and those grown conventionally. One study did find that organic tomatoes had higher levels of vitamin C, carotenoids (lycopene and β-carotene) and polyphenols (except chlorogenic acid) (expressed on a FW basis; but carotenoids not significant when expressed on DW basis), but there was no significant difference between the two farming practices with respect to their effects on vitamin C and lycopene plasma concentrations when the tomatoes were consumed as part of a normal diet [54]. There is stronger evidence that phytochemical levels are influenced by stage of maturity of the fruit at harvest, light quality, controlled irrigation, cultivar, and the impact of the growing season [55, 56]. The lycopene content of tomatoes grown in greenhouses either in the summer or winter has been found to be lower than in tomatoes grown outside. Also, tomatoes picked green and ripened in storage – a very common practice for out-of-season tomatoes – were found to have substantially lower levels of lycopene than 'vine-ripened' tomatoes [57].

Bell peppers

The carotenoid content of bell peppers is an important determinant of their colour. Red peppers contain capsanthin and, to a lesser extent, capsorubin. Red peppers contain very little lutein, whereas this carotenoid predominates in yellow and green peppers. The yellow colouration of lutein is masked in green peppers by the high chlorophyll content. Yellow peppers also contain zeaxanthin, and this is also the predominant carotenoid in orange peppers. Degree of freshness may be an important factor in carotenoid content since green bell peppers obtained on the day of harvest had far higher levels of α- and β-carotene than supermarket bought peppers that had incurred 7–14 days' storage and transportation [58].

Peppers are an excellent source of vitamin C – in fact, this vitamin was first isolated from paprika-type peppers in the 1930s by Szent-Gyorgyi. One hundred grams of red pepper contain about 90 mg of vitamin C. Being water soluble, vitamin C is lost during water blanching and subsequent canning. Peppers also contain high levels of vitamin E.

Peppers are also rich in flavonoids including quercetin and luteolin, with levels varying widely between cultivars. Total flavonoid content generally declines as the fruit ripens, and in one study immature green peppers had a 4- to 5-fold higher level of flavonoids compared to the same cultivar after it had matured and become red [58].

Hot pepper varieties of pepper contain capsaicinoids. These are alkaloids and they have been shown to lower cholesterol levels.

Aubergines

The purple skin of aubergines (American, eggplant) is due to anthocyanins. Aubergines also contain around 11 mg/100 g of lignans (www.phenol-explorer.eu).

5.2.6 Legumes

Legumes were amongst the earliest plants to be cultivated in the Mediterranean. Farming in the Levant region (Eastern Mediterranean) is thought to have originated with a group of 'founder crops' which consisted of legumes (peas, lentil, chickpea and bitter vetch) and grains (einkorn wheat, emmer wheat and barley) [59]. Legumes

Table 5.5 Consumption of pulses in Mediterranean countries and the UK in 1961 and 2003 (FAOSTAT).

	Consumption (g/per capita/per day)	
	1961	2003
Egypt	16.44	24.66
France	5.48	5.48
Greece	19.18	10.96
Italy	10.96	13.70
Morocco	10.96	16.44
Spain	24.66	13.70
Tunisia	5.48	21.92
Turkey	24.66	27.40
United Kingdom	5.48	10.96

are particularly suited to the harsh growing conditions of parts of the Mediterranean since they fix nitrogen and so can grow in poor soils whilst at the same time enriching it, and many are drought tolerant and so are suitable for growing even in the more arid areas.

Legumes that are mainly grown for their dried seeds are often referred to as 'pulses', whereas the broader definition of legumes also includes green beans and green peas. Pulses are very important in Mediterranean cuisine and are consumed in quite high amounts and on a regular basis, Turkey ranking highest amongst Mediterranean countries (Table 5.5).

In Egypt, *ful mudammas,* based on mashed fava (broad) beans, is considered the national dish, and it is eaten at many different times through the day, including breakfast, lunch or supper. The technique of mashing pulses is common in many countries and aids digestion. Chickpeas are particularly popular in Turkey and Spain (where they are known as *garbanzos*). In Spain, *cocido*, a stew of meat, chickpeas, and vegetables, is one of the Spanish national dishes. In Southern France, *panisse* is still popular in Provence and *la socca* in the Nice region, and these are made of chick-pea flour and olive oil (plus water for *panisse*). Lentils are another type of pulse popular throughout the Mediterranean. Pulses can be stored for extended periods with little loss of nutritional value, and hence the nutritional value will be unaltered by export to non-producing countries such as the UK.

Pulse dishes are often strongly flavoured with spices (especially in North Africa) or herbs (Italy). For example, *falafel* is a North African dish of fritters made with mashed broad beans or chickpeas and large quantities of cumin and coriander. Hence a high consumption of pulses often goes hand-in-hand with a high intake of herbs or spices – an important point nutritionally, although not one that is generally scored for in epidemiological food studies, including Mediterranean diet scores.

Pulses dishes are often complemented with grain dishes and this will ensure intake of a complete range of amino acids (pulses contain low levels of methionine and grains are relatively deficient in lysine). Chickpeas are rich in tryptophan which is converted in the body into serotonin. Serotonin improves mood and gives a feeling of satiety, and it has been speculated that this may have contributed to the reasons for selecting chickpeas early on for domestication [59].

Table 5.6 Nutrient content of common Mediterranean pulses per 100 g cooked (USDA database).

	Chickpea	Lentil	Broad (fava) bean
Protein, g	8.9	9.0	7.6
Fat, total, g	2.6	0.4	0.4
saturated, g	0.27	0.05	0.16
monounsaturated, g	0.58	0.06	0.08
polyunsaturated, g	1.12	0.18	0.16
LA, g	1.11	0.14	0.15
ALA, g	0.04	0.04	0.01
Fibre, total dietary, g	7.6	7.9	5.4
Vitamins			
Folate, μg	172	181	104
Vitamin B_2, mg	0.06	73	89
Niacin, mg	0.53	1.06	0.71
Vitamin B6, mg	0.14	0.18	0.07
Vitamin B12, mg	0.29	0.64	0.16
Vitamin A, IU	27	8	15
Vitamin E, mg	0.35	0.11	0.02
Vitamin K, μg	4.0	1.7	2.9
β-carotene, μg	16	5	9
Minerals			
Ca, mg	49	19	36
Zn, mg	1.5	1.3	1.0
Fe, mg	2.9	3.3	1.5
Mg, mg	48	36	43

Constituents

Pulses are good sources of many nutrients. A serving of 100 g of chickpeas would provide almost the recommended daily requirement of folate, as well as various other vitamins (especially B vitamins) and minerals (Table 5.6). Pulses have a good protein content (Table 5.6), but they are often referred to as 'poor man's meat'; as incomes improve, diets tend to switch from pulses to meat, a trend seen in some Mediterranean countries such as Spain and Greece (see Table 5.5).

Pulses are also a good source of dietary fibre. The outer seed coat comprises most of the insoluble fibre, together with some phyto-estrogens, whereas the central part (comprising the cotyledons for the embryo) contains soluble fibre. Pulses also contain oligosaccharides such as raffinose, stachyose and verbascose. These oligosaccharides are something of a double-edged sword: on the one hand they act as prebiotics stimulating the growth of beneficial gut bacteria, but on the other they generate flatulence in some people which decreases their appeal, although the preparation method can have a strong influence on this.

Data on Italian pulses from INRAN (Istituto Nazionale di Ricerca per gli Alimenti e la Nutrizione) indicate higher values for ALA than data from the USDA database. Based on these values, it was estimated that pulses can make a significant contribution to the overall daily recommended intake of ALA ($\geq 0.5\%$ total energy) in the Italian diet. For example, the ALA content of a typical bean soup from Southern Italy was estimated at 640 mg ALA per serving [60]. Chickpeas are exceptional amongst

Mediterranean pulses in containing relatively high levels of fat, constituting about 15% of total energy [61]. (Only soybeans have higher amounts.)

Pulses are also a good source of some phytochemicals, including phytosterols and lignans. For example, the major phytosterol β-sitosterol was found at levels of up to 160 mg/ 100 g in chickpeas and 123 mg/100 g in lentils [62].

Despite their very low GI and favourable nutrient profiles, only a limited number of epidemiological studies have assessed the health benefits of Mediterranean legumes (most studies focus on soya beans), probably because their consumption is very low nowadays. There is some limited evidence for protection against metabolic syndrome and risk of CVD (see Chapters 10 and 11).

5.3 Wheat products

Grains or cereals have been cultivated in the Mediterranean region since the beginning of agriculture. Wheat constitutes one the three fundamental foodstuffs of Mediterranean countries (along with wine and olives). It is used not only for making bread, but is also processed from a paste of flour and water to make pasta, or made into bulgur wheat, popular in the Eastern Mediterranean, or couscous which is widely consumed in the Maghreb. Other grains are also grown in Mediterranean countries including rice, which is grown in Spain, Italy and the Camargue region of France, and maize which is ground into cornmeal and used to make polenta in Italy and countries on the Adriatic. However, wheat is by far the most prevalent grain grown in Mediterranean countries (Table 5.7) and bread accompanies most meals and would traditionally have been made from relatively unrefined grain. Further discussions will be limited to this grain.

Wheat grain consists of an outer layer of bran (10–14%), a middle layer called the endosperm (80–85%), and an inner germ layer (2.5–3%) (Figure 5.6). Bioactive constituents are not evenly distributed amongst these layers, and refining removes most of the bran and germ layers and hence many of the nutritionally important constituents present in these layers are lost (Table 5.8).

Table 5.7 Wheat and cereal food supply in Mediterranean countries and the UK in 2005 (FAOSTAT).

Country	Wheat supply (g/capita/day)	Cereal supply (g/capita/day)
Egypt	382	667
France	290	341
Greece	381	413
Italy	406	435
Morocco	486	706
Spain	236	262
Tunisia	544	568
Turkey	490	571
United Kingdom	269	308

The outer bran and inner germ are the main sources of fibre. Wheat grain contains 9–17 g fibre/100 g edible portion compared to <6 g/100 g typical of vegetables. Wheat grain is a major dietary source of insoluble fibre (e.g. cellulose, hemicellulose), but contain relatively low levels of soluble fibre (β-glucan and arabinoxylans) (about 1:5 soluble to insoluble) [63]. Cereal fibre increases satiety and hence may reduce obesity, and some dietary fibres are fermentable and contribute to colonic health. Cereal

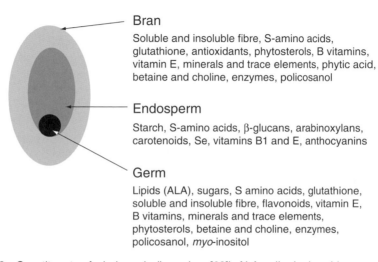

Bran

Soluble and insoluble fibre, S-amino acids, glutathione, antioxidants, phytosterols, B vitamins, vitamin E, minerals and trace elements, phytic acid, betaine and choline, enzymes, policosanol

Endosperm

Starch, S-amino acids, β-glucans, arabinoxylans, carotenoids, Se, vitamins B1 and E, anthocyanins

Germ

Lipids (ALA), sugars, S amino acids, glutathione, soluble and insoluble fibre, flavonoids, vitamin E, B vitamins, minerals and trace elements, phytosterols, betaine and choline, enzymes, policosanol, *myo*-inositol

Figure 5.6   Constituents of whole grain (based on [63]). ALA: α-linolenic acid.

Table 5.8   Nutrients in wholemeal and white flour [64]. Crown copyright.

Nutrient	Nutrient per 100 g flour		% lost after refining
	Wholemeal flour	White flour	
Protein (g)	12.7	9.4	26
Fat (g)	2.2	1.3	41
Carbohydrate (g)	63.9	77.7	<0
Fibre (g)	8.6	3.6	58
Sodium (mg)	3	3	0
Potassium (mg)	340	150	56
Magnesium (mg)	120	20	83
Phosphorus (mg)	320	110	66
Iron (mg)	3.9	1.5	62
Zinc (mg)	2.9	0.6	79
Manganese (mg)	3.1	0.6	81
Selenium (μg)	53	4	92
Thiamin (mg)	0.46	0.1	78
Riboflavin (mg)	0.09	0.03	67
Niacin (mg)	5.7	1.7	70
Vitamin B6 (mg)	0.5	0.15	70
Folate (μg)	57	22	61
Vitamin E (mg)	1.4	0.3	79

fibres also lower the glycaemic index of a meal and improve glucose tolerance at a subsequent meal: lunch after a low GI breakfast or breakfast after a low GI dinner – the so-called 'second-meal effect' [63].

Whole grain wheat is also a good source of phenolics. The relatively high daily consumption of wheat makes it a significant dietary source of plant lignans. These are converted into mammalian lignans which have been linked to protection against hormone-dependent cancers (see Chapter 12). Up to 90% of the total phenolics in wheat bran comprises ferulic acid [65]. Ferulic acid has antioxidant properties and inhibitory activity in experimental models of carcinogenesis [66]. Most ferulic acid in wheat bran is bound to hemicelluloses and other constituents, and this is expected to reduce its absorption [67], although it may slowly be released from fibre by colonic bacteria and so afford protection in the colon [68].

Cereals are also a major source of phytosterols and were the second major source in the Spanish diet after oils (30% and 39% of total, respectively) [37]. Phytosterols have cholesterol-lowering properties. Whole grain is also an important dietary source of unsaturated fats, folates, magnesium, potassium, vitamin E, flavonoids and selenium.

In conclusion, whole grain wheat contains a complex mixture of bioactive constituents. This mixture suggest (1) the possibility for bioactive substances to interact synergistically and (2) influences of the cereal matrix on the bioavailability of compounds.

5.4   Fruits

Fruits are tasty to encourage eating and so disseminate the seed within. To ensure that the fruit is only eaten when the seed is ready, fruit is hard and unappetising when unripe, and soft and tasty when ripe. The softening process is exemplified by the breakdown of pectic polysaccharides, whereas taste changes are associated with an increase in sugars and a reduction in bitter-tasting phytochemicals – such as the conversion of bitter limonoids in citrus fruits into tasteless glycoside derivatives. Ripe fruits signal when they are ready to be consumed by developing an attractive colour and smell. The emphasis on seasonal, naturally ripened fruits in the MedDiet ensures that they are consumed with the complex mix of phytochemicals that give them their authentic smells and tastes.

5.4.1   Citrus fruits

Citrus fruits rank first in terms of world fruit production, and about 12% of this production comes from the Mediterranean region (behind Brazil, the US and China) (Table 5.9).

All citrus varieties are thought to originate from three parent species, namely the citron (also known as cedrat), mandarin (or tangerine) and pumello, although the taxonomy of citrus species is controversial [69]. The citron reached the Mediterranean from the Himalayas by 300 BC [69]. It is a very large type of citrus fruit with a thick skin, and the aromatic rind is used after being candied. It plays an important role in Jewish culture. Pumellos are not widely grown in Mediterranean countries.

A wide variety of oranges, mandarins, limes and lemons are now consumed in Mediterranean countries, as elsewhere. These varieties are the result of inter-breeding,

Table 5.9 Production and consumption of citrus fruits (FAOSTAT).

	Production (thousand tonnes)		Consumption (g/per capita/per day)	
	Oranges, mandarins	Lemons, limes	Oranges, mandarins	Lemons, limes
Egypt	1800	335	68	8
France	0.1	0.6	112	3
Greece	778	92	140	22
Italy	2293	547	106	25
Morocco	750	22	63	0
Spain	2599	499	90	30
Tunisia	141	31	33	5
Turkey	1427	652	49	11
United Kingdom	0	0	115	3

some of these varieties having been developed centuries ago, whereas others are more recent. The bitter orange (also called sour or Seville orange) was introduced by the Moors in the 11th century. The juice is squeezed like lemon juice over fish. It is also used to make marmalade where its bitterness is counter-balanced with the sweetness of sugar. Sweet oranges – possibly a cross between pumellos and mandarins – became established in the Mediterranean in the 15th century and are eaten on their own or in salads. Blood oranges are the most commonly consumed orange in Italy, the red coloration being due to anthocyanins. The rind of oranges is candied and is a widely-used ingredient in Mediterranean cooking.

There are many varieties of lemons. They are used not only for juice, but are also preserved in salt to make a condiment that is popular in N. African cuisines. It is only the rind of preserved lemons that is consumed. True lemonade, as opposed to its industrial imitator, is made using both the rind and juice of lemons. Some alcoholic drinks are based on citrus peel, such as *limoncello*, an Italian liqueur made from lemon rind.

Constituents

Citrus fruits provide many important nutrients including vitamin C, soluble fibre (pectin), folates, B vitamins, minerals (e.g. potassium, calcium, phosphorus, magnesium, copper) and a wide variety of phytochemicals. These constituents are not evenly distributed between the juice, fruit segments and peel, and so consumption of the constituents will vary accordingly. For example, the rind contains most of the fibre and also has higher levels of some phytochemicals than the juice.

Vitamin C
The vitamin C content of citrus fruits is a major contributor to human health. Orange juice contains 40–70 mg/100 ml vitamin C, and grapefruits, tangerines and lemons contain 20–50 mg/100 ml. Since most oranges and orange juice are eaten fresh there is no loss of vitamin C. A 225 ml glass of orange juice contains approximately 125 mg

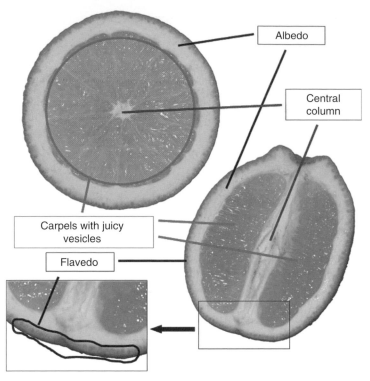

Figure 5.7   Main tissues in oranges (Wikipedia).

of vitamin C which provides the recommended daily intake (30–100 mg). The peel is also rich in vitamin C, containing five times more in the outer skin (flavedo) and three times more in the albedo (the thick white spongy layer) than the juice on a per weight basis (see Figure 5.7). Vitamin C plays a key role in collagen formation, and hence the prevention of scurvy, and it is an important water-soluble antioxidant vitamin. The antioxidant capacity of oranges may be due to both vitamin C and other constituents such as phytochemicals since drinking blood orange juice was found to be more protective against oxidative damage to DNA than consuming an equivalent amount of pure vitamin C [70].

Fibre
Consuming the segmented fruit or peel of citrus fruit is a source of fibre, particularly pectin, which constitutes 65–70% of the total fibre. Lemon peel constitutes about 5% of the fresh weight of a lemon compared to 2.5–4% for the pulp [71].

Phytochemicals
Citrus fruits contain a wide range of phytochemicals, including flavonoids (flavanones and flavones) and various terpenes (limonene, limonoids and carotenoids) [72–74] (see Table 5.10).

Flavonoids were originally isolated from paprika, and later from lemon juice, by Szent-Gyorgyi and colleagues in 1936 who named them citrin or substance P since

Table 5.10 Some major phytochemicals in citrus fruits.

	Examples	Typical sources
Flavonoids		
Flavanones (glycosides)	Naringin	bitter orange
	Narirutin	sweet orange, tangerine
	Hesperidin	sweet orange, tangerine, lemon
	Neohesperidin	bitter orange
	Eriocitrin	lemon
Flavones	Nobiletin	orange juice
	Tangeretin	orange juice
Monoterpenes	(+)-Limonene	orange
	(−)-Limonene	lemon
Limonoids	Limonin	citrus juices
Carotenoids	Violaxanthin	orange
	β-carotene	clementine, mandarin
	β-cryptoxanthin	mandarin, orange
	Zeaxanthin	orange

they reduced capillary fragility and permeability [75]. A wide range of beneficial effects have now been attributed to citrus flavonoids including protection against atherosclerosis and cancer, although most of this evidence comes from cell culture and animal models [76].

Many different groups of flavonoids are present in citrus fruits. Flavanones are the major class of flavonoids found in citrus fruits and most are present as glycosides. Bitter oranges have a distinct flavanone composition dominated by naringin and neohesperidin that impart the bitter taste. Hesperidin and narirutin are the main flavanones in sweet oranges and tangerines. There are various reports of anti-proliferative activity of flavanones against cancer cell lines, but because flavanones are subject to extensive metabolism these observations need following up in animal studies [76] Citrus rind is of particular interest since its flavanone content is far higher than that of the juice.

Citrus fruits also contain flavones, principally nobiletin and tangeretin. These flavones contain several methoxyl groups and these polymethoxylated flavones occur exclusively in citrus fruits. It has been suggested that polymethoxylated flavones will have superior activity compared to other flavonoids, for example as chemopreventative agents, since the methoxyl groups make them more resistant to metabolic degradation [77]. However, there is no human data to support these claims.

Several different types of terpenes occur in citrus fruits, including simple monoterpenes as well as the more complex limonoids and carotenoids. Monoterpenes are important aroma compounds in citrus fruits [78]. The major monoterpene is d-limonene which comprises 80–95% of the essential oil in citrus peel. This monoterpene has attracted interest for its potential to prevent or treat cancer, particularly breast cancer, when given as a supplement (http://clinicaltrials. gov). A major active metabolite of limonene in the body is perillic acid (see Figure 5.8), and drinking 'Mediterranean-style' lemonade made from blending whole lemons in water was found to result in the appearance in the plasma of this metabolite [79]. It is not yet known if limonene as a single agent may be an

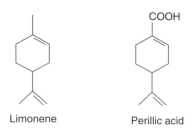

Figure 5.8   Structures of limonene and perillic acid.

effective anti-cancer agent in humans, or if it might interact with other dietary components in a beneficial way.

Limonoids are triterpenes and are responsible for bitterness in unripe citrus fruits. During ripening, the bitter aglycones are converted into tasteless glycosides[2]. However, the aglycones remain in the seed, and they impart a strong bitter taste to the seeds which will reduce the likelihood that they will be chewed and thus damaged during consumption. Both the glycones and aglycones have a range of anti-cancer and cholesterol-lowering activities in animal models, although there are no human studies [80].

Citrus fruits contain a wider variety of carotenoids than any other fruit. The main carotenoids in orange, mandarin and clementine juices are lutein, zeaxanthin, β-cryptoxanthin, β-carotene and violaxanthin [74]. Mandarin and clementine (a hybrid between mandarin and orange) are especially rich in β-cryptoxanthin, which is nutritionally important since this xanthophyll has pro-vitamin A activity.

5.4.2   Apples and related fruits

This group of fruits is part of the Rose family (belonging to the sub-family *Maloideae*) and not only includes apples but also pears, medlars and quinces. The botanical term for the fruit is a pome. Apples originated in Central Asia, and Turkey is still one of the top producers in the world (Table 5.11). There are more than 7500 varieties of pome. The European pear (there is a separate East Asian species) also originated in Central Asia and has given rise to a large number of cultivars that are popular in Mediterranean countries, not only eaten fresh but also poached in red wine. Quinces require a hot summer to ripen and Turkey is the top producer in the world. Most quinces are too astringent to eat fresh and are either cooked or made into a jam; in fact the word 'marmalade' originated from the Portuguese 'marmelada', meaning quince jam. Medlars, like quince, can only be eaten raw after 'bletting', i.e. left after ripening to start to decay and ferment. They are popular in the Eastern Mediterranean.

Only the pulp of quinces and medlars are consumed whereas the peel of apples and pears is also eaten. This is significant since fruit peel usually contains far higher levels of phytochemicals than the pulp. The main phenolic in quince pulp was found to be chlorogenic acid [81].

In experimental studies apples have anti-proliferative, antioxidant and cholesterol-lowering effects [82, 83]. Apples contain a range of bioactive substances including vitamin C, soluble fibre, potassium and high levels of various phenolics (Table 5.12). Apples are a major dietary source of phenolics in North European countries and the

---

[2] By contrast, for flavanones it is the *aglycones* that are tasteless.

Table 5.11 Production (FAOSTAT 2007) and consumption (FAOSTAT 2003) of pomes.

	Production (thousand tonnes)			Consumption (g/per capita/per day)
	Apples	Pears	Quinces	Apples
Egypt	545	39	0.04	16
France	2144	203	2.5	27
Greece	260	75	4	38
Italy	2073	840	0.6	27
Morocco	427	44	35	22
Spain	678	518	15	38
Tunisia	102	55	4	25
Turkey	2458	356	95	82
United Kingdom	263	21	0	60

Table 5.12 Nutrient content of apples [83]. Reproduced with permission. © Georg Thieme Verlag KG, Stuttgart, New York.

Constituent	Concentration per 100g FW
Fibre (pectin) (g)	2 (0.5)
Potassium (mg)	144
Calcium (mg)	7
Magnesium (mg)	6
Phosphorus (mg)	12
Vitamin C (mg)	12
Organic fruit acids (g)	0.5
Total phenolics (mg)	66–212
○ hydroxycinnamic acids (mg)	5–38
○ flavan-3-ols (mg)	12–41
○ procyanidins (mg)	39–162
○ quercetin glycosides (mg)	3–8
○ anthocyanins (red apples (mg))	0–4

US [82], although their contribution to total phenolic intake in the MedDiet will be less. Some of the main phenolics in apples are hydroxycinnamic acids (chlorogenic, coumaric and caffeic), quercetin glycosides, flavan-3-ols (catechin, epicatechin) and their polymeric forms the procyanidins, and chalcones, especially phloridzin which is not found in many other plant foods. Procyanidins comprise 63–77% of all phenolics [83]. Chlorogenic acid levels are higher in the flesh, whereas the peel contains several-fold more flavan-3-ols, procyanidins and phloridzin. Quercetin glycosides occur exclusively in the peel. Phloridzin competes with glucose for uptake from the gut and may have an effect on lowering the glycaemic index of a meal. Apples are a moderate source of vitamin C, but it was estimated that <1% of the total antioxidant activity of apples comes from vitamin C, and that the major contributor is antioxidant phytochemicals, particularly chlorogenic acid, caffeic acid and epicatechin [84]. In addition to phenolics, the waxy peel of apples contains lipophilic triterpenoids (especially ursolic acid) which have antiproliferative activity.

Pears contain many of the phytochemicals present in apples, including high levels of chlorogenic acid, as well as procyanidins and quercetin glcyosides. The main

Table 5.13   Production of stone fruits (FAO STAT, 2007).

	Production (thousand tonnes)			
	Apricots	Cherries	Peaches & nectarines	Plums (& sloes)
Egypt	78	–	365	18
France	127	48	365	249
Greece	79	63	784	10
Italy	212	145	1719	176
Morocco	105	6	77	79
Spain	88	73	1160	191
Tunisia	24	5	101	12
Turkey	558	398	539	241
United Kingdom	–	1	–	14

difference is the presence of high levels of the phenolic arbutin (which is only present in the peel), and the absence of phloridzin [85].

Most pome fruits are rich in pectin, and hence can be made into jams. As these fruits ripen and soften there is a partial breakdown of the pectic polysaccharides [71]. Apple pectin has attracted a lot of interest for its chemopreventative properties. Pectin may act by binding carcinogens in the gut and diluting carcinogens by increasing faecal bulk. In addition, pectin is fermented in the colon producing short chain fatty acids, such as butyrate, which are thought to reduce the development of colon cancer. Procyanidins from apples are also fermented by colonic bacteria. Apple juice does not retain the procyanidins present in the intact fruit, suggesting that intact apples will have superior health benefits, and this is borne out by epidemiological evidence [83].

5.4.3   Stone fruits

Many of the classic Mediterranean fruits, including apricot, nectarine, peach, cherry, damson and plum, are members of the genus *Prunus* (Table 5.13). They are classified botanically as drupes, i.e. they consist of an outer fleshy part containing a stone within which is the seed. Strictly speaking, almonds are also drupes, but their hardened outer flesh means that they are usually categorised with nuts. It is thought that the apricot, cherry and plum were introduced into the Mediterranean basin by Alexander the Great in the 3rd century BC from Central Asia, whereas peaches were introduced from China [69].

Apricots are an excellent source of β-carotene which can represent up to 85% of the total carotenoids. They can be an important source of provitamin A activity when animal sources of vitamin A are not consumed, with 250 g of fresh apricots providing 100% of the RDA of vitamin A. β-carotene is responsible for the orange hue of apricots; hence, consumers choosing bright orange apricots will also be choosing ones with high provitamin A levels [86]. It is thought that β-carotene in fruits is loosely dispersed and readily bioavailable, unlike in tomatoes where the carotenoid lycopene is tightly trapped inside the cells. The tradition in Mediterranean countries of consuming fruits at the end of a meal containing olive oil or other fats

Table 5.14 Grape consumption in
Mediterranean countries and the UK
(FAOSTAT 2003).

	Consumption (g/per capita/per day)
Egypt	35.62
France	5.48
Greece	93.15
Italy	52.06
Morocco	19.18
Spain	8.22
Tunisia	19.18
Turkey	73.97
United Kingdom	27.40

could conceivably further enhance the bioavailability of lipophilic carotenoids in the gut, although there is no experimental evidence for this. Apricots also contain high levels of chlorogenic acid and flavonols (catechin and epicatechin), and quercetin glycosides and procyanidins are also present.

Peaches contain lower levels of nutrients than some other fruits, (such as β-carotene, vitamin C (4 mg/100 g) and total phenolics (36 mg/100 g), but this is compensated for somewhat by the popularity of this fruit during the summer months [87].

Chlorogenic acids (comprising mainly neochlorogenic acid) and the anthocyanidin pigment cyanidin together comprised 88% of the total antioxidant phenolics in plums [88]. Cherries are also a very rich source of anthocyanidin pigments and chlorogenic acids.

5.4.4 Grapes

Although the majority of grapes in Mediterranean countries are made into wine, quite high amounts of the fresh fruit are consumed in some countries (Table 5.14). Grapes are also turned into juice or dried to make currants, raisins and sultanas. Sultanas are from a type of white grape and come mainly from Turkey. According to legend, the sultana was invented when the Sultan of the Ottoman empire discovered his wizened grapes after having left them in the sun after fleeing a tiger attack. Raisins are dried white grapes usually of the variety 'Muscatel'; the main Mediterranean producers are Turkey and Greece. Currants are dried, black, seedless grapes, and derive their name from Corinth in Greece where they were originally produced. Currants and raisins are widely used in Mediterranean cooking in both sweet and savoury dishes.

Over 1600 compounds have been identified in grapes, including phenolics (anthocyanins, catechins, ellagic acid, quercetin, resveratrol) and carotenoids (lutein, lycopene) [89]. Grape variety and growth conditions influence phytochemical levels, and only red grapes contain anthocyanins (with levels up to 15 mg/100 g in one study [90]). Phenolics are concentrated in the skin where they act as a barrier to UV irradiation, and hence thick-skinned varieties grown under an intense sun tend to have higher levels of phenolics; levels of up to 36 mg/100 g have been reported [90]. Muscat grapes are claimed to be the oldest grape variety and are a particular delicacy due to their floral taste, which is due to terpenes – mainly linalool, geraniol and nerol [91]).

The health benefits of grapes have been overshadowed by research on wine. Generally, the levels of phenolics are lower in table grapes than grapes used for wine making. This may partly be related to variety, but table grapes are also picked younger, and before phenolic production is at its maximum. In addition, grapes and grape products lack the multitude of chemicals generated during the fermentation of wine. Grape juice, rather than grapes, has been used in many of the human studies – especially using juice made from Concord grapes which are mainly grown in the US. Some of these studies have found that risk factors for CVD such as platelet aggregation, endothelial function, high blood pressure and elevated LDL-cholesterol can be reduced following consumption of grape juice [89]. There remains a relative paucity of information on the effects of consuming grapes themselves.

5.4.5   Other berries

Consumption of berries predates agriculture since they were one of the foods of early hunter-gatherers. As such, they occupy a special position in human nutrition since their ancient association with humans is likely to have influenced the evolution of human nutrition. However, berries have been subject to intense breeding programmes, and many of the berries available today probably bear little resemblance to those of pre-agricultural times.

Although many types of berries are more suited to cooler climates, strawberries are widely grown in Mediterranean countries. Strawberries contain a variety of phenolics including anthocyanins, the flavonols quercetin and kaempferol, catechin, p-coumaric acid, lignans and significant amounts of ellagic acid, some of which is present as ellagitannins. Studies suggest that these phytochemicals may act synergistically in *in vitro* models for cancer, neurodegenerative diseases and inflammation. Strawberries are also rich in minerals, vitamin C and folate, with one Italian study reporting folate values between 13 and 96 μg/ 100 g FW depending on cultivar [92].

5.4.6   Pomegranates

Pomegranates require a long, hot summer to mature and are grown in Tunisia, Turkey, Egypt, Spain, Southern France and Morocco. Whereas many Mediterranean fruits and vegetables have undergone significant changes due to selective breeding, this is not the case with pomegranates, which have changed very little throughout the history of man. The name pomegranate derives from the Latin *pomum* = apple and *granatus* = seed. The Spanish city Granada derives its name from the Spanish word for pomegranate and the pomegranate is the city's symbol.

In Mediterranean cuisine, pomegranate seeds are sprinkled on salads. The whole fruit is squeezed to make fresh pomegranate juice, and this also extracts some tannins, giving the juice its characteristic mildly astringent taste. The juice of sour pomegranates is reduced to make pomegranate molasses, and these are added to cooked dishes.

A wide variety of phytochemicals have been identified in the fresh juice [93]. The main constituents are hydrolysable tannins – in particular, an ellagitannin called punicalagin, procyanidins and anthocyanins (which give the juice its red colour). The constituents of the molasses have not been analysed. Pomegranate juice has a very high antioxidant activity in *in vitro* assays, with hydrolysable tannins accounting for 92% of the antioxidant activity. Punicalagin, the main hydrolysable tannin, has a molecular weight of over 1000 daltons and so does not enter the body intact. This compound is metabolised in the gut to ellagic acid and related breakdown products known as urolithins, which are mostly produced by the metabolic activity of colonic bacteria. The seeds of pomegranate are unusual in that the seed oil contains >60% of a fatty acid called punicic acid, a type of conjugated linolenic acid.

Pomegranate juice has been shown to have anti-atherosclerotic, anti-hypertensive, antioxidant, and anti-inflammatory effects in animal models and in some human studies, and has beneficial effects against animal models of cancer [93, 94]. Hence pomegranate juice is of interest in relation to CVD and cancer in humans. Since there is good evidence that the phytochemicals in pomegranate juice act together [93], on-going clinical trials are using the whole juice. Eighteen clinical trials of pomegranate juice and other pomegranate products against cancer and a wide range of other conditions are listed at http://clinicaltrials.gov/ct2/results?term=pomegranate.

5.4.7 Figs

Cultivation of figs may have predated that of grains and legumes, making it one of the very first crops to be domesticated. The fig tree tolerates a wide range of conditions and is grown in many Mediterranean countries; the top producers are Turkey and Egypt. There are many fig cultivars and these vary in colour from green to yellow to reddish and purple. Figs are eaten fresh in Mediterranean countries, although about 40% of the crop is dried. Figs are a rich source of fibre, with a high content of soluble fibre, and minerals (including Fe, Ca, K). Purple varieties contain anthocyanins, and these varieties were also found to contain the highest levels of other polyphenols [95]. In a small human study, consuming dried figs was shown to increase plasma antioxidant capacity [96].

5.4.8 Dates

Dates have been cultivated since ancient times in North Africa. Egypt is the top producer in the Mediterranean basin. Although the Arabs spread the date into Spain, consumption is still mainly in Egypt, Algeria and Tunisia, and here daily consumption can be high. Dates contain glucose and fructose, as well as dietary fibre which is mainly present as insoluble fibre [97]. Dates are also a good source of carotenoids and phenolics [98].

5.4.9 Olives

The olive is *the* emblematic Mediterranean tree. Wild olives have been collected for thousands of years and the first cultivation of olive trees is thought to have been during the Minoan period (1500–3000 BC) in Crete. Cultivation then spread to the rest of Greece and to North Africa and Asia Minor. Olive cultivation was very important to the Romans and spread as the Roman Empire expanded. The potential health benefits of consuming olives has been somewhat overshadowed by olive oil, as demonstrated by the fact that whereas olive oil consumption is evaluated in

Table 5.15   Consumption of olives (FAOSTAT, 2003).

	Consumption (g/per capita/per day)
Egypt	10.96
France	2.74
Greece	32.88
Italy	5.48
Morocco	2.74
Spain	8.22
Tunisia	5.48
Turkey	10.96
United Kingdom	0.00

epidemiological studies of the MedDiet, olive consumption is not. However, olives contain high levels of antioxidants and other constituents with potential health benefits.

Greece has the highest production of black olives for direct consumption, and consumption of olives is also highest in Greece (Table 5.15). Egypt is noteworthy because, although there is quite a high consumption of olives, the use of olive oil has traditionally been very limited. Olives are commonly consumed in Mediterranean countries with anise-flavoured drinks or wine drunk before a meal. Olives, particularly black olives, are also used in various Mediterranean recipes, including salads and fish and meat dishes.

Processing of olives

The olive is the fruit of the olive tree, and botanically speaking it is a drupe, i.e. a fruit with a single stone. The outer skin, or epicarp, of the olive is covered with a water-impermeable layer of wax that protects it from fungal and insect attack (Figure 5.9). Initially the skin is green due to chlorophyll, but it later changes to black as the balance of pigments shifts towards anthocyanins (mainly cyanidin glycosides).

About 10% of olive production is for 'table olives', and the remainder is processed for oil (see Chapter 6). Olives off the tree are too astringent and bitter to be edible and must be processed prior to consumption as table olives. Green (unripe) and black (ripe olives) are subject to different processes. The less ripe the olive, the stronger is the treatment needed to eliminate bitterness. In ancient times, only black olives were eaten, and it is said that the way to render olives edible was a chance finding. Women used to pour ashes around olive trees to improve soil fertility. A child, unaware of the olive's bitterness, chewed an olive that had stayed in the humid ashes, much to the astonishment of the child's parents, hence discovering both the gustative quality of olives and the way to prepare them in this manner. Indeed, to this day the basic principle to eliminate bitterness is to treat olives with a salt base (the level of potassium base is high in wood ashes).

Various methods are used today to produce table olives. In the so-called Spanish method, green olives – the usual type – or 'cherry' olives (the next stage of ripeness

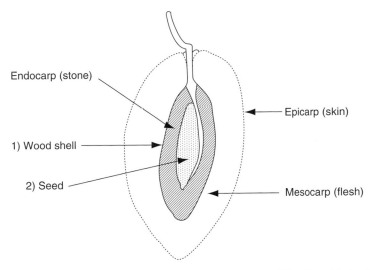

Figure 5.9   Cross section of olive fruit [99]. With permission from Wiley-VCH Verlag GmbH & Co. KGaA.

when the olives are purple) are harvested. Green olives are treated with sodium hydroxide solution – so-called lye treatment – for 8–12 h, whereas weaker potassium base is sufficient for the half-ripe purple olives. This step removes the bitter compound oleuropein. The olives are then washed, mostly with water, in conditions that avoid oxidation, and fermented in brine (5–9% NaCl). For black olives, fermenting in brine for one to three months, without using a base, can be sufficient to eliminate bitterness. Rinsing is necessary, mostly with water, in conditions that avoid oxidation. To avoid the use of sodium base, olives in brine might be inoculated with *Lactobacillus plantarum* and kept at 22 °C for 10 to 150 days. The olives are firmer and crunchier, and they retain more phenolics (mainly hydroxytyrosol). Whichever processing procedure has been used, olives are subsequently kept in a light pickling brine, sometimes with herbs, chilli peppers or garlic, or in olive oil. They can be treated at 60 °C for 5 to 10 min in pickling brine without alterations to their organoleptic properties. This is important when herbs are present in order to avoid microbial contamination. One of the best green olives is the *Lucques*. Black olives might be kept either in pickling brine or in olive oil, and among the most famous black olives are Greek Kalamata olives and *Caillette* olives from Nice, France.

Another method, used particularly to produce black olives in Greece and in Nimes (Southern France), is to pack the ripe black olives with dry salt. This shrivels the olives and they remain fairly salty and bitter. In a third method, the Californian method, olives are harvested while green or just starting to change colour, and then treated several times with NaOH. The olives are then washed in water and aerated, which darkens them, and the colour is 'fixed' using ferrous gluconate. The olives are subsequently canned or bottled in brine and sterilised to preserve them [100].

Constituents

The pulp or flesh (mesocarp) of the fresh, unprocessed olive fruit contains variable amounts of oil, about 15% in green olives and up to about 30% in black olives. Olives with low oil content are generally favoured for table production. Olives also

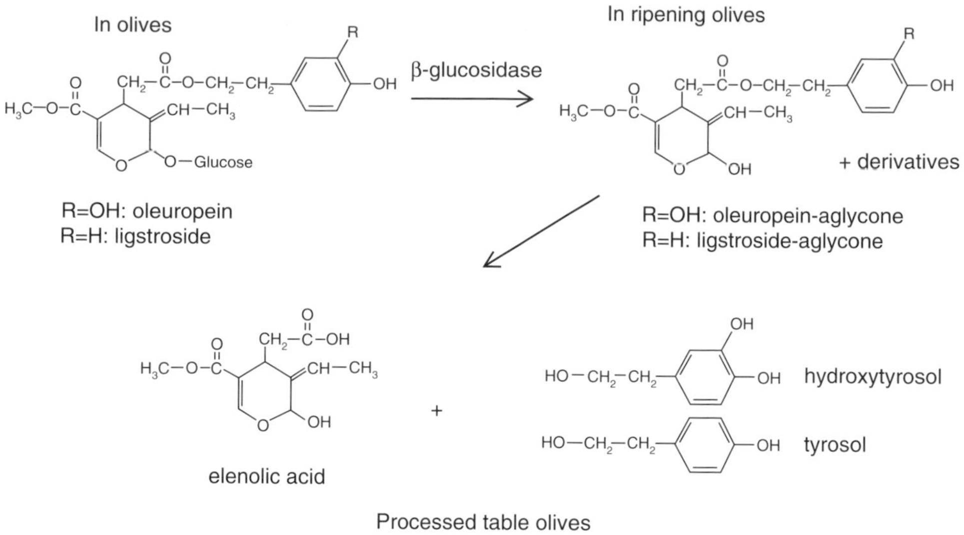

Figure 5.10   Changes in phenolics in olives and olive oil (redrawn from [104]).

contain a number of non-lipid components, including a number of phenolics. In general, phenolics increase during maturation on the tree from the green stage to the 'cherry' stage, but then decline rapidly when the olives turn black [101]. The main phenolic present in the unripe olive fruit is the bitter-tasting compound oleuropein. Smaller quantities of the related compound ligstroside are also present. In the unripe fruit these phenolics are mainly present as glycosides, and during ripening some of the glycosides are broken down into the aglycones. In general, small fruit cultivars contain a higher oleuropein content than large cultivars. During ripening of the immature fruit to the still green mature fruit, the levels of oleuropein decline and the levels of the structurally related compounds hydroxytyrosol and tyrosol increase. Levels of oleuropein decline further if ripe green olives are left on the tree to mature to black olives, and hence black olives do not need the processing with NaOH that is required for green olives. The black maturation phase is also characterised by the appearance of anthocyanins.

The processing of olives for consumption results in significant changes in their phenolic content, although it does not significantly alter the triglyceride composition. The major change is conversion of most or all of the oleuropein into tyrosol and hydroxytyrosol (Figure 5.10). In one study of Greek olives, hydroxytyrosol, tyrosol, and luteolin were the main phenolics in most of the olives examined. High levels of hydroxytyrosol were found mainly in Kalamata olives and Spanish-style green olives (250–760 mg/kg) [102]. Hydroxytyrosol is a major antioxidant in virgin olive oil, and may contribute to its cardioprotective effects [103] (and see Chapter 11).

Olive processing procedures can have a major influence on the final levels of phenolics present in table olives. Firstly, the use of NaOH softens the wax cuticle of the olives and allows water-soluble phenolics such as hydroxytyrosol and tyrosol to leach into the brine. Thus, avoiding NaOH treatment can result in olives with a higher content of water-soluble phenolics. Secondly, and of particular significance, is the aeration and ferrous gluconate step used in the Californian method. This results

Table 5.16 Content of triterpenes in olives and olive oil (based on [105]).

	Maslinic acid (mg/kg)	Oleanolic acid (mg/kg)
Olive fruit	681	420
Virgin olive oil	194	244
Extra virgin olive oil	64	57

in the oxidation and polymerisation of hydroxytyrosol (indeed it is this reaction that is responsible for the browning of the olives) [100]. No intact hydroxytyrosol remains in olives processed by the Californian method, and this could potentially have a major detrimental impact on the health benefits of these olives due to the possible health effects of this phenolic (see Chapter 11). Some hydroxytyrosol leaches into the brine during the production of Californian style olives, although the level of water-soluble phenolics in the final packing brine is not known – but using this solution, for example in cooking stocks, could be a good idea.

Olives also contain the triterpenes oleanolic and maslinic acid. These substances are located in the skin of olives. Although significant quantities are lost when olives are processed in brine for use as table olives, far greater losses occur when olives are processed into oil (Table 5.16). These triterpenes act as anti-microbial agents for the olive fruit, and have been reported to inhibit the growth of human colon cancer cells *in vitro* [105].

In conclusion, the limited number of studies on table olives has found that they contain a range of phenolics and other phytochemicals with interesting actions, and levels are strongly influenced by olive type and processing method (as well as growth condition, etc). However, the health benefits of olive consumption have not been evaluated, possibly because the high content of salt might be deleterious, especially for subjects with high blood pressure.

5.5   Herbs and spices

Many of the best known herbs, such as sage, rosemary, oregano and thyme, originate in the Mediterranean, and they are still often collected from the wild. Other herbs and spices were introduced by occupying nations. Herbs and spices are a defining feature of Mediterranean cuisines. Paprika is widely used in North Africa and was introduced into Spain by the Moors. In Spain, it is often used in place of pepper and it is also used in the manufacture of sausages such as chorizo. The practice of using the pollen-capturing stigmas from crocus flowers – saffron – was also introduced by the Arabs to Spain. The main herbs in Spanish cuisine are parsley, oregano, rosemary and thyme (http://spanishfood.about.com). In Greek cuisine, oregano, mint, dill and bay leaves, basil, thyme and fennel and sesame seeds are consumed. Many Greek recipes, especially in the northern parts of the country, use 'sweet' spices such as cinnamon and cloves, not only in desserts but also in meat stews or vegetable dishes. Italian cooking uses a lot of herbs such as basil, parsley, rosemary, thyme, fennel, sage, but rather fewer spices, although chilli pepper is occasionally used. By contrast, Moroccan cuisine emphasises a wide variety of spices such as saffron,

Table 5.17 Terpenes and aromatic compounds in the essential oils of some Mediterranean herbs and spices [106] [107]. With permission from John Wiley & Sons.

Herb or spice	Major constituents with typical composition (%)
Basil (sweet)	(+)-Linalool (up to 55), methyl chavicol (up to 70)
Caraway seeds	(+)-Carvone (50–70), limonene (47)
Cardamom seeds	α-Terpenyl acetate (25–35), cineole (25–45), linalool (5)
Coriander seeds	(+)-Linalool (60–75), γ-terpinene (5), α-pinene (5), camphor (5)
Dill seeds	(+)-Carvone (40–65)
Ginger rhizome	Zingerberene (34), β-sesquiphellandrene (12), β-phellandrene (8), β-bisabolene (6)
Juniper berries	α-Pinene (45–80), myrcene (10–25), limonene (1–10), sabinene (0–15)
Lavender (fresh flowering tops)	Linalyl acetate (25–45), linalool (25–38)
Lemon (dried peel)	Limonene (60–80), β-pinene (8–12), γ-terpinene (8–10), citral (2–3)
Orange (bitter) (dried peel)	Limonene (92–94), myrcene (2)
Orange (sweet) (dreid peel)	Limonene (90–95), myrcene (2)
Orange flower (neroli)	Linalool (36), β-pinene (16), limonene (12), linalyl acetate (6)
Oregano (Turkish)	Carvacrol (51–85), borneol (1–8), p-cymene (5–12), γ-terpinene (2–14)
Peppermint leaves	Menthol (30–50), menthone (15–32), menthyl acetate (2–10), menthofuran,
Rose (attar of rose)	Citronellol (36), geraniol (17), 2-phenylethanol (3), straight chain hydrocarbons (25)
Rosemary (fresh flowering tops)	Cineole (15–45), α-pinene (10–25), camphor (10–25), β-pinene (8)
Sage (fresh flowering tops)	Thujone (40–60), camphor (5–22), cineole (5–14), β-caryophyllene (10), limonene (6)
Thyme (fresh flowering tops)	Thymol (40), p-cymene (30), linalool (7), carvacrol (1)

cinnamon, cumin, turmeric, ginger, pepper and paprika, as well as aniseed, sesame seed, coriander, parsley and mint. Herbs and spices used in Lebanon and Turkey have much in common since both were part of the Ottoman empire until the early 20th century. Parsley and mint are main ingredients in *tabbouleh*, a salad that uses bulgur wheat. *Za'atar*, a mixture of dried thyme (or oregano), toasted sesame seeds and salt, is used as a seasoning for meats and vegetables. Aniseed-flavoured drinks are popular in many Mediterranean countries and mint tea is a national drink in Morocco (see Chapter 7).

Herbs and spices contain a diverse range of potentially beneficial phytochemicals. Some of the phytochemicals found in herbs and spices are also found in fruits and vegetables, such as the red carotenoid capsanthin which is present in both paprika and red bell peppers. Terpenes are responsible for the characteristic aroma of many herbs and spices (Table 5.17). Many terpenes are stored in specialised structures in plant cells and are released by cutting or grinding. Some terpenes, such as limonene, are pharmacologically active in experimental systems.

It has been argued that the amounts of phytochemicals obtained from eating herbs and spices are too low to have any health benefits. At present, there is insufficient quantitative data on consumption levels to draw any firm conclusions regarding this point. But it is clear that levels can vary widely between countries and between individuals, and in Mediterranean countries many herbs and spices are consumed life-long in quantities that are significantly higher than in many non-Mediterranean countries. For example, Italians and Greeks consume a lot of parsley and oregano, and basil consumption can be high when made into sauces such as *pesto* in Italy and *pistou* in France. Aniseed-flavoured aperitifs are frequently drunk in rather high amounts. The Oldways organisation acknowledged the importance of herbs and spices by including them on their 2009 version of the MedDiet food pyramid (http://www.oldwayspt.org/med_pyramid).

Herbs and spices are rarely eaten on their own, and so it is appropriate to consider effects in combination with other foodstuffs. In one study, it was found that including herbs such as marjoram with olive oil in salad dressings significantly increased the antioxidant capacity of salads [108]. Marinades of herbs for meat and fish are popular in Mediterranean cuisine, and marinades of rosemary, thyme and sage have been shown to reduce the formation of potentially dangerous oxidation products during cooking [109].

Perhaps even more so than fruits and vegetables, the levels of phytochemicals in herbs varies with growth conditions. Herbs are usually low-growing soft plants with little physical protection and phytochemicals are produced in order to discourage animals from eating them or to inhibit microbial attack.

Herbs and spices have a long tradition in Mediterranean countries not only as flavouring but also as medicines. A study of the herbal market in Thessaloniki in Northern Greece found that the majority of the herbs for sale were collected from the wild and would have been familiar to the Greek physician Dioscorides from the 1st century AD [110]. Although the medicinal use of herbs is outside the scope of this book, many excellent books are available (e.g. [111]).

5.6 Nuts and seeds

5.6.1 Nuts

Nuts are a common snack food in Mediterranean countries and they are also used in many sweet and savoury dishes. The word 'nut' is used here in its culinary, rather than botanical, sense and so includes, for example, almonds (technically a drupe) and peanuts (a legume). The FAO food balance sheets (FAOSTAT, 2004) show that, in 2001, Lebanon and Greece were the countries in the Mediterranean region with the highest supply of nuts, an annual average of 16.5 and 11.9 kg/person, respectively. Spain ranked third with 7.3 kg per capita available for consumption, followed by Israel and Italy. Other countries of the Mediterranean region such as Libya, Turkey and Tunisia also have high levels of nut supply.

Walnuts and almonds grow and are consumed in many Mediterranean countries. The French word for walnut is *noix* and simply translates as 'nut'. Some regions have particular favourites: pistachios are very popular in Eastern Mediterranean countries. In Spain, walnuts, almonds, hazelnuts and peanuts are the most widely consumed nuts [112]. Chestnuts were once a staple food and energy source (they are rich in starch) in many mountainous regions where wheat could not grow such as Corsica and the Cévennes region in Southern France.

Peeling, toasting, frying or salting enhances the flavour and aroma of many nuts eaten in snacks, although some are also eaten raw with an aperitif. Pine nuts are

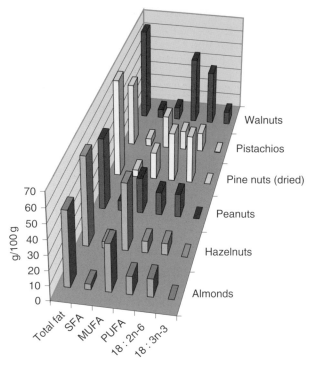

Figure 5.11   Average fatty acid compositon of nuts (g/100 g) [114]. Data for raw nuts, except when specified.

consumed in the popular *pistou* (Provence) or *pesto* (Italy), in pastries, on salads or with spinach and raisins – a popular combination in several Mediterranean countries. Almonds and walnuts are used in various East Mediterranean pastries with honey such as *baklava*. Almonds are used in Spanish cooking to make a soup known as *ajoblanco* and walnuts are made into a sauce called *taratoor* that is used for meat and fish. Ground almonds are used in many sweet dishes, and one of the pillars of Catalan cuisine is a sauce based on ground almonds called *picada*.

Nuts are particularly rich in nutrients. With the exception of chestnuts, they contain high levels of protein, fats (mostly unsaturated), dietary fibre, vitamins (e.g. folates, niacin, vitamin E, vitamin B6), minerals (e.g. copper, magnesium, potassium, zinc) and phytochemicals. Some nuts are rich sources of certain nutrients – pine nuts: linoleic acid; walnuts: α-linolenic acid; hazelnuts: manganese; peanuts: niacin; pistachios: β-sitosterol; almonds: α-tocopherol [113]. Most nuts have high levels of MUFA and relatively low levels of SFA (Figure 5.11).

Nuts also contain numerous types of phytochemicals (Figure 5.12). Nuts are a good source of phystosterols which are found in the fatty acid fraction. Nuts also contain variable levels of phenolics including both flavonoids and non-flavonoids. The stilbene resveratrol – better known as a constituent of red wine – is present in peanuts and pistachios, but not other nuts. Nuts are also a good source of proanthocyanidins (condensed tannins).

Many phenolics have antioxidant activity. Most antioxidant phenolics in nuts are located in the skin, known as the pellicle, and the overall antioxidant capacity of nuts is greatly reduced when the pellicle is removed – by 95% in the case of walnuts

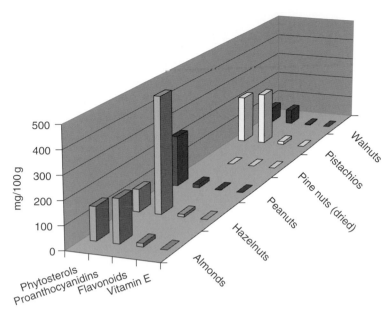

Figure 5.12 Antioxidant phytochemicals (mg/100 g) in nuts (redrawn from [115]). With permission from Wiley-VCH Verlag GmbH & Co. KGaA.

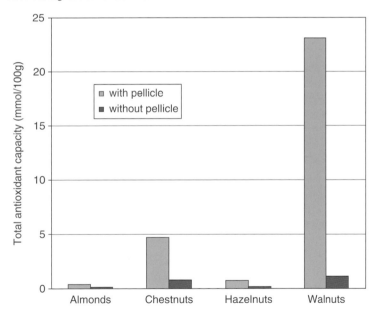

Figure 5.13 Total antioxidant capacity* in nuts with or without pellicle (redrawn from [116]). *Determined by the FRAP assay. Reprinted with permission from Macmillan Publishers Ltd, copyright Nature.

(Figure 5.13) [116]. Polyphenol antioxidants in the pellicle provide a protective antioxidant barrier against oxidation of the unsaturated fats in the nuts. Buying nuts in their shells may also help retain antioxidant activity [116].

Nuts have favourable effects on risk factors for CVD (see Chapter 11). In part this may be due to their fat content, but phytochemicals in nuts also have potential cardioprotective effects, possibly due to the antioxidant activity of phenolics or the cholesterol-lowering properties of phytosterols. There is also interest in proanthocyanidins for possible cardioprotective effects [117]. However, proanthocyanidins, which are polymeric forms of flavanols, are not absorbed intact and it is not clear if they are metabolised by colonic bacteria, after which they may be absorbed. Otherwise, any therapeutic action will be restricted to the gut itself. The high levels of some antioxidants (vitamin E, selenium, flavonoids) may also inhibit carcinogenesis, although there is no conclusive epidemiological evidence supporting this hypothesis [118].

5.6.2 Seeds

Sunflower and pumpkin seeds are popular aperitif foods in many Mediterranean countries. Sesame seeds are sprinkled on bread in Greece and elsewhere. Sesame seeds are also ground to a paste called *tahini* that is widely used in Mediterranean countries, for example as an ingredient in *hummus*. Roasted sesame seeds are used as a condiment, for example as an ingredient in *za'atar*.

Seeds are a particularly rich source of phytosterols with β-sitosterol concentrations of 232 mg/100 g reported for sesame seeds [119]. Although β-sitosterol is usually the main phytosterol in plants, it was found to represent only a small proportion (5%) of the total phytosterols in pumpkin seeds [119]. Sesame seeds are an exceptionally good source of lignans. Linseed is generally regarded as the richest source of plant lignans – mainly due to the high content of secoisolariciresinol. However, when the lipophilic sesamin type lignans were included in analysis of total lignans, the content in sesame seeds was found to be even higher than that of linseeds [120] (see Chapter 2). Sesame seeds also have vitamin E activity which is produced from an interaction between γ-tocopherol with sesame lignans [121]. Despite the promising phytochemical profile of seeds, there is a paucity of information on their possible health benefits.

References

1. Garcia-Closas, R., Berenguer, A., Gonzalez, C.A. *Changes in food supply in Mediterranean countries from 1961 to 2001. Public Health Nutr*, 2006. **9**(1): 53–60.
2. Wright, C.A., *Mediterranean vegetables*. 2001: Harvard Common Press.
3. Buchner, F.L. et al. *Variety in fruit and begetable consumption and the risk of lung cancer in the European Prospective Investigation into Cancer and Nutrition*. Cancer Epidemiol Biomarkers Prev, 2010.
4. Jin, J. et al. Analysis of phytochemical composition and chemoprotective capacity of rocket (Eruca sativa and Diplotaxis tenuifolia) leafy salad following cultivation in different environments. *J Agric Food Chem*, 2009. **57**(12): 5227–34.
5. Verkerk, R. et al. Glucosinolates in Brassica vegetables: The influence of the food supply chain on intake, bioavailability and human health. *Mol Nutr Food Res*, 2008. **53** Suppl 2: S219–S265.
6. Cartea, M., Velasco, P. Glucosinolates in Brassica foods: bioavailability in food and significance for human health. *Phytochem Rev*, 2008. **7**: 213–229.
7. Higdon, J.V. et al. Cruciferous vegetables and human cancer risk: epidemiologic evidence and mechanistic basis. *Pharmacol Res*, 2007. **55**(3): 224–36.
8. van den Berg, H. et al. The potential for the improvement of carotenoid levels in foods and the likely systemic effects. *Journal of the Science of Food and Agriculture*, 2000. **80**: 880–912.
9. Edenharder, R. et al. Isolation and characterization of structurally novel antimutagenic flavonoids from spinach (Spinacia oleracea). *J Agric Food Chem*, 2001. **49**(6): 2767–73.
10. Genannt Bonsmann, S.S. et al. Oxalic acid does not influence nonhaem iron absorption in humans: a comparison of kale and spinach meals. *Eur J Clin Nutr*, 2008. **62**(3): 336–41.

11. Kosar, M. et al. Effect of brining on biological activity of leaves of Vitis vinifera L. (Cv. Sultani Cekirdeksiz) from Turkey. *J Agric Food Chem*, 2007. **55**(11): 4596–603.
12. Barreiro-Hurle, J., Colombo, S., Cantos-Villar, E. Is there a market for functional wines? Consumer preferences and willingness to pay for resveratrol-enriched red wine. *Food Quality and Preference*, 2008. **19**: 360–371.
13. Douillet-Breuil, A.C. et al. Changes in the phytoalexin content of various Vitis spp. in response to ultraviolet C elicitation. *J Agric Food Chem*, 1999. **47**(10): 4456–61.
14. Rivera, D. et al. Gathered Mediterranean food plants–ethnobotanical investigations and historical development. *Forum Nutr*, 2006. **59**: 18–74.
15. Trichopoulou, A. et al. Nutritional composition and flavonoid content of edible wild greens and green pies: a potential rich source of antioxidant nutrients in the Mediterranean diet. *Food Chemistry*, 2000. **70**: 319–323.
16. Nebel, S., Pieroni, A., Heinrich, M. Ta chorta: wild edible greens used in the Graecanic area in Calabria, Southern Italy. *Appetite*, 2006. **47**(3): 333–42.
17. Salvatore, S. et al. Antioxidant characterization of some Sicilian edible wild greens. *J Agric Food Chem*, 2005. **53**(24): 9465–71.
18. Ghirardini, M.P. et al. The importance of a taste. A comparative study on wild food plant consumption in twenty-one local communities in Italy. *J Ethnobiol Ethnomed*, 2007. **3**: 22.
19. Manios, Y. et al. Dietary intake and biochemical risk factors for cardiovascular disease in two rural regions of Crete. *J Physiol Pharmacol*, 2005. **56 Suppl 1**: 171–81.
20. Heinrich, M., Muller, W., Galli, C. Local Mediterranean food plants and nutraceuticals. *Forum of Nutrition, ed. I. Elmadfa*. Vol. 59. 2006, Basel: Karger.
21. Vardavas, C.E.A. The antioxidant and phylloquinone content of wildly grown greens in Crete. *Food Chemistry*, 2006. **99**: pp. 813–821.
22. Trichopoulou, A. et al. Traditional foods: Why and how to sustain them. *Trends in Food Science & Technology*, 2006. **17**: 498–504.
23. Reiter, R.J. et al. Melatonin in edible plants (phytomelatonin): identification, concentrations, bioavailability and proposed functions. *World Rev Nutr Diet*, 2007. **97**: 211–30.
24. Srinivasan, V. et al. Melatonin in Alzheimer's disease and other neurodegenerative disorders. *Behav Brain Funct*, 2006. **2**: 15.
25. Simopoulos, A.P. et al. Purslane: a plant source of omega-3 fatty acids and melatonin. *J Pineal Res*, 2005. **39**(3): 331–2.
26. Vardavas, C.I. et al. Lipid concentrations of wild edible greens in Crete. *Food Chemistry*, 2006. **99**: 822–834.
27. Simopoulos, A.P. The importance of the omega-6/omega-3 fatty acid ratio in cardiovascular disease and other chronic diseases. *Exp Biol Med* (Maywood), 2008. **233**(6): 674–88.
28. USDA. *USDA Database for the Flavonoid Content of Selected Foods Release 2.1*. 2007.
29. Patel, D., Shukla, S., Gupta, S. Apigenin and cancer chemoprevention: progress, potential and promise (review). *Int J Oncol*, 2007. **30**(1): 233–45.
30. Dilis, V., Vasilopolou, E., Trichopoulou, A. The flavone, flavonol and flavan-3-ol content of the Greek traditional diet. *Food Chemistry*, 2007. **105**: 812–821.
31. Deli, J., Matus, Z., Toth, G. Carotenoid composition in the fruits of Asparagus officinalis. *J Agric Food Chem*, 2000. **48**(7): 2793–6.
32. Sun, T., Powers, J., Tang, J. Evaluation of the antioxidant activity of asparagus, broccoli and their juices. *Food Chemistry*, 2007. **105**: 101–106.
33. Kuhnle, G. et al. Phytoestrogen content of fruits and vegetables commonly consumed in the UK based on LC–MS and 13C-labelled standards. *Food Chemistry*, 2009. **116**(2): 542–554.
34. Mitchell, S.C. Food idiosyncrasies: beetroot and asparagus. *Drug Metab Dispos*, 2001. **29**(4 Pt 2): 539–43.
35. Wang, M. et al. Analysis of antioxidative phenolic compounds in artichoke (Cynara scolymus L.). *J Agric Food Chem*, 2003. **51**(3): 601–8.
36. Lattanzioa, V. et al. Globe artichoke: A functional food and source of nutraceutical ingredients. *J Functional Foods*, 2009. **1**(2): 131–144.
37. Jimenez-Escrig, A., Santos-Hidalgo, A.B., Saura-Calixto, F. Common sources and estimated intake of plant sterols in the Spanish diet. *J Agric Food Chem*, 2006. **54**(9): 3462–71.
38. Vargas, A.J., Burd, R. Hormesis and synergy: pathways and mechanisms of quercetin in cancer prevention and management. *Nutr Rev*, 2010. **68**(7): 418–28.
39. Nemeth, K., Piskula, M.K. Food content, processing, absorption and metabolism of onion flavonoids. *Crit Rev Food Sci Nutr*, 2007. **47**(4): 397–409.

40. Dragoni, S. et al. Red wine alcohol promotes quercetin absorption and directs its metabolism towards isorhamnetin and tamarixetin in rat intestine *in vitro*. *Br J Pharmacol*, 2006. **147**(7): 765–71.
41. Slimestad, R., Fossen, T., Vagen, I.M. Onions: a source of unique dietary flavonoids. *J Agric Food Chem*, 2007. **55**(25): 10067–80.
42. Corzo Martınez, M., Corzo, N., Villamiel, M. Biological properties of onions and garlic. *Trends in Food Science & Technology*, 2007. **18**: 609–625.
43. Nishijima, T. et al. Chronic ingestion of apple pectin can enhance the absorption of quercetin. *J Agric Food Chem*, 2009. **57**(6): 2583–7.
44. Pittler, M.H., Ernst, E. Clinical effectiveness of garlic *(Allium sativum)*. *Mol Nutr Food Res*, 2007. **51**(11): 1382–5.
45. Cavagnaro, P.F. et al. Effect of cooking on garlic (Allium sativum L.) antiplatelet activity and thiosulfinates content. *J Agric Food Chem*, 2007. **55**(4): 1280–8.
46. Fujisawa, H. et al. Antibacterial potential of garlic-derived allicin and its cancellation by sulfhydryl compounds. *Biosci Biotechnol Biochem*, 2009. **73**(9): 1948–55.
47. Canizares, P. et al. Thermal degradation of allicin in garlic extracts and its implication on the inhibition of the in-vitro growth of Helicobacter pylori. *Biotechnol Prog*, 2004. **20**(1): 32–7.
48. Shukla, Y., Kalra, N. Cancer chemoprevention with garlic and its constituents. *Cancer Lett*, 2007. **247**(2): 167–81.
49. Benavides, G.A. et al. Hydrogen sulfide mediates the vasoactivity of garlic. *Proc Natl Acad Sci USA*, 2007. **104**(46): 17977–82.
50. Arnault, I., Auger, J. Seleno-compounds in garlic and onion. *J Chromatogr A*, 2006. **1112**(1–2): 23–30.
51. Jenab, M. et al., Variations in lycopene blood levels and tomato consumption across European countries based on the European Prospective Investigation into Cancer and Nutrition (EPIC) study. *J Nutr*, 2005. **135**(8): 2032S–6S.
52. Garcia-Closas, R. et al. Dietary sources of vitamin C, vitamin E and specific carotenoids in Spain. *Br J Nutr*, 2004. **91**(6): 1005–11.
53. Slimestad, R., Fossen, T., Verheul, M.J. The flavonoids of tomatoes. *J Agric Food Chem*, 2008. **56**(7): 2436–41.
54. Caris-Veyrat, C. et al. Influence of organic versus conventional agricultural practice on the antioxidant microconstituent content of tomatoes and derived purees; consequences on antioxidant plasma status in humans. *J Agric Food Chem*, 2004. **52**(21): 6503–9.
55. Juroszek, P. et al. Fruit quality and bioactive compounds with antioxidant activity of tomatoes grown on-farm: comparison of organic and conventional management systems. *J Agric Food Chem*, 2009. **57**(4): 1188–94.
56. Dorais, M., Ehret, D., Papadopoulos, A. Tomato (*Solanum lycopersicum*) health components: from the seed to the consumer. *Phytochem Rev*, 2008. **7**: 231–250.
57. Shi, J., Le Maguer, M. Lycopene in tomatoes: chemical and physical properties affected by food processing. *Crit Rev Food Sci Nutr*, 2000. **40**(1): 1–42.
58. Wildman, R. *Handbook of nutraceuticals and functional foods*. 2007, Boca Raton: CRC Press.
59. Kerem, Z. et al. Chickpea domestication in the Neolithic Levant through the nutritional perspective. *Journal of Archaeological Science*, 2007. **34**: 1289–1293.
60. Marangoni, F., Martiello, A., Galli, C. Dietary fat intake of European countries in the Mediterranean area: An update. *World Rev Nutr Diet*, 2007. **97**: 67–84.
61. Messina, M.J. Legumes and soybeans: overview of their nutritional profiles and health effects. *Am J Clin Nutr*, 1999. **70**(3 Suppl): 439S–450S.
62. Anon, *EuroFIR BASIS*. http://ebasis.eurofir.org Date accessed 4 November 2009.
63. Fardet, A. New hypotheses for the health-protective mechanisms of whole-grain cereals: what is beyond fibre? *Nutr Res Rev*, 2010. **23**(1): 65–134.
64. Holland, B., McCance, R.A., Widdowson, E.M. *McCance and Widdowson's the composition of foods*. 5th rev. Extended by B. Holland, (eds). Cambridge: Royal Society of Chemistry, 1991. In progress.
65. Naczk, M., Shahidi, F. Phenolics in cereals, fruits and vegetables: occurrence, extraction and analysis. *J Pharm Biomed Anal*, 2006. **41**(5): 1523–42.
66. Yang, C.S. et al. Inhibition of carcinogenesis by dietary polyphenolic compounds. *Annu Rev Nutr*, 2001. **21**: 381–406.
67. Manach, C. et al. Polyphenols: food sources and bioavailability. *Am J Clin Nutr*, 2004. **79**(5): 727–47.

68. Vitaglione, P., Napolitano, A., Fogliano, V. Cereal dietary fibre: a natural functional ingredient to deliver phenolic compounds into the gut. *Trends Food Sci Technol*, 2008. **19**: 451–463.

69. Janick, J. The origin of fruits, fruit growing, and fruit breeding. *Plant Breeding Rev*, 2005. **25**: 255–320.

70. Guarnieri, S., Riso, P., Porrini, M. Orange juice vs vitamin C: effect on hydrogen peroxide-induced DNA damage in mononuclear blood cells. *Br J Nutr*, 2007. **97**(4): 639–43.

71. Prasanna, V., Prabha, T.N., Tharanathan, R.N. Fruit ripening phenomena–an overview. *Crit Rev Food Sci Nutr*, 2007. **47**(1): 1–19.

72. Peterson, J. et al. Flavanones in grapefruit, lemons, and limes: A compilation and review of the data from the analytical literature. *Journal of Food Composition and Analysis*, 2006. **19**: S74–S80.

73. Peterson, J. et al. Flavanones in oranges, tangerines (mandarins), tangors, and tangelos: a compilation and review of the data from the analytical literature. *Journal of Food Composition and Analysis*, 2006. **19**: S66–S73.

74. Dhuique-Mayer, C. et al. Varietal and interspecific influence on micronutrient contents in citrus from the Mediterranean area. *J Agric Food Chem*, 2005. **53**(6): 2140–5.

75. Armentano, et al. Über den Einfluß von Substanzen der Flavongruppe auf die Permeabilität der Kapillaren. Vitamin P. *Dtsch. Med. Wschr*, 1936. **62**: 1325.

76. Tripoli, E. et al. Citrus flavonoids: Molecular structure, biological activity and nutritional properties: A review. *Food Chemistry*, 2007. **104**: 466–479.

77. Walle, T. Methoxylated flavones, a superior cancer chemopreventive flavonoid subclass? *Semin Cancer Biol*, 2007. **17**(5): 354–62.

78. Moufida, S., Marzouk, B. Biochemical characterization of blood orange, sweet orange, lemon, bergamot and bitter orange. *Phytochemistry*, 2003. **62**(8): 1283–9.

79. Chow, H.H., Salazar, D., Hakim, I.A. Pharmacokinetics of perillic acid in humans after a single dose administration of a citrus preparation rich in d-limonene content. *Cancer Epidemiol Biomarkers Prev*, 2002. **11**(11): 1472–6.

80. Manners, G.D. Citrus limonoids: analysis, bioactivity, and biomedical prospects. *J Agric Food Chem*, 2007. **55**(21): 8285–94.

81. Magalhaes, A.S. et al. Protective effect of quince (Cydonia oblonga Miller) fruit against oxidative hemolysis of human erythrocytes. *Food Chem Toxicol*, 2009. **47**(6): 1372–7.

82. Boyer, J., Liu, R.H. Apple phytochemicals and their health benefits. *Nutr J*, 2004. **3**: 5.

83. Gerhauser, C. Cancer chemopreventive potential of apples, apple juice, and apple components. *Planta Med*, 2008. **74**(13): 1608–24.

84. Bandoniene, D., Murkovic, M. On-line HPLC-DPPH screening method for evaluation of radical scavenging phenols extracted from apples *(Malus domestica L.)*. *J Agric Food Chem*, 2002. **50**(9): 2482–7.

85. Galvis Sanchez, A., Gil-Izquierdo, A., Gil, M. Comparative study of six pear cultivars in terms of their phenolic and vitamin C contents and antioxidant capacity. *Journal of the Science of Food and Agriculture*, 2003. **83**: 995–1003.

86. Ruiz, D. et al. Carotenoids from new apricot (Prunus armeniaca L.) varieties and their relationship with flesh and skin color. *J Agric Food Chem*, 2005. **53**(16): 6368–74.

87. Cantin, C.M., Moreno, M.A., Gogorcena, Y. Evaluation of the antioxidant capacity, phenolic compounds, and vitamin C content of different peach and nectarine [*Prunus persica (L.) Batsch*] breeding progenies. *J Agric Food Chem*, 2009. **57**(11): 4586–92.

88. Chun, O.K. et al. Contribution of individual polyphenolics to total antioxidant capacity of plums. *J Agric Food Chem*, 2003. **51**(25): 7240–5.

89. Pezzuto, J.M. Grapes and human health: a perspective. *J Agric Food Chem*, 2008. **56**(16): 6777–84.

90. Cantos, E., Espin, J.C., Tomas-Barberan, F.A. Varietal differences among the polyphenol profiles of seven table grape cultivars studied by LC-DAD-MS-MS. *J Agric Food Chem*, 2002. **50**(20): 5691–6.

91. Sanchez-Palomo, E., Diaz-Maroto, M.C., Perez-Coello, M.S. Rapid determination of volatile compounds in grapes by HS-SPME coupled with GC-MS. *Talanta*, 2005. **66**(5): 1152–7.

92. Tulipani, S., Mezzetti, B., Battino, M. Impact of strawberries on human health: insight into marginally discussed bioactive compounds for the Mediterranean diet. *Public Health Nutr*, 2009. **12**(9A): 1656–62.

93. Seeram, N.P., Schulman, R.N., Heber, D. Pomegranates: ancient roots to modern medicine. *Medicinal and aromatic plants – industrial profiles*; Vol. 43. 2006, Boca Raton: CRC/Taylor & Francis.

94. Basu, A., Penugonda, K. Pomegranate juice: a heart-healthy fruit juice. *Nutr Rev*, 2009. **67**(1): 49–56.

95. Solomon, A. et al. Antioxidant activities and anthocyanin content of fresh fruits of common fig *(Ficus carica L.)*. *J Agric Food Chem*, 2006. **54**(20): 7717–23.

96. Vinson, J.A. et al. Dried fruits: excellent in vitro and in vivo antioxidants. *J Am Coll Nutr*, 2005. **24**(1): 44–50.

97. Al-Farsi, M.A., Lee, C.Y. Nutritional and functional properties of dates: a review. *Crit Rev Food Sci Nutr*, 2008. **48**(10): 877–87.

98. Al-Farsi, M. et al. Comparison of antioxidant activity, anthocyanins, carotenoids, and phenolics of three native fresh and sun-dried date *(Phoenix dactylifera L.)* varieties grown in Oman. *J Agric Food Chem*, 2005. **53**(19): 7592–9.

99. Bianchi, G. Lipids and phenols in table olives. *Eur J Lipid Sci Technol*, 2003. **105**: 229–242.

100. Marsilio, V., Campestre, C., Lanza, B. Phenolic compound change during California-style ripe olive processing. *Food Chem*, 2001: 55–60.

101. Conde, C., Delrot, S., Geros, H. Physiological, biochemical and molecular changes occurring during olive development and ripening. *J Plant Physiol*, 2008. **165**(15): 1545–62.

102. Blekas, G. et al. Biophenols in table olives. *J Agric Food Chem*, 2002. **50**(13): 3688–92.

103. Raederstorff, D. Antioxidant activity of olive polyphenols in humans: a review. *Int J Vitam Nutr Res*, 2009. **79**(3): 152–65.

104. Vissers, M.N., Zock, P.L., Katan, B. Bioavailability and antioxidant effects of olive oil phenols in humans: a review. *Eur J Clin Nutr*, 2004. **58**(6): 955–65.

105. Juan, M.E. et al. Olive fruit extracts inhibit proliferation and induce apoptosis in HT-29 human colon cancer cells. *J Nutr*, 2006. **136**(10): 2553–7.

106. Dewick, P.M. *Medicinal natural products: a biosynthetic approach*. 2nd ed. 2002, Chichester: Wiley. xii.

107. Leung, A.Y., Foster S. *Encyclopedia of common natural ingredients used in food, drugs, and cosmetics*. 2nd ed. 2003, New York; Chichester: Wiley. xxxv.

108. Ninfali, P. et al. Antioxidant capacity of vegetables, spices and dressings relevant to nutrition. *Br J Nutr*, 2005. **93**(2): 257–66.

109. Murkovic, M., Steinberger, D., Pfannhauser, W. Antioxidant spices reduce the formation of heterocyclic amines in fried meat. *Z Lebensm Unters Forsch A*, 1998. **207**: 477–480.

110. Hanlidou, E. et al. The herbal market of Thessaloniki (N Greece) and its relation to the ethnobotanical tradition. *J Ethnopharmacol*, 2004. **91**(2–3): 281–99.

111. Barnes, J., Anderson, L., Phillipson, J. *Herbal medicines*. 3rd ed. 2007, London: Pharmaceutical Press.

112. Aranceta, J. et al. Nut consumption in Spain and other countries. *Br J Nutr*, 2006. **96 Suppl 2**: S3–11.

113. Chen, C.Y., Blumberg, J.B. Phytochemical composition of nuts. *Asia Pac J Clin Nutr*, 2008. **17 Suppl 1**: 329–32.

114. Ros, E., Mataix, J. Fatty acid composition of nuts–implications for cardiovascular health. *Br J Nutr*, 2006. **96 Suppl 2**: S29–35.

115. Lopez-Uriarte, P. et al. Nuts and oxidation: a systematic review. *Nutr Rev*, 2009. **67**(9): 497–508.

116. Blomhoff, R. et al. Health benefits of nuts: potential role of antioxidants. *Br J Nutr*, 2006. **96 Suppl 2**: S52–60.

117. Corder, R. et al. Oenology: red wine procyanidins and vascular health. *Nature*, 2006. **444**(7119): 566.

118. Gonzalez, C.A., Salas-Salvado, J. The potential of nuts in the prevention of cancer. *Br J Nutr*, 2006. **96 Suppl 2**: S87–94.

119. Phillips, K.M., Ruggio, D.M., Ashraf-Khorassani, M. Phytosterol composition of nuts and seeds commonly consumed in the United States. *J Agric Food Chem*, 2005. **53**(24): 9436–45.

120. Smeds, A.I. et al. Quantification of a broad spectrum of lignans in cereals, oilseeds, and nuts. *J Agric Food Chem*, 2007. **55**(4): 1337–46.

121. Yamashita, K. et al. Sesame seed lignans and gamma-tocopherol act synergistically to produce vitamin E activity in rats. *J Nutr*, 1992. **122**(12): 2440–6.

6 Olive Oil and Other Fats

Summary

- The MedDiet has a unique fatty acid composition, and this is particularly related to the use of olive oil as the main dietary fat.
- Olive oil consists of a saponifiable fraction and an unsaponifiable fraction. The saponifiable fraction consists predominantly of the monounsaturated fatty acid (MUFA) oleic acid, but olive oil also contains a balanced proportion of saturated fatty acids (SFAs) and polyunsaturated fatty acid PUFAs.
- The unsaponifiable fraction (approx. 1–2%) comprises various microconstituents including squalene, triterpenic alcohols, sterols (essentially β-sitosterol), tocopherols and phenolics (mainly oleuropein and its metabolite, hydroxytyrosol). These constituents have antioxidant and other properties. The phenolics are low or absent in non-virgin olive oils.
- Nuts and seeds are important sources of fats in the MedDiet: almonds and sesame seeds provide linoleic acid (LA), and walnuts are a particularly good source of α-linolenic acid (ALA).
- Mediterranean animals grazed naturally produce milk and meat richer in PUFAs than that of equivalent animals given feed.
- Milk from the main dairy animals – goats and sheep – is richer in medium chain FAs than cow's milk, and these fatty acids are associated with a lower risk of CVD than longer chain fatty acids (C12 to C18).
- Industrially produced trans fatty acids (TFAs) are virtually absent from a traditional MedDiet, and TFAs from natural sources do not appear to contribute significantly to risk of coronary heart disease when consumed in normal amounts.
- Oily fish is the main contributor of long chain n-3 PUFAs.

6.1 Overview

Dietary fats are usually composed of saturated fatty acids (SFAs), monounsaturated fatty acids (MUFAs) and polyunsaturated fatty acids (PUFAs). The MUFAs complement a limited amount of SFAs and a necessary amount of n-6 PUFAs and n-3 PUFAs, of which two are essential, namely the n-6 PUFA linoleic acid (LA) and the n-3 PUFA α-linolenic acid (ALA) [1]. Both plant sources and moderate and specific animal sources of these FAs are present in the MedDiet, and these satisfy the balanced FA requirement. Olive oil is the main source of lipid and provides not only MUFAs but

The Mediterranean Diet: Health and Science, First Edition. Richard Hoffman and Mariette Gerber.
© 2012 Richard Hoffman and Mariette Gerber. Published 2012 by Blackwell Publishing Ltd.

also a balanced proportion of SFAs and PUFAs together with other beneficial nutrients and microconstituents, which makes it unique from other sources of MUFAs.

6.2   Olive oil

6.2.1   Consumption and production

Mediterranean countries are the highest producers, consumers and exporters of olive oil in the world. Greece has the highest per capita consumption, followed by Italy and Spain (Table 6.1). Olive oil consumption in some non-Mediterranean countries such as Germany, US, UK and Japan is now increasing [2]. Although olive oil is the main fat used in the MedDiet, and consumption in Mediterranean countries is still high, less expensive vegetable oils are becoming more popular. Some countries, such as Turkey, have traditionally used a wide variety of fats (including sunflower oil and butter). Although Egypt has quite a high consumption of olives, the use of olive oil has traditionally been very limited. However, attempts are being made to encourage its use in order to reduce the consumption of clarified butter.

Of particular significance in the overall context of the MedDiet is the ability of olive oil to greatly increase the palatability of foods, both by improving the texture and by enhancing flavour. Very popular in Greece are *lathera* dishes which consist of vegetables cooked in an olive oil-based sauce often including tomatoes and garlic. As noted by Dr Antonia Trichopoulou, a leading authority on the MedDiet, 'It would have been impossible to consume the high quantities of vegetables and legumes, which characterize the Mediterranean diet, were it not for olive oil that is traditionally used in the preparation of these dishes'[3]. Olive oil is not only used for cooking, but also appears raw in many dishes such as *aiolli* and other dips, and in vegetable marinades. It is also added as a flavouring at the end of the long, slow cooking of soups and stews such as *pistou*. Olive oil is also used in dough, batter and various pastries. Bread with oil is elemental Mediterranean cuisine, and a fascinating book has evocatively described how *pa amb oli* ('bread with oil') is rooted in Catalan culture [4].

Table 6.1   Supply and production of olive oil.

	Food supply (g/per capita/per day)[1]	Production (1000 tonnes)[2]
Egypt	0.31	7.5
France	4.63	4.7
Greece	43.58	327.2
Italy	38.31	510.0
Morocco	7.96	85.0
Portugal	13.30	36.3
Spain	32.34	1236.1
Tunisia	9.36	170.0
Turkey	1.98	72.0
United Kingdom	2.37	0

[1]FAOSTAT, 2007.
[2]International Olive Oil Council, 2007/8.

In 1996, there were more than 8 million hectares of olive trees in the world; there were over 9 million in 2000, and this is expected to rise to more than 10 million in 2010 of which 57% are in the European Union [2]. The world production of olive oil in 2007 was 2.72 million tonnes, of which Europe produced 78.67%; Spain was the number one producer with 43.3%, followed by Italy, 20.2% and Greece, 13.5%, and far behind these countries are Portugal, 1.1%, Croatia, 0.17% and France, 0.15% (see Table 6.1). Other producers are the countries of the Maghreb, Turkey and the Middle East. In the Americas, only Argentina is significant, with 0.37% of world production [2].

6.2.2 Origin and varieties of olive trees

Olive trees have been part of Mediterranean agriculture for centuries, as shown by their representation in the tombs of ancient Egypt. The original species *Olea europaea* may have been domesticated 3700 years BC in the Fertile Crescent[1]. However, recent genetic studies show that the indigenous ancestor of *O. europaea* (known as autochthonous oleastre) was present in the West as well as in the East of the Mediterranean Basin. After the glaciations, there was diversification in the West (Maghreb, Corsica, Sicily, Southern France), whereas only one genotype survived in the East (Figure 6.1) [5]. There are now six main subspecies of *O. europaea*: one subspecies of *O. europaea* is found all around the Mediterranean, two further south, two further west and one, *Olea cuspidate*, further east (in Asia, Southern Arabia, South and East Africa). Besides being established in Europe, the Spanish and Portuguese imported olive trees into North and South America, and increasing numbers are being grown in Japan and Australia.

Approximately 1000 varieties of olive trees exist in Europe. As an example, in Southern France alone there are 43 varieties including *Tanche* (Haute-Provence), *Caillette* (Nice region), *Salonenque* (Marseille region and Provence), *Picholine* (Languedoc and Corsica), *Negrette* (Nîmes region), *Lucques* (Languedoc) and *Olivière* (Roussillon). The AOC (Appellation d'Origine Contrôlé) designated olive oils of France are generally made of several cultivars, e.g. olive oil from Nîmes is made of *Picholine* and *Negrette* as principal varieties, together with several other secondary local or ancient varieties.

6.2.3 Olive oil production

Main process

Olive oil is usually made from olives at veraison (i.e. as they turn from green to purple), when oil levels are usually at their maximum, or from ripe olives, that is to say black olives (there is no difference between the olive trees that produce green and black olives). In Tuscany and Sardinia (Italy), olives are harvested from the trees before being fully black, either by hand or mechanically, whereas in Corsica the olives are harvested at full maturity, after they have fallen onto nets dispersed around the trees.

---

[1] Middle East corresponding to Israel, Palestine, Lebanon and parts of Syria, Jordan, Iraq, Egypt and South West of Turkey.

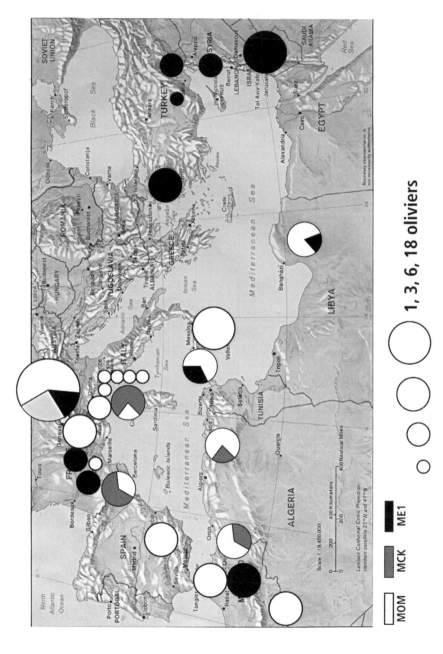

Figure 6.1 Distribution of olive genotypes (MOM, MCK, ME1) (modified from [5]). The numbers refer to the number of trees tested. With permission from Springer Science + Business Media (Springer).

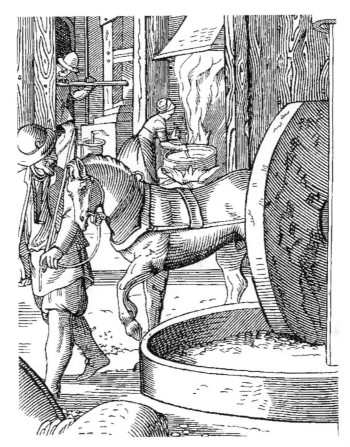

Figure 6.2 The manufacture of olive oil in the 16th century (drawn and engraved by J. Amman) (Wikipedia Commons).

The oil is present in lipovacuoles that are part of the cells in the olive pulp. The principle of oil production is first to extract the liquid part from the pulp, and then to separate the aqueous phase from the lipid phase. Only mechanical steps are used to produce the final product. The olives should be treated as soon as possible after harvest, and in conditions that avoid fermentation, namely a cool place and aerated baskets or boxes. First, olive tree leaves are eliminated, and then the olives are washed and crushed. In ancient times, crushing was done between two to six millstones that were rotated using animals (Figure 6.2), and millstones are still sometimes used, although today they are driven by motors. The rotation is rather slow (15–20 revolutions per minute) and lasts 20–40 minutes. However, pulping is mainly achieved nowadays by metal hammers, knives or plates rotating at high speed (1200–3000 rpm). Millstones are more efficient and produce oil with a better aromatic quality, and at a lower temperature (27° C). However, the modern apparatus is faster and avoids the risk of oxidation, since the emulsion obtained passes continuously towards the next apparatus that slowly kneads the paste. The temperature should not exceed 29° C at this stage, but should be sufficient to disintegrate the emulsion, preparing the paste for a good extraction.

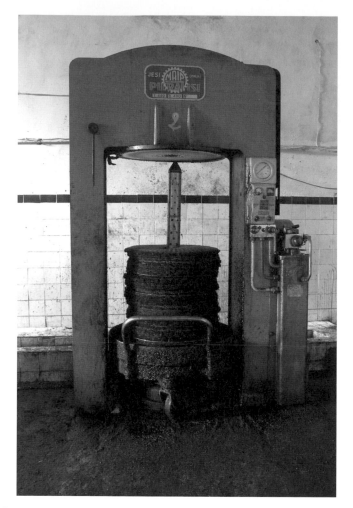

Figure 6.3   Olive press showing fibre discs (Wikipedia).

Two main techniques are used for extracting the oil from the paste: pressure or centrifugation. Pressure is exerted after spreading olive paste on discs, which are stacked on top of each other so that discs and olive paste are organised in alternate layers (Figure 6.3). These are then placed into a press. The discs were originally made of osier or coco fibre, but are now made from synthetic fibre. The first pressing gives the best oil (known as the first cold pressing), and the quality of subsequent oils depends on the number of pressings. Until a few decades ago, quality was not as important a requirement as it is today, and the paste was pressed and pressed again, and forced with hot water producing inferior quality oils. However, these procedures are no longer used.

Centrifugation (along a horizontal axis) is a more recent method used to separate the oil from the solids. A small quantity of water remains with the oil, and decantation or centrifugation is necessary to get rid of it. (Solid and liquid wastes remain from the extraction, and these can be used as a fertiliser.) After, this step, the oil is now ready for consumption, although it may still be turbid. To avoid oxidation, it is left under a nitrogen atmosphere to settle down, and may or may not be filtered.

Supplementary technologies

A few supplementary technologies have been proposed, such as washing the olives in water at 70° C in order to decrease bitterness [6]. This action might be of interest for marketing less bitter olive oils in countries not culturally used to olive oil consumption. However composition is affected: there are increases in chlorophyll and carotenoids, and a decrease in phenolic compounds, noticeably of the phenolic oleuropein, which is the main phytochemical responsible for the bitterness. Similarly, storage of olives at 5° C before extraction decreases bitterness, and this is associated with a decrease in total phenolics with increasing ripeness during storage [7].

Fine talcum powder increases the efficiency of extracting the oily phase by coalescing small oil droplets into larger ones. This procedure is allowed in most European countries, but not in France. The use of cellulolytic or pectolytic enzymes, which break the cell walls and facilitate oil extraction, is no longer permitted in Europe.

The use of de-stoned olives for olive oil extraction has major advantages: there is less acidity and peroxidation, because of a better resistance to oxidation, and no change in organoleptic properties (i.e. the oil's flavour, bouquet and colour) [8]. Another advance in technology, proposed to work with a paste obtained from de-stoned olives, is the use of heat exchangers. The use of heat exchangers has been demonstrated to improve the efficiency of oil production, content of phenolic compounds (hence an increased resistance to oxidation) and of aromatic compounds that form part of the organoleptic quality [9].

Storage and preservation

Filtration is sometimes used since it generally ensures better preservation without modifying organoleptic quality. However, filtration decreases the phenolic content and organoleptic quality when oils contain moisture [10]. Higher quality oils tend to be more stable. The limit for optimal preservation is approximately 18 months in the dark and in a large airtight bottle, and after this time the acidity increases and the oil loses its organoleptic character of extra-virgin oil.

6.2.4 Traceability and European regulations

FA composition is one criteria for traceability of origin. The degradation of oleic triglyceride to free FA is an indicator of quality, measured by the % acidity (i.e. grams of oleic acid per 100 g of olive oil). Olive oil is an unusual product in that it is characterised not only by its chemical properties but also by its organoleptic ones. These are on a scale of 1 to 10 and use terms such as 'fruity' (ripe, green, black, more descriptively: artichoke, tomato leaf, almond, green apple etc.), 'bitter' and 'hot'. There are some organoleptic characteristics that disqualify an olive oil from the extra-virgin category including 'rancid', 'mouldy', and 'tasting of the lees' (a result of fermentation of the pulp).

In 1992, the EU set the criteria for the different categories of olive oil (CEE 2081/92 regulations). There are several categories, schematically classified as (1) virgin and (2) non-virgin oils:

1. **Virgin oils:** these are prepared from the fruit of olive trees by only physical or mechanical processes, within thermal limits that ensure there is no alteration to

the product, and without any processes other than washing, decantation, centrifugation and filtration. Oils extracted by solvent or re-esterification, and resulting from mixing with other oils, are excluded. Several classes are described for virgin oils:
 – Extra virgin olive oil (EVOO): organoleptic note >6.5, acidity ≤1%
 – Virgin olive olive oil (VOO): organoleptic note >5.5, acidity ≤2%
 – Current virgin olive oil: organoleptic note >3.5, acidity ≤3.3%
 – Lampante[2] virgin olive oil: organoleptic note <3.5, acidity >3.3%
2. **Non-virgin oils:** these are refined oils (extracted by a solvent, acidity: ≤0.5%), olive oil (mix of refined and virgin oils, acidity: ≤1.5%), pulp residue, olive oil (raw, or after refining, acidity: ≤0.5%, or after mixture of refining pulp residue, olive oil and virgin olive oil, acidity: ≤1.5%).

The description as 'first pressing at low temperature' is reserved for extra virgin oil extracted by pressure at a temperature kept at or below 27° C (EU N°1019, 2002). Using the above information, the consumer can use the description on the label to learn to select a good quality olive oil from the shelf.

6.2.5   Biochemical composition

VOO is composed of a lipid fraction – also referred to as a glycerol fraction or saponifiable fraction (comprising about 98–99%), and an unsaponifiable (non-saponifiable) fraction. The major component of the saponifiable fraction is oleic acid, and the high content of this MUFA was originally regarded as the main reason for the heath benefits of olive oil. However, there is now considerable evidence that the unsaponifiable fraction also has important health properties. Some seed oils, such as rapeseed, are rich in oleic acid, but these do not contain many of the unsaponifiable components – especially phenolics – found in olive oil.

Saponifiable fraction

The major fatty acid in olive oil is oleic acid (comprising a minimum of approximately 55% up to a maximum of approximately 83%), together with smaller amounts of other fatty acids such as palmitic acid, linoleic acid and stearic acid (Table 6.2).
 The FA composition of olive oil varies with the cultivar, and this can be illustrated by considering some popular cultivars grown in France. *Tanche* olives give an oil with the highest proportion of MUFA (81.4%) and the lowest percentage of SFA (11.7%), and *Salonenque* olives give an oil with the lowest proportion of MUFA (68.4%) and the highest proportion of SFA (17.8%) and PUFA (13.8%, mainly LA, 13.2% and ALA, 0.59%). *Picholine* has the highest proportion of ALA (average content 0.8%, up to 1.1%) and *Olivière* has the best ratio of linoleic/linolenic acid (between 6.5 and 4.5). Some local varieties show extreme characteristics, like *Bechude* (from the Ardèche region) which is very low in SFA (<10%), very high in MUFA (approx. 86%) but also rather low in PUFA (4.15%, with a ratio of LA:ALA of 7). These details illustrate the good balance between SFA and PUFA, whatever their respective proportion in olive oils, and also that when consumed in high

---

[2] Means slightly rancid, an organoleptic character that might be found pleasant (Corsica).

Table 6.2 Fatty acid composition of olive oils (1400 samples from 46 varieties) (based on [11]).

Fatty acid Composition	Name	Median	25% quartile	75% quartile
C16:0	Palmitic	11.80	10.90	12.70
C16:1 *n*-9	Hypogeic	0.12	0.11	0.14
C16:1 *n*-7	Palmitoleic	0.81	0.62	1.08
C17:0	Margaric	0.08	0.05	0.12
C17:1 *n*-8	Margaroleic	0.15	0.10	0.25
C18:0	Stearic	2.20	1.90	2.70
C18:1 *n*-9	Oleic	72.60	68.90	75.10
C18:1 *n*-7	Vaccenic	2.30	2.00	2.70
C18:2 *n*-6	Linoleic	7.90	6.50	10.1
C18:3 *n*-3	α-Linolenic	0.65	0.60	0.70
C20:0	Arachidic	0.37	0.34	0.42
C20:1 *n*-9	Gondoic	0.2	0.25	0.31
C22:0	Behenic	0.11	0.10	0.12
C24:0	Lignoceric	0.05	0.04	0.05
	Saturated FA	14.8	14.0	15.6
	Monounsaturated FA	76.6	73.4	79.1
	Polyunsaturated FA	8.6	7.2	10.8

amounts, olive oil is a sizeable contributor to total ALA intake. In addition, most of the SFAs are situated in the sn-1/sn-3 external positions of the triglyceride molecule (less than 10% of the palmitic acid is in sn-2 position versus about 70% of LA and 50% of MUFA). This reduces the absorption of SFA, and ensures a better absorption of LA and MUFA [12].

Unsaponifiable fraction

The unsaponifiable fraction includes various triterpenes (mostly squalene), sterols (mostly β-sitosterol) and tocopherols (mostly vitamin E) [12]. These compounds are extractable with solvents and so are present in non-virgin olive oils. VOOs also contain a range of phenolics (especially oleuropein and its metabolite, hydroxytyrosol). These are only present in significant amounts in VOO, and are probably important for many of its health benefits.

Squalene is present in olive oils at about 0.5% w/w, which is much higher than in other oils (Table 6.3). Consequently, the MedDiet is probably associated with a significantly higher consumption of squalene than most other dietary patterns. Regular consumption of squalene is claimed to have a wide range of health benefits, ranging from preventing heart disease and diabetes to arthritis and cancer, and although there have been positive results with animal studies, the relevance of these findings to humans has not been established [13]. Olive oils also contain the triterpenes oleanolic and maslinic acid, although levels are lower than in olives (see Chapter 5).

Olive oil contains carotenoids (which chemically are tetraterpenes), mainly lutein and β-carotene. These carotenoids, together with chlorophyll, are responsible for the colours of olive oils, which range from yellow-green to greenish-gold. Plant sterols are present in olive oil in quite high amounts (100–200 mg/100 g). The main plant sterols are β-sitosterol, campesterol and delta-5-avenasterol, and levels vary with

Table 6.3 Squalene content of olive oil and other oils.

Oil	Squalene (mg/100g)
Olive	136–708
Corn	19–36
Peanut	13–49
Soybean	7–17
Sunflower	8–19
Rapeseed	28

variety, cultivation conditions and processing. Plant sterols are well known for their ability to reduce cholesterol uptake in the gut, and this may possibly afford protection against CVD (see Chapter 11). Olive oil also contains the antioxidant α-tocopherol (vitamin E), with levels between 100–350 mg/kg depending on the quality of the oil and its origin [13]. Lower amounts of other tocopherols are also present.

Olive oil is less prone to oxidation than other oils when frying at high temperatures, and in part this is probably due to the high levels of antioxidants in olive oil, such as α-tocopherol, squalene and delta-5-avenasterol [13]. The relatively low amounts of oxidation-prone polyunsaturated fatty acids (PUFAs) in olive oil are probably also important for the high degree of resistance of olive oil to oxidation. Indeed, although sunflower oil has a higher level of vitamin E than olive oil, it is more prone to oxidation due to its high level of PUFAs.

Phenolics are a major component of the unsaponifiable fraction of VOO. At least 36 phenolics have been identified and these include:

- phenolic acids
- tyrosol, hydroxytyrosol and their derivatives (these derivatives are known as secoiridoids – chemically defined as having elenolic acid in their structure – and include the glycosides oleuropein and ligstroside, and their aglycone derivatives) and oleocanthal
- flavonoids including luteolin and apigenein
- lignans such as pinoresinol and acetoxypinoresinol.

Estimates of the phenolic content of various EVOOs range from 50–800 mg/kg with an average of 180 mg/ kg [14]. This equates to approx. 9 mg of olive oil phenols per day based on a daily consumption of 50 g. The phenolic contents of VOOs can vary widely, and this reflects the influence of many factors including olive variety, growth conditions, maturity of fruit at harvest and manufacturing processes [15]. Storage of oils (especially in clear bottles exposed to the light) reduces the phenolic content. The 'shelf life' of VOO has been found to correlate with its phenolic content [13]. Frying with VOO also reduces phenolic content [16], and this emphasises the important role that consumption of raw olive oil may play in the MedDiet.

Phenolics in VOO have high bioavailability, and studies suggest that they have important health benefits. Hydroxytyrosol is a good antioxidant and is thought to be a major phenolic that contributes to the health benefits of VOO (see Chapter 11).

Although levels of hydroxytyrosol and tyrosol in VOO are relatively low – about 7.7 mg/kg and 11.3 mg/kg respectively – the overall level of all of the various derivatives of these compounds in VOO is about 59 mg/kg [17]. There is evidence that some of these derivatives, such as oleuropein, can be converted into tyrosol and hydroxytyrosol in the body [18]. Hence, the overall 'pool' of tyrosol and hydroxytyrosol in the body may be due to various compounds present in VOO. Excessive oleuropein in olive oil will give it a bitter taste, although a certain level is considered desirable.

A number of other physiological actions, besides antioxidant activity, have been demonstrated for phenolics in VOO. Animal studies have shown that the phenolic fraction from olive oil reduces cholesterol synthesis in the liver by inhibiting HMG-CoA reductase, the key enzyme in cholesterol synthesis [19]. Pinoresinol-rich olive oil has inhibitory effects on colon cancer cells *in vitro*, although the relevance of this to humans has not been ascertained [20].

Some EVOOs have a distinct peppery bite at the back of the throat and this effect is due to oleocanthal. A similar peppery sensation is caused by the anti-inflammatory drug ibuprofen, a non-steroidal anti-inflammatory drug. This similarity between oleocanthal and ibuprofen provoked an examination of the anti-inflammatory actions of oleocanthal. It was duly found that oleocanthal has anti-inflammatory actions that are similar to those of ibuprofen, namely by inhibiting the pro-inflammatory enzymes cyclo-oxygenase-1 (COX-1) and COX-2 [21]. It has been estimated that a daily dose of 50 g of olive oil would only confer the equivalent of about 10% of the recommended ibuprofen dose for adult pain relief and so normal olive oil consumption may be insufficient to relieve a headache [21]. Since a low dose of aspirin, also a COX inhibitor, reduces platelet aggregation and also has long-term benefits on cardiovascular health, it is possible that oleocanthal could contribute to the long-term health benefits of consuming olive oil. Olecocanthal is moderately heat stable and so some is present even after using olive oil for cooking [22]. It should be noted that there are wide variations in the content of oleocanthal between olive oils (8.4–298.1 mg/kg [15]), but it is possible that regular consumption of an olive oil rich in oleocanthal could contribute to the anti-inflammatory effects of the MedDiet.

6.3 Other fat sources

6.3.1 Nuts and seeds

Nuts are eaten as a dessert, and also used in pastries and for cooking. They are an important source of FAs in the MedDiet (see also Section 5.6). Almonds provide LA (10 g/100 g) (together with other nutrients such as fibre, 15 g/100 g and calcium and magnesium, each 250 mg/100 g). Walnuts are a sizeable contributor to PUFA intake (LA 30 g/100 g, ALA 6 g/100 g). Although the walnut tree is not considered to be a typical Mediterranean plant, it is present in front of many houses, or in community places in rural regions such as in Crete and in Southern France [23].

Sesame seeds are also a source of LA (10 g/100 g) (as well as fibre (11 g/100 g), and lignans), and are mainly used in pastries (e.g. *halva* in the Southern bank of the Mediterranean) and as a paste in a few – but emblematic – culinary recipes such as *hummus*.

Table 6.4   Fat composition of various meats (based on [24, 25]).

	% of FA in total fat				
	SFA	**MUFA**	**Total PUFAs**	**LA**	**ALA**
Lamb	52.1	40.5	5.8	5.0	0.8
Pork	43.2	47.6	9.2	8.6	0.6
Beef	56.4	40.3	3.2	2.5	0.7

6.3.2   Herbs and spices

Herbs and spices are commonly used in the MedDiet, in culinary recipes, salads and infusions (see Chapter 2). Most of these plant ingredients are rich in ALA. Purslane and dandelions, used in salads, pies and soups, are the richest sources (see also Chapter 5) [23].

6.3.3   Meat and dairy

There is only moderate consumption of animal products, whether dairy or meat, in the MedDiet. The geographical characteristics of the Mediterranean favour small livestock with specialised feeding habits: sheep and goats can take advantage of the hilly landscape and of Mediterranean grazing, whereas pigs prefer open wild spaces such as in holm-oak forest.

The plasma and adipose tissue FA composition of animals (and humans) reflects their intake of the non-synthesisable FAs (*n*-6 PUFAs and *n*-3 PUFAs). Thus, because the pasture of Mediterranean animals used to produce dairy and meat is richer in PUFAs than that of the equivalent animal given animal feeds, their FA profile is healthier. This is especially true for pigs running in open spaces in Corsica and Sardinia – their meat is leaner, and their fat is made up of 40 to 50% of MUFA (Table 6.4).

The importance of the food chain. i.e. from animal feed to animal to human, can be illustrated with a dietary intervention study which analysed the LC-PUFA composition of platelets taken from subjects who had eaten meat either from grass-fed animals or from animals that had been fed concentrates [26]. The former group were found to have significantly higher levels of LC-PUFAs in their platelets than subjects who ate meat from animals fed a concentrate (Table 6.5). This suggests that meat consumed from animals raised in a traditional Mediterranean way would result in a relatively higher consumption of LC-PUFAs than from animals fed a concentrate.

In a traditional MedDiet, there is a relatively low consumption of SFAs derived from meat and cow's milk, and a relatively high consumption of SFAs from cheese and yogurt made from goat and sheep milk. This results in the types of SFAs consumed as part of a MedDiet being quantitatively different to those in a North European diet since SFAs in milk from goat and sheep are richer in medium chain FAs (MCFAs), i.e. <12 carbon atoms (<12C). These MCFAs include caproic acid (C6:0), caprylic (C8:0), capric (C10:0) (the names drive from the Latin *caper* for a goat), and lauric (C12:0). Their concentrations (%) in sheep, goat and cow milk, respectively, have been estimated as: caproic: 2.9, 2.4, 1.6; caprylic: 2.6, 2.7, 1.3; capric: 7.8, 10.0, 3.0; lauric: 4.4, 5.0, 3.1 [28]. For example, fresh goat cheese with 40% fat comprises 15% <12C FAs whereas these FAs only constitute 7% in a comparable cow's milk cheese.

Table 6.5 Fatty acids composition of platelets in human subjects (% total) fed meat from either grass-fed or concentrate-fed animals. (Adapted with permission from Cambridge University Press [27].)

Fatty acid (% total in platelets)	Grass-fed animals		Concentrate-fed animals		
	Base-line	Post-intervention	Base-line	Post-intervention	p[1]
EPA	4.96	5.75	4.88	4.58	<0.01
DHA	4.96	5.75	4.93	4.58	<0.01

[1]Difference between groups at post-intervention with base-line value as covariate in ANOVA. EPA – eicosapentaenoic acid; DHA – docosahexaenoic acid.

Similarly, the fat content of Roquefort cheese (a fatty cheese made from sheep's milk) comprises 15% <12C FA and 23 % palmitic acid. By comparison, a cow's milk fatty cheese comprises 33% palmitic acid [24].

MCFAs are absorbed directly in the gut without re-esterification and are not metabolised in the same way as long chain SFAs [29]. There is some evidence that MCFAs do not raise cholesterol levels to the same extent as longer chain FAs (i.e. C12:0–C16:0). MCFAs do not accumulate in adipose tissue (in contrast to palmitic acid) and are known for being non-atherogenic [30]. It is, however, difficult to establish whether or not consuming goat and sheep milk products is associated with a lower risk of CVD than dairy produce made with cow milk since food sources contain a mixture of FAs. The peculiar composition of animal fat in the Mediterranean has for long been ignored when describing the advantages of the MedDiet, despite this being a specific feature of this dietary pattern. This may be because it is difficult to evaluate in present models of the MedDiet. Low levels of the LC-PUFAs eicosapentaenoic acid (EPA) and docosahexaenoic acid (DHA) have also been found in Greek feta cheese [31] (see below).

LA consumed by cows, goats and sheep is converted by bacteria in the rumen of these animals into various isomers, referred to as conjugated linoleic acid (CLA), via the *trans* fatty acid (TFA) vaccenic acid (11-*trans* octadecenoic acid). CLA then finds its way into the milk and meat of these animals. Quite high levels of CLA have been detected in aged Greek cheeses and feta [32]. CLA is so-named because it contains 2 double bonds adjacent to each other (i.e. the bonds are conjugated). The main CLA in ruminant milk is 9*cis*, 11*trans* linoleic acid. CLA has attracted a lot of interest because of promising effects in cell and animal models of cancer and other diseases. However, the doses used in these experiments have been quite high, and results from human studies at normal nutritional intake have not found any clear association between CLA intake and protection against breast cancer [33].

Industrially-produced TFAs have adverse effects on risk factors for CVD, by lowering HDL-cholesterol and raising LDL-cholesterol. Industrial TFAs are produced by the partial hydrogenation of vegetable fats, and are not a significant part of a traditional MedDiet. However, a TFA that is present in the MedDiet is vaccenic acid (see above), and occurs in ruminant milk at concentrations ranging between 0.4–4.0% [34]. Hence, there is interest in establishing whether or not naturally-occurring TFAs from ruminants have the same adverse effects on markers for CVD as industrially-produced TFAs [35, 36]. Although establishing possible adverse effects of these TFAs is complex, a major review summing up these studies has concluded that 'total TFA from natural sources, in actual amounts consumed in diets, do not contribute importantly to risks of coronary heart disease' [37].

Industrial- and naturally-occurring trans fatty acids (TFAs)

With the development of the food industry, there has been an increased intake in Western populations of TFAs as a proportion of total fatty acid intake. By contrast, natural TFAs constitute a relatively small component of the human diet, and are mainly found in dairy products. *Cis* and *trans* are terms that refer to the arrangement of hydrogen atoms in the double bond, for example of unsaturated fatty acids. In the *cis* arrangement, the hydrogen atoms in the double bond are on the same side, resulting in a kinked geometry. In the *trans* arrangement, the hydrogen atoms in the double bond are on opposite sides, and the chain is straight overall. A few decades ago, the food industry applied a technological process to vegetable oils, namely partial hydrogenation, in order to harden them and obtain a butter substitute with little SFA. This technology gives rise to TFA isomers in a different position to natural ruminant ones. In natural ruminant TFAs the double bond is mainly at C11 (vaccenic acid) [38, 39], whereas technologically-produced TFAs contain mixtures of isomers in which the *trans* bond may occur anywhere between the 4th and 10th carbons [40]. The most common TFA in partially hydrogenated vegetable oils is a trans isomer of oleic acid referred to as elaidic acid (trans-18:1 n9/Δ9), constituting between 1–65% of total fatty acids.

Not only is dietary ALA obtained directly from wild greens, but this fatty acid can also be obtained indirectly from animals that feed on wild greens. This is because ALA from plants is preserved through the food chain. Hence, herbivores, such as goats, sheep and chickens, eating wild greens will incorporate ALA into their fat. Moreover, there is a low level of conversion of ALA by herbivores into the longer chain *n*-3 fatty acids EPA and DHA. Hence, eating milk, butter and cheese, meat or eggs from herbivores consuming wild greens will contribute to the *n*-3 fats in a traditional MedDiet. One study found that there were low levels of EPA and DHA in Greek feta (which is made from sheep and/or goats milk) (14 mg/100 g and 5 mg/100 g respectively) whereas none was detected in a Cheddar cheese made from milk from cows – which have a high grain diet [41]. However, it should be noted that these levels of EPA and DHA are still significantly lower than the levels of EPA and DHA in oily fish (which are > 1 g/100 g) which will still represent the major source of these fatty acids for most Mediterranean people.

6.3.4 Eggs

Egg yolks contain ALA, the chickens obtaining their ALA from their diet. One study found that the yolk of eggs from Greek chickens allowed to roam and eat naturally had far higher levels of ALA than levels present in eggs sold in an American supermarket (6.9 mg ALA/g egg yolk and 0.52 mg ALA/g respectively) [31]. Egg yolks also contain low levels of LC *n*-3 PUFAs including EPA and DHA, and the overall levels of *n*-3 PUFAs in the Greek eggs were far higher than in the supermarket eggs (17.7 mg/g egg yolk and 1.7 mg/g respectively). These differences were attributed to the higher dietary consumption of *n*-3 PUFAs by the Greek chickens (from grass, purslane, various insects, etc).

6.3.5   Fish and shellfish

The other source of animal FA in the MedDiet is from marine sources, namely fish and seafood. Fish is the main contributor of LC *n*-3 PUFAs. These FAs from fish and seafood are not essential in the strict sense, since theoretically ALA, present in plants, is the precursor of EPA (20:5 *n*-3), which is further desaturated to DHA (22:6 *n*-3). However, the efficiency of the desaturation of ALA through the elongases and the desaturases $\Delta 5$ and $\Delta 6$ towards EPA and DHA is very poor in humans, especially for the final product, DHA. Therefore, EPA and DHA are considered essential, especially for the role of DHA in neurological development of the foetus, the infant and the child. These FAs occur predominantly in fatty fish, and in the Mediterranean three good sources of LC *n*-3 FA are sardines, anchovies and mackerel. Levels of EPA and DHA in preserved anchovies have been estimated at 466 and 886 mg/100 g, respectively, with even higher levels of EPA and DHA in fresh mackerel (662 and 886 mg/100 g, respectively) and fresh sardines (638 and 1269 mg/100 g respectively) [42]. It is worth noting that fatty fish are also the main source of dietary vitamin D (8–20 µg/100 g).

The EPA and DHA content of oily fish is dependent on their diet since oily fish are themselves poor converters of ALA into EPA and DHA. Phytoplankton, on the other hand, are good converters, and hence oily fish will contain high levels of EPA and DHA if they have consumed a diet rich in plankton, or if they have consumed other fish [43]. Farmed fish will only contain significant amounts of EPA and DHA if their feed contains these fatty acids [43]. A study found that oily fish from the warm waters of the Mediterranean contained lower levels of *n*-3 fatty acids than fish from colder, more northerly waters [44]. However, the season and stage of the reproductive cycle of the fish are probably more important factors that influence fatty acid content [45].

Fish and other seafood are not only popular dishes in some regions close to the Mediterranean shore but fish is also eaten in the hinterland, since here there exists a strong tradition of salting, marinating and smoking fillets from fatty fish. Cod – a non-fatty fish – is also preserved, salted and used in many cooking recipes. Cod is also transformed into a dish called '*brandade*', which can be kept for a long period of time. These aspects help ensure a convenient consumption of LC *n*-3 FAs.

References

1. FAO/OMS. Interim summary of conclusions and dietary recommendations on total fat & fatty acids, 2010.
2. Anon. International Olive Oil Council. www.internationaloliveoil.org
3. Trichopoulou, A.V. Dilis, olive oil and longevity. *Mol Nutr Food Res*, 2007. **51**(10): 1275–8.
4. Graves, T. *Bread and oil: Majorcan culture's last stand*. 2006: Grub Street.
5. Besnard, G. et al. Olea europaea (Oleaceae) phylogeography based on chloroplast DNA polymorphism. *Theor Appl Genet*, 2002. **104**(8): 1353–1361.
6. Garcia, J.M. et al. Hot water dipping of olives (Olea europaea) for virgin oil debittering. *J Agric Food Chem*, 2005. **53**(21): 8248–52.
7. Yousfi, K., Cayuela, J.A., Garcia, J.M. Reduction of virgin olive oil bitterness by fruit cold storage. *J Agric Food Chem*, 2008. **56**(21): 10085–91.

8. Mulinacci, N. et al. Analysis of extra-virgin oil from stoned olives. *J Sci Food Agric*, 2005. **85**(4): 662–670.

9. Amirantea, P. et al. Advance technology in virgin olive oil production from traditional and de-stoned pastes: Influence of the introduction of a heat exchanger on oil quality. *Food Chem*, 2006. **98**(4): 797–805.

10. Petit C. et al. Effet de la filtration sur la qualité et stabilité de l'huile d'olive vierge. *Le Nouvel Olivier*, 2006. **54**: 3–10.

11. Moutier, N. et al. Idetification et caractérisation des variétés d'olivier cultivées en France. *Naturalia publications*, 2004. **1**.

12. Léger, C., Descomps, B. Olive oil, olive oil by-products and olive fruit Mediterranean diet and health. Current news and prospects., ed. P. Besancon. 2001, Paris: John Libbey Eurotext, pp. 53–68.

13. Boskou, D. Olive oil. *World Rev Nutr Diet*, 2007. **97**: 180–210.

14. Vissers, M.N., Zock, P.L., Katan, M.B. Bioavailability and antioxidant effects of olive oil phenols in humans: a review. *Eur J Clin Nutr*, 2004. **58**(6): 955–65.

15. Cicerale, S. et al. Chemistry and health of olive oil phenolics. *Crit Rev Food Sci Nutr*, 2009. **49**(3): 218–36.

16. Gomez-Alonso, S. et al. Changes in phenolic composition and antioxidant activity of virgin olive oil during frying. *J Agric Food Chem*, 2003. **51**(3): 667–72.

17. Phenol-Explorer, http://www.phenol-explorer.eu.

18. Vissers, M.N. et al. Olive oil phenols are absorbed in humans. *J Nutr*, 2002. **132**(3): 409–17.

19. Tripoli, E. et al. The phenolic compounds of olive oil: structure, biological activity and beneficial effects on human health. *Nutr Res Rev*, 2005. **18**(1): 98–112.

20. Fini, L. et al. Chemopreventive properties of pinoresinol-rich olive oil involve a selective activation of the ATM-p53 cascade in colon cancer cell lines. *Carcinogenesis*, 2008. **29**(1): 139–46.

21. Beauchamp, G.K. et al. Phytochemistry: ibuprofen-like activity in extra-virgin olive oil. *Nature*, 2005. **437**(7055): 45–6.

22. Cicerale, S. et al. Influence of heat on biological activity and concentration of oleocanthal–a natural anti-inflammatory agent in virgin olive oil. *J Agric Food Chem*, 2009. **57**(4): 326–30.

23. Gerber, M., Corpet, D. Food, lifestyle and cardio-vascular disease in Europe. *Rivista di Anthropologia*, 1998. **S76**: 419–430.

24. McCance, R.A. et al. *McCance and Widdowson's The composition of foods*, 4th revised and extended by A.A. Paul and D.A.T. Southgate for the Ministry of Agriculture, Fisheries and Food and the Medical Research Council. 1978, London: H.M.S.O.; Amsterdam; Oxford: Elsevier/North-Holland Biomedical Press.,

25. Favier, J.C. et al. *TEC-DOC*. 1995, Paris: Lavoisier.

26. McAfee, A.J. et al. Red meat from animals offered a grass diet increase platelet n-3 PUFA in healthy consumers. *Proc Nut Soc*, 2010. **69**(OCE4): E335.

27. McAfee, A.J. et al. Red meat from animals offered a grass diet increases plasma and platelet n-3 PUFA in healthy consumers. *Br J Nutr*, 2010: 1–10.

28. Park, Y.W. et al. Physico-chemical characteristics of goat and sheep milk. *Small Ruminant Research*, 2007. **68**: 88–113.

29. Sanz Sampelayo, M.R. et al. Influence of type of diet on the fat constituents of goat and sheep milk. *Small Ruminant Research*, 2007. **68**: 42–63.

30. Hu, F.B. et al. Dietary saturated fats and their food sources in relation to the risk of coronary heart disease in women. *Am J Clin Nutr*, 1999. **70**(6): 1001–8.

31. Simopoulos, A.P. The Mediterranean diets: what is so special about the diet of Greece? The scientific evidence. *J Nutr*, 2001. **131**(11 Suppl): 3065S–73S.

32. Zlatanosa, S. et al. CLA content and fatty acid composition of Greek Feta and hard cheeses. *Food Chemistry*, 2002. **78**: 471–477.

33. Larsson, S.C., Bergkvist, L., Wolk, A. Conjugated linoleic acid intake and breast cancer risk in a prospective cohort of Swedish women. *Am J Clin Nutr*, 2009. **90**(3): 556–60.

34. Turpeinen, A.M. et al. Bioconversion of vaccenic acid to conjugated linoleic acid in humans. *Am J Clin Nutr*, 2002. **76**(3): 504–10.

35. Chardigny, J.M. et al. Do trans fatty acids from industrially produced sources and from natural sources have the same effect on cardiovascular disease risk factors in healthy subjects? Results of the trans Fatty Acids Collaboration (TRANSFACT) study. *Am J Clin Nutr*, 2008. **87**(3): 558–66.

36. Motard-Belanger, A. et al. Study of the effect of trans fatty acids from ruminants on blood lipids and other risk factors for cardiovascular disease. *Am J Clin Nutr*, 2008. 87(3): 593–9.
37. Willett, W., Mozaffarian, D. Ruminant or industrial sources of trans fatty acids: public health issue or food label skirmish? *Am J Clin Nutr*, 2008. 87(3): 515–6.
38. Jakobsen, M.U. et al. Intake of ruminant trans fatty acids and risk of coronary heart disease – an overview. *Atheroscler Suppl*, 2006. 7(2): 9–11.
39. Jakobsen, M.U. et al. Intake of ruminant trans fatty acids in the Danish population aged 1–80 years. *Eur J Clin Nutr*, 2006. 60(3): 312–8.
40. Mozaffarian, D. et al. Trans fatty acids and cardiovascular disease. *N Engl J Med*, 2006. **354**(15): 1601–13.
41. Simopoulos, A.P. What is so special about the diet of Greece? The scientific evidence. *World Rev Nutr Diet*, 2005. **95**: 80–92.
42. Sirot, V. et al. Lipid and fatty acid composition of fish and seafood consumed in France: CALIPSO study. *J Food Comp Anal*, 2008. **21**: 8–16.
43. Sargent, J.R. Fish oils and human diet. *Br J Nutr*, 1997. **78 Suppl 1**: S5–13.
44. Tornaritis, M. et al. Fatty acid composition and total fat content of eight species of Mediterranean fish. *Int J Food Sci Nutr*, 1993. **45**: 135–139.
45. Bandarra, N. et al. Seasonal changes in lipid composition of sardine (Sardina pilchardus). *J Food Sci*, 1997. **62**(1): 40–42.

7 Wine and Other Drinks

Summary

- Wine, especially red, is widely consumed in non-Muslim Mediterranean countries.
- The major bioactive ingredients in wine are alcohol (8–15%) and phytochemicals, mostly polyphenols. Red wine contains approx. 7-fold more polyphenols than white wine.
- Alcohol is converted by alcohol dehydrogenase into acetaldehyde, a putative carcinogen, and then into acetate. After high consumption, alcohol is also converted into acetaldehyde by cytochrome P450.
- Wine in Mediterranean countries is consumed in moderate amounts (women are low consumers) and almost always with a meal, and this pattern of consumption influences the metabolism of alcohol and may have an important impact on the health risk/benefit balance of wine consumption compared with consuming alcohol in different ways.
- Aniseed-based spirits are widely consumed by men in non-Muslim Mediterranean countries. Major phytochemical constituents are anethole (from star anise) and glycyrrhizic acid (from liquorice).
- Tea is an important drink, especially in Muslim Mediterranean countries. Green tea is particularly popular in Morocco, and is a rich source of polyphenols including epigallocatechin gallate. Herbal teas are consumed throughout the Mediterranean.
- Turkish and espresso are the most widely consumed styles of coffee. Phenolics, especially chlorogenic acid, the alkaloid caffeine, and the diterpene alcohols cafestol and kahweol are major constituents in coffee.

7.1 Wine

7.1.1 Introduction

In many countries bordering the north shore of the Mediterranean sea, wine – most often red – usually accompanies the main meal, particularly for men. Children in some Mediterranean societies are introduced to watered-down wine from an early age. Binge drinking is not a part of Mediterranean culture, and drinking on an empty

The Mediterranean Diet: Health and Science, First Edition. Richard Hoffman and Mariette Gerber.
© 2012 Richard Hoffman and Mariette Gerber. Published 2012 by Blackwell Publishing Ltd.

Table 7.1   Some common red grape cultivars.

Country	Grape cultivar
France	Cabernet Sauvignon
	Cabernet Franc
	Merlot
	Grenache
	Pinot noir
	Syrah
Italy	Sangiovese
	Trebbiano Toscano
	Berbera
	Nebbiolo
Spain	Tempranillo
Portugal	Touriga National

stomach is also considered undesirable. Alcohol is highly calorific, and in the past wine was an important source of energy.

Wine was established by the time of the ancient Greeks in the Minoan and Mycenaean cultures and spread throughout the Mediterranean region. Today, France, Italy and Spain are the top three wine-producing countries in the world, and Languedoc-Roussillon on the French Mediterranean coast is the single largest wine-producing region. Greece and Portugal are also important wine-producing countries. Far less wine is produced in other Mediterranean countries, mainly for religious reasons. France, Italy and Spain have relatively high per capita consumption of wine – although the Vatican state has the highest per capita consumption in the world!

7.1.2   Production

Wine is essentially fermented grape juice. Many grape varieties are used to make wine in Mediterranean countries, although far fewer than the 15,000 grapevine cultivars that have been named worldwide. Grape variety, together with variations in the growth conditions and wine-making (vinification) skills of the wine maker, are responsible for the huge range of wines that not only differ widely in taste but also in their phytochemical composition. This latter attribute could conceivably influence the health benefits of the wine, although to what extent is still a matter of debate. Many of the best-known grape cultivars were developed in France, reflecting both the long tradition of wine making in this country and its influential position in the wine world. Some widely-occurring red grape cultivars from different countries are shown in Table 7.1.

Wine is made by fermenting the juice of grapes (known as the 'must'), followed by maturing of the wine [1]. After removing the leaves, stems (usually) and other extraneous material, the grapes are crushed, and maceration of the must and crushed grapes is allowed to proceed. Maceration involves the release of various compounds from the pulp, seeds and skins and is facilitated by hydrolytic enzymes released from the ruptured cells. For white wines, maceration is only allowed to proceed for a few hours, and the juice that is released ('free-run') is combined with juice produced by pressing the grapes, and the two are then fermented together. This procedure extracts only low levels of phytochemicals from the skin and seeds (known as the pomace).

Table 7.2 Some phenolics in red and white French wines (from [4]).

Component	Red wine (mg/L)	Dry white wine (mg/L)
Total phenol content	2155	414
Flavan-3-ols, total	177	59
○ catechin	41	15
○ epicatechin	29	12
○ procyanidins	106	31
Anthocyanins (mainly malvidin glucoside)	22	n.d.
Gallic acid	30	4
Caffeic acid	11	3
Caftaric acid*	51	33

*The tartrate ester of caffeic acid; n.d.: not detected.

For red wines, maceration is allowed to proceed for far longer and occurs simultaneously with fermentation. Alcohol, mostly ethanol, produced by the fermentation acts as a solvent helping extract phenolics from the skin (such as pigmented anthocyanins) and tannins from the seeds and skin. Ethanol also helps solubilise flavour compounds from the pulp and skin. After partial or complete fermentation, the free-run is collected and may be combined with pressings from the grapes. After completing fermentation, the wine may be subject to a second fermentation known as malolactic fermentation. This improves taste by converting tart-tasting malic acid into softer-tasting lactic acid, although it is not commonly used in Mediterranean regions since grapes grown in these hot conditions tend to be lower in malic acid than grapes grown in more northerly regions. Wine is allowed to mature either in stainless steel vats or oak barrels – an important source of tannins – prior to bottling.

7.1.3 Composition

Wine is a solution of phytochemicals and other components such as organic acids and sugars, dissolved in 8–15% ethanol. Fermentation of grape juice must and subsequent maturing of the wine causes changes to the chemicals in the must, and so wine should not be thought of as just grape juice with added alcohol. Nevertheless, some studies have shown beneficial effects of grape juice similar to those seen with wine, and these studies are important in order to establish whether or not non-drinkers can obtain health benefits linked to wine consumption by drinking grape juice. The main phytochemicals in wine are phenolics, with red wine containing significantly higher levels of phenolics than white wine, especially flavonoids (Table 7.2). It has been estimated that a typical bottle of red wine contains about 1.4 g of phenolics compared to about 0.2 g in a bottle of white wine [2], with an overall range of 0.7–1.9 g/bottle for red and 0.14–0.22 g/bottle for white [3]. The higher level – and greater variety – of phenolics in red wine compared to white wine is the result of the partial fermentation of red wine in the presence of the skin and seeds since these are major sources of phenolics. The ageing of wine generates many more phenolics. These can be formed by the fermentation products reacting with each other and also with phytochemicals in the oak barrels, when these are used, and also with oxygen that can diffuse into the wine barrel. These phenolics will not be present in grape juice.

More than 200 different phenolics have been identified in red wine, as well as many other phytochemicals. Some of the phenolics found in red wine are also present in various fruits and vegetables. However, the wide variety in red wine sets it apart from most other foods since these tend to be rich in a single or small number of phenolics. In addition, whereas many flavonoids in fruits and vegetables are present as glycosides, some glycosides present in must are hydrolysed during vinification, and this may increase their bioavailability. Although aglycones are less soluble, the presence of alcohol increases their solubility. Red wine also contains some phytochemicals not commonly found in other foodstuffs in the MedDiet, including resveratrol and the oxidation reaction products resulting from vinification. Resveratrol concentrations in red wine have been found to vary between 0–11 mg/bottle with lower concentrations usually being present in white wine (0–1.5 mg/bottle) [5]. Resveratrol has sparked much interest for its potential health-enhancing effects [6].

Anthocyanins give red wine its colour. They are located in the skins of grapes, and these are present during the production of red wine but not of white wine. The anthocyanin pigments complex with catechins, such as procyanidins, during vinification to form products termed co-pigments. This reaction stabilises both the anthocyanins and catechins. Co-pigments are particularly prominent in aged wines and change the red colour to a more tawny colour. Procyanidins contribute 'mouth-feel' to wine.

Hydroxycinnamic acids, such as caffeic acid, are found mainly in the pulp of the grape, and since the pulp is used in the production of both red and white wine, overall levels do not differ significantly between the two types. Tyrosol is not present in grapes but is formed from tyrosine during fermentation. Estimates range from 5–62 mg/bottle of red wine and 9–27 mg/bottle of white wine. Tyrosol is also present in olive oil, so the MedDiet is a particularly good source of this antioxidant phytochemical. The related compound hydroxytyrosol is also present at low levels in wine, and amounts of hydroxytyrosol in the body are significantly increased following wine consumption due to the induction by ethanol of endogenous production from dopamine [7]. Phytochemicals acquired by the wine during maturing in oak barrels include various tannins such as ellagic acid.

Factors affecting polyphenol levels

'Terroir' describes how the type of soil, weather conditions, grapes and wine-maker's savoir-faire contribute to give a wine its specific personality. It is a word coined by the French and it has been at the heart of wine production in France, although other countries consider it less important. Terroir may contribute to differences between wines in a number of ways. The quality of the grapes – and hence the wine made from them – is improved by relatively poor growth conditions. This includes not too much water or nutrients since nutrients and water encourage leaf growth rather than channelling energy into producing phenolics. These growth conditions are in turn influenced by the structure, mineral content and water retention of the soil. The importance of soil structure was demonstrated in a study that found that wine made from grapes grown on soil with poor water retention had significantly higher levels of polyphenols than wine made at a neighbouring vineyard where the soil had higher water retention [8]. Other aspects of the vineyard are also important, such as its elevation, slope and orientation. These influence the microclimate of the vineyard in terms of temperature, humidity, sunlight and rainfall. A south-facing slope increases exposure to autumn sunlight and hence extends the growing season, and this allows time for greater accumulation of phenolics and flavour compounds. Resveratrol levels in wine can be significantly influenced by growth conditions. The fungus *Botrytis cinerea* infects grapes more in wet years and this fungus triggers resveratrol production; hence, levels of resveratrol are correspondingly higher in wines made in wetter years [8].

7.1.4   Metabolism of wine

Alcohol metabolism

Following wine consumption, the ethanol is converted into acetaldehyde by alcohol dehydrogenase (ADH), a constitutive enzyme that is present in the liver, gastric epithelium and other tissues of the body. Acetaldehyde in turn is converted into acetate by acetaldehyde dehydrogenase (ALDH). At low levels of consumption, most ethanol that enters the liver is metabolised and does not enter the systemic circulation, but when alcohol intake is high, acetaldehyde can accumulate before it is broken down. Acetaldehyde is a mutagen and is linked to pro-carcinogenic effects of heavy alcohol consumption (see Chapter 12). Heavy alcohol consumption leads to levels of ethanol in the body that are sufficiently high to induce the ethanol-metabolising enzyme cytochrome CYP2E1 (a member of the P450 enzyme family) present in the liver and gi tract. This enzyme not only oxidises ethanol into acetaldehyde but it also generates ROS that are thought to be carcinogenic. Most ROS are inactivated by glutathione and other antioxidants, but this can deplete glutathione levels in the liver. ADH, ALDH and CYP2E1 exist in various isoforms that are polymorphic, and individuals may be at increased cancer risk if they express isoforms of these enzymes that result in a net accumulation of acetaldehyde (either through increased production or by slower rates of breakdown) [9]. The relative contributions of different isoforms of ADH (ADH1B and ADH1C) and of ALDH in the metabolism of ethanol and acetaldehyde, respectively, are shown in Figure 7.1.

Polyphenol metabolism

The bioavailability of wine phenolics is an important consideration when assessing their potential health benefits. A number of phenolic compounds have been detected in plasma and urine after either acute (single intake) or chronic consumption of wine – the latter scenario clearly being more relevant in the context of the MedDiet [10]. However, levels of phenolics are usually quite low, and most are present in the body as conjugates. Some scientists have therefore questioned whether phenolics from wine consumption are relevant to health, since, based on cell culture models, the plasma levels of phenolics are too low to be biologically active, and the conjugates are usually less active than the parent compound. This debate has been particularly prominent in relation to resveratrol (see below).

Interactions

Unlike for fruits and vegetables, wine is unusual in that the phenolics are being presented to the body in a solution of alcohol. Hence, it is of interest to determine if this solvent influences the bioavailability of wine phenolics. A study that compared

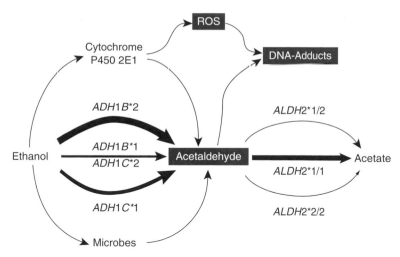

Figure 7.1 Patterns of alcohol metabolism and their roles in carcinogenesis [9]. The thickness of the arrows represents the relative contribution of different isoforms of alcohol dehydrogenase (ADH) and acetaldehyde dehydrogenase (ALDH) in the metabolism of ethanol and acetaldehyde respectively. Microbes in the gut can also convert ethanol into acetaldehyde. Acetaldehyde and reactive oxygen species (ROS) can form DNA adducts that increase the risk of cancer.

the absorption of three phenolics (resveratrol, catechin and quercetin) dissolved either in aqueous solution (grape juice or vegetable juice) or in an alcoholic solution (white wine) concluded that absorption was 'broadly equivalent' irrespective of which matrix the phenolics were dissolved in [11]. Interestingly, a study with isolated rat gut found that red wine promoted the absorption of quercetin and directed its metabolism towards products (namely isorhamnetin and tamarixetin) [12] which have potential protective effects against cancer and CVD. However, the relevance of this in humans in relation to red wine modifying the metabolism of dietary flavonoids and subsequent health effects has not been established.

7.1.5   Consumption patterns and health

It has long been recognized that the problems with alcohol relate not to the use of a bad thing, but to the abuse of a good thing.

Abraham Lincoln [13]

The distinction between excess consumption and consumption in moderation is essential when evaluating the health effects of alcoholic drinks, including wine. There is now ample evidence that the health effects of moderate alcohol consumption are quite distinct from those resulting from excess alcohol consumption or in abstainers. Hence, in the context of the MedDiet it is only relevant to consider the effects of moderate alcohol consumption, and not be detracted by the undoubted adverse effects of excess alcohol consumption. As memorably stated in 1926 by Pearl: 'one cannot judge the role of diet by starvation or excess' [14].

The alcohol intake that is regarded as maximal for minimal health risk varies quite widely between countries (see Table 7.3). However, levels of consumption are not the only important consideration in relation to alcoholic drinks: the type of

Table 7.3 Maximum recommended daily intake of alcohol by country (from http://www.wineinmoderation.eu).

Country	Maximum recommended daily intake (g)*	
	Men	Women
France	30	20
Italy	40	30
Spain	42	28
	30	30
United Kingdom	32	24
United States	28	14

*In the UK one unit is 8 g of alcohol.

Table 7.4 Characteristics of alcohol consumption as part of the MedDiet.

Type of consumption	Mediterranean diet	Other contexts
Main type of alcohol	Wine (more frequently red)	Wide range of alcoholic beverages
Amount	Low to moderate	Low to high
Pattern	With a meal and family	May be on an empty stomach in a wide range of social contexts

alcoholic drink and the context in which it is drunk are also important. Wine, the main alcoholic drink in Mediterranean countries, is consumed daily as part of a family meal or social gathering. Hence consumption can take place over several hours, and becoming drunk would be frowned upon. Some of the distinguishing features of alcohol consumption as part of a Mediterranean dietary pattern compared to drinking in other contexts are summarised in Table 7.4.

There is increasing evidence that consumption patterns of alcoholic drinks affect health outcomes [15–17]. This gives rise to potential confounding factors when comparing epidemiological data from studies undertaken in different cultures that have different drinking patterns. This issue was emphasised in the closing remarks to a 2007 conference on alcohol: 'We should no longer define "moderate drinking" as a daily, weekly, or monthly average amount below a certain number of drinks or grams of alcohol. We must include in such a definition the drinking pattern, so that studies across cultures are more comparable' [18]. Aspects of drinking of particular relevance to the MedDiet will now be considered.

Wine versus other alcoholic beverages

A reductionist perspective of 'wine = alcohol' is probably inappropriate. Many of the phenolics in red wine, and white wine to a lesser extent, have been demonstrated to have beneficial effects in cell culture and animal models of age-related diseases. Although the relevance of these studies to humans remains unclear, wine phenolics could potentially confound comparisons with other alcoholic drinks containing the same amount of alcohol.

Although wine is an integral part of many MedDiets, the contribution of wine to total alcohol intake varies widely even between alcohol-drinking Mediterranean countries. For example, wine constituted 88–94% of total alcohol consumed in Italy, but this fell to 56% in Greece [19]. Generally, wine consumption represents a higher proportion of total alcohol for women compared to men. Some studies suggest that wine consumption is decreasing in Southern Europe and increasing in Northern Europe [20].

Moderate levels of consumption

The EPIC study on patterns of alcohol consumption in 10 European countries found that whereas in Mediterranean countries women consumed much less total ethanol than men, in central and northern Europe the total ethanol consumption of women was only a little less than that of men [19]. Consumption levels are important in the context of whether or not there is a threshold effect of benefit or risk. This especially arises in the context of cancer, where some studies suggest that there is no minimum amount of alcohol not associated with an increase risk of certain cancers, whereas other studies suggest that there is no cancer risk below a certain threshold (see Chapter 12).

Levels of alcohol consumption are prone to misreporting by some participants in food questionnaires, and measuring metabolites of resveratrol in urine has been suggested as a useful objective biomarker for wine consumption [21].

Consumption patterns

It is common knowledge that drinking on an empty stomach increases the rate of inebriation. Drinking without consuming food may also have important health consequences. An Italian study found that drinking wine outside of a meal was associated with a higher all-cause mortality compared to drinking with a meal [22]. Other studies have shown that alcohol consumption outside a meal is associated with a higher risk of hypertension and metabolic syndrome than drinking with a meal [16, 23–25].

These studies suggest that interpreting epidemiological data based solely on units of alcohol consumed over a given time may not give the full picture if these studies do not taking drinking patterns into consideration. The average weekly alcohol intake of someone enjoying a glass or two of red wine every day could be similar to someone who binge drinks on Friday and Saturday night, but the health consequences may be quite different. Drinking patterns are also important when extrapolating data from experimental studies since changes in biochemical markers in human subjects given a single dose of wine may not reflect the consequences of consuming wine daily over many years.

The differing consequences of consuming alcohol with or without a meal are linked to the role of food in slowing the rate of alcohol absorption from the gut. Ethanol in the gut is most rapidly absorbed from the duodenum and jejunum, and since food (protein, fat or carbohydrate do not appear to be any different in this regard [26]) slows the rate of gastric emptying, consumption of food with alcohol will delay ethanol absorption. This results in a lower peak blood alcohol concentration (BAC) and also, usually, a quicker return of BAC to baseline levels [26]. This potentially has important pathological implications since at low BAC ethanol is metabolised by alcohol dehydrogenase alone, whereas at higher BAC ethanol is also metabolised by cytochrome P450 2E1 (CYP2E1). Metabolism of ethanol by CYP2E1 generates ROS and may lead to additional pathological effects not produced by a low BAC. Hence, it is possible that it is not only the level of alcohol consumption that is important, but also factors that influence the resulting BAC. As has been noted: 'Drinking large amounts outside mealtimes may be particularly harmful because the alcohol is absorbed quickly as the stomach is empty and metabolising enzymes will be quickly saturated' [19].

Consuming wine with a meal may have other benefits besides slowing down the rate of alcohol absorption. Wine may aid the digestion of food by stimulating the production of gastrin, and the delay in gastric emptying favours acid hydrolysis and improved digestion [27]. The antimicrobial properties of wine have been known for thousands of years. Various phenolics found in wine have bacteriostatic and fungistatic properties and studies have demonstrated protection against bacterial diarrhoea [28].

The consequences of the Mediterranean way of wine consumption may also have other knock-on effects. Apart from restraining the likelihood of drunkenness, and the corresponding high BAC, intertwining drinking and eating in a family gathering can make for a more leisurely and relaxed meal, and this may enhance biofeedback mechanisms for satiety and thus reduce overall food consumption. Not smoking while drinking may also reduce the likelihood of cancers of the aerodigestive tract, since smoking significantly enhances the risk of these cancers due to high alcohol consumption (see Chapter 12).

Other possible confounding factors associated with wine consumption

There is a high correlation between wine drinking and other aspects of the MedDiet, and this increases the difficulty in analysing the wine/alcohol component separate from other food components. Related to this, is the possibility that wine drinkers in general have a healthier lifestyle than non-wine drinkers, and hence epidemiological studies showing a beneficial health effect in this group might instead be due to another aspect of this healthier lifestyle. In relation to eating habits, it was found that Danish wine drinkers were more likely to also purchase various 'healthy' foods such as olives, fruit and vegetables and poultry [29]. However, in contrast to this study, Spanish wine drinkers were not found to consume healthier foods than non-wine drinkers [30, 31]. These observations suggest cultural differences between these two populations, and may be because North Europeans who purchase wine tend to also be health-conscious and so purchase other foods perceived to be healthier, whereas consumption of wine in Spain spans more socially diverse groups.

Another potential confounding factor in epidemiological studies on wine consumption is that the non-drinking cohort may include so-called 'sick-quitters', that is individuals who no longer drink – and so are included in the group of abstainers – but who have stopped drinking for health reasons and hence are more likely to have underlying health problems. Inclusion of this group may skew the abstainers to an overall less healthy profile than for true abstainers. This group was not corrected for in many early studies.

7.1.6 The resveratrol controversy

The large number of phytochemicals in wine makes it difficult to establish whether any individual compounds are particularly important for the potential health benefits of wine consumption. It has been suggested that 'the beneficial effects of red wine should be attributed to the combined effects of several phenolics rather than individual compounds, and an astute pattern of consumption – i.e. regular moderate rather than binge drinking' [32]. Indeed, several studies have shown synergistic beneficial effects (for example, increased antioxidant activity) when wine phenolics are combined [33]. However, other investigators take a less cautious approach, and have promoted specific phenolics or groups of phenolics. The wine phenolic that has attracted the most attention in this regard is resveratrol.

Resveratrol has a wide range of beneficial effects in various cell culture and animal models including protection against heart disease, cancer and Alzheimer's disease, and extending the lifespan of normal and obese animals [34, 35]. There is consumer interest in information on resveratrol levels in wine and a willingness to pay a premium for wines with demonstrable health benefits [36]. Hence, establishing whether resveratrol in wine has health benefits would be of benefit to both the consumer and the producer.

Resveratrol and ageing

The best-documented way of increasing lifespan is to restrict calorie intake. Calorie-restricted diets (which include all essential nutrients but contain 30% fewer calories than the typical diet) extend the lifespan of rodents by as much as 50%. Monkey studies currently in progress have shown significantly positive results as well. Resveratrol has been found to activate the same specific 'longevity gene' that gets switched on by calorie restriction (a gene known as Sirt1) [37]. Hence, there is now interest in resveratrol and related compounds as anti-ageing agents for humans.

Despite the experimental data, it is unclear whether resveratrol in wine is relevant to human health, since far higher levels are usually used experimentally than are achievable in human plasma – usually cultured cells are incubated with micromolar concentrations, whereas plasma concentrations in subjects after wine consumption are in the nanomolar range [35]. A similar discrepancy exists for *in vivo* studies: the amounts of resveratrol given to animals would be equivalent to tens of milligrams or grams when scaled up to humans, whereas dietary intake of resveratrol is far lower. Dietary intake was estimated for the Spanish cohort of the EPIC study at between 48 and 2504 µg/day in men (25th–75th percentiles) and 0–148 µg/day in women (these estimates also included the resveratrol glycoside piceid) [38]. The wide variability of intake between individuals largely reflected variability in red wine consumption, which was the main source of resveratrol. Based on these discrepancies between data from humans and from experimental models, some commentators argue that the health benefits of wine are extremely unlikely to be due to the resveratrol content[1] [40].

Despite these reservations, many scientists persist with their interest in resveratrol, and continue to consider that resveratrol from red wine may be biologically relevant (e.g. [41]). Is this dogged determination justified? The best answer at present may be

[1] However it should be noted that high doses of pure resveratrol are being evaluated as an anti-cancer agent [39].

a 'possibly', since many aspects of the pharmacology of resveratrol remain to be elucidated. Some of these unresolved issues are listed in the box below; many of these issues are also relevant when evaluating the biological relevance of other dietary phenolics.

Unanswered questions about resveratrol

1. *Are resveratrol metabolites active?* Resveratrol is rapidly metabolised in both rodents and humans, but despite this it still exerts biological effects *in vivo*. Hence it is possible that resveratrol metabolites exert biological effects.
2. *Is the metabolism of resveratrol modified by other dietary factors?* A major metabolite of resveratrol is resveratrol sulphate. Quercetin is a potent inhibitor of resveratrol sulphation. Hence, it is possible that dietary quercetin (which is found in red wine itself or other foods such as onions) could reduce the metabolism of resveratrol resulting in more parent compound.
3. *Are resveratrol metabolites circulating stores for resveratrol?* It is possible that resveratrol sulphate could act as a circulating 'store' of resveratrol, and that free resveratrol is liberated by sulphatases inside cells. Indeed, this has been demonstrated in a study using breast tissue (both malignant and non-malignant) which showed that resveratrol sulphate is readily converted back to resveratrol [42]. This would be analogous to the known metabolism of oestrone sulphate which is a major circulating form of oestrogen and which is cleaved to free oestrogen in cancer cells [43].
4. *Does resveratrol concentrate in some tissues?* Although *plasma* concentrations of resveratrol are measured, resveratrol is concentrated in some tissues in the body and so may achieve pharmacologically relevant concentrations only in some tissues [35].
5. *Does resveratrol accumulate in the body with chronic ingestion?* Animal studies are short term, whereas people consume red wine over many years, and this could possibly lead to an accumulation of resveratrol in the body [44].
6. *What are the most relevant targets for resveratrol in the body?* The anti-ageing effects of resveratrol may be the most relevant since they can occur at nanomolar concentrations of resveratrol, whereas the effects on the cardiovascular system and on the heart require higher concentrations [45].

7.2 Aniseed-flavoured spirits

7.2.1 Consumption

An aperitif of an aniseed-based spirit, maybe accompanied by a few olives or pistachios, is one of the drinks that form part of the social fabric of many countries bordering the north shore of the Mediterranean sea. Aniseed-flavoured spirits are mainly drunk by men and include *anis* in Spain, *pastis* and *anisette* in Mediterranean France, *sambuca* in Italy, *ouzo* in Greece, and *raki* in Turkey. The production of alcoholic infusions of herbs in the Mediterranean region has a long tradition, and medicinal herbs have been collected for thousands of years. Pedlars sold medicinal herbs in Mediterranean France in the Middle Ages, and by the 17th and 18th centuries apothecaries were set up selling herbs in the form of distilled products – which would help preserve them. In the 19th century, some of these apothecaries became pharmacists, whereas others became distillers such as Henri Pernod in the South of France.

7.2.2 Composition

Aniseed-flavoured spirits are produced by flavouring and distilling alcohol (ethanol) with natural extracts in varying proportions of star anise, anise, liquorice, fennel and other herbs. The aniseed flavour is mainly due to the monoterpene anethole which is soluble in the alcohol base but comes out of solution when water is added, giving a milky colour. An average drink is made by diluting about $2\,cm^3$ spirit with 5–10 times this volume with water. EU law states that pastis must contain between 1.5–2.0 g/l of anethole and 0.05–0.5 g/l of glycyrrhizic acid from liquorice [46].

7.2.3 Physiological effects

Aniseed-flavoured spirits are generally drunk as an aperitif and have a calmative effect on the digestive system. Several of the phytochemicals in aniseed-flavoured spirits have potential therapeutic benefits, although no studies have explicitly examined the effects on health of consuming these drinks. Anethole has anti-tumour activity in animal models [47]. Liquorice has numerous well-documented health benefits including protection against peptic ulcers. Liquorice also contains the isoflavan glabridin which has multiple effects, including acting as a phytoestrogen [48]. Alcohol has been found to enhance the uptake by the gut of some flavonoids in wine by relaxing the cells lining the gut, but it is not known if the alcohol in herb-based drinks could also increase the uptake of phytochemicals in these drinks.

7.3 Tea

7.3.1 Consumption

Tea is an important part of daily life in many Muslim Mediterranean countries, and it is offered as a sign of friendship and hospitality in countries where alcohol is not permitted – 'tea-totallers', so to speak. Tea is considered to be the national drink of Egypt and, along with Turkey and Morocco, these Mediterranean countries have amongst the highest per capita consumption of tea in the world. Black tea is drunk in Egypt and Turkey, usually either before or after a meal. Turkish and Egyptian teas are often made very strong, and milk may be added in Egypt, whereas this not traditional in Turkey. Green tea is mainly consumed in Morocco and other countries of the Maghreb (Tunisia and Algeria), often with mint and sugar, sometimes with pine kernels, and normally without milk. Green tea is drunk at any time of the day, and also during a meal. Green tea is a rich source of polyphenols and may provide some of the health benefits of red wine.

Herbal teas, widely consumed throughout the Mediterranean, are now recognised as an important component of the MedDiet and are represented in a new version of

Table 7.5 Polyphenol content of tea [51]. With permission from Elsevier.

Compound	Black tea (mg/100g dry tea)	Green tea (mg/100g dry tea)
Total catechins[1]	3937	15667
– Catechin	167	24
– Epicatechin	316	793
– Epicatechin-3-gallate	923	1755
– Epigallocatechin	1257	1712
– Epigallocatechin-3-gallate	1393	8975
Theaflavins	568	ND
Thearubigins	12490	ND
Flavonols	367	406

[1] Including other minor catechins.
ND: no data.

the MedDiet pyramid [49]. Whereas tea is an infusion of the leaves of *Camellia sinensis*, herbal teas are infusions (tisanes) of various parts of plants (flowers, stems, etc) other than from *Camellia sinensis*. Herbal teas are consumed throughout the Mediterranean and many are taken medicinally. For example, Mountain tea, a popular herbal tea in Greece and other Eastern Mediterranean countries, is made using the dried leaves and flowers of *Sideritis* plants (ironwort), a member of the *Lamiaceae* family, and is taken against the common cold. Other members of the *Lamiaceae* family of herbs used to make herbal teas include *Origanum dictamnus* (in Southern Greece), wild oregano, sage and mint [50]. Thyme and rosemary are popular teas in Southern France and are recommended for their beneficial effects on digestion and respiratory problems, respectively. Other plant sources include mallow, chamomile, *Tilia* (lime or linden tree), yarrow and artichoke [50].

7.3.2 Composition

Fresh tea leaves are very rich in polyphenols, mainly catechins (up to 30% of the dry weight). These catechins are oxidised by the enzyme polyphenol oxidase (PPO) during the processing of tea leaves, and the extent of oxidation varies depending on the type of tea that is being produced. Green teas are withered by air and then either pan-fried or steamed to inactivate PPO prior to being dried. Hence, dried green tea retains many of the polyphenols present in fresh tea leaves. The most abundant catechin in green tea is epigallocatechin gallate (EGCG), constituting about 50–75% of the total catechins (Table 7.5). Also present are epigallocatechin (EGC), epicatechin-3-gallate (ECG), epicatechin, catechin and other related molecules. A typical cup of green tea contains about 650 mg of water-extractable material of which about one-third is catechins of various sorts.

Tea leaves for producing black tea are crushed prior to being dried and this brings the catechins into contact with PPO. The catechins are oxidised to various products (the process is referred to as fermentation), including oligomers known as theaflavins and polymeric thearubigins. These account for 2–6% and 15–20% respectively of the dry weight of black tea infusions (Table 7.5). Theaflavins are major taste compounds in black tea. Teas also contains variable levels of other flavonoids, fluorine and caffeine (about 3%). Herbal teas contain a wide range of antioxidant phenolic compounds [50].

Brewing

The levels of EGCG and other catechins extracted from green tea increase with brewing time and brewing temperature [52]. Moroccan green tea is traditionally prepared by adding boiling water to the tea leaves, which may then be brewed for up to 15 min[2]. This produces a bitter tea, presumably rich in bitter-tasting catechins, and Moroccan tea is sweetened to make it more palatable. Second and third brews are produced by adding fresh leaves and mint, and these brews are less bitter. A famous Moroccan saying describes these teas:

> *Le premier verre est aussi amer que la vie,*
> *le deuxième est aussi fort que l'amour,*
> *le troisième est aussi doux que la mort.*
> The first glass is as bitter as life,
> the second glass is as strong as love,
> the third glass is as gentle as death.

By contrast, tea in Asia is traditionally brewed at a lower temperature (about 80C) and for a shorter time in order to reduce bitterness. Most epidemiological studies on the health benefits of green tea have been carried out using tea prepared according to Asian principles. It is not known if tea prepared according to Moroccan traditions has different health benefits, although the content of catechins – the presumed main active ingredient (see below) – may well be different.

7.3.3 Physiological effects

Tea is perceived as a low calorie, healthy drink [53]. Tea polyphenols are good antioxidants *in vitro*, and prevention of DNA damage and lipid peroxidation may contribute to the anti-tumour and anti-cardiovascular effects following tea consumption seen in animal, and some human studies (see Sections 11.3.3 and 12.3.3). Since tea flavonoids are considered to be the major bioactive components, it is of interest to consider factors that influence plasma levels. As discussed above, tea preparation has a significant influence on the extraction of EGCG and other catechins from green tea. Black tea may be drunk with milk, and although milk proteins may complex with flavonoids and so reduce their solubility, the influence of milk on the bioavailability of the flavonoids remains inconclusive [54]. Generally speaking, the absorption of flavonoids is related to their molecular weights [55]. It is thought that most green tea catechins are absorbed to some extent. Although EGCG, with its relatively high molecular weight, is absorbed relatively poorly compared to other catechins, this may be partly compensated for by the relatively large amounts present. Theaflavins and thearubigins – the main catechins in black tea – have high molecular weights and are only absorbed to a limited extent. The poor absorption of high molecular weight catechins is probably a major factor reducing systemic effects of

---

[2] A first rinse of the tea leaves with boiling water may be discarded prior to adding more boiling water.

black tea, although it is possible that high molecular weight polyphenols in black tea could have protective effects in the gut.

7.4   Coffee

7.4.1   Consumption

Although not unique to the MedDiet, regular and moderate consumption of coffee is widespread in countries of the Mediterranean basin. Coffee is consumed throughout the day and is a traditional ending to a main meal. Coffee originates in Ethiopia and Yemen, and consumption spread from the Arab world first to Istanbul (Turkey) and then to Italy and other European countries. The two most popular coffees in Mediterranean countries are 'Turkish' coffee and espresso. Turkish coffee (also known as Cypriot, Greek or Armenian coffee) is the most popular coffee throughout the Middle East, North Africa and the Arab world, Caucasus, and the Balkans. It is prepared by boiling finely powdered roast coffee beans in a pot, sometimes with sugar, and served in a cup, where the dregs settle. Milk is not added. Espresso is the main type of coffee in most of southern Europe, notably Italy, France, Portugal and Spain, and, like Turkish coffee, it is generally drunk without milk. Coffees may be flavoured with spices such as cinnamon or cardamom. Filter coffee and instant coffee are less popular in Mediterranean countries than in North European countries and the US.

Although there have been a number of studies on the relationship between coffee drinking and risk of CVD, cancer and neurological disorders, results from these studies have often been contradictory, and these are discussed in subsequent chapters. There are a number of potential confounding factors in some of these studies such as smoking and alcohol, as well as differences between countries in terms of the type of coffee consumed, and brewing method.

7.4.2   Composition and physiological effects

Preparation techniques affect the final composition of coffee. Brewing with a paper filter produces clear, light-bodied coffee, which is free of sediments but lacking in some coffee oils and essences which are trapped in the paper filter. Instant coffee (usually from robusta beans) loses flavour as the essential oils evaporate over time. The percentage of caffeine in instant coffee is less, and bitter flavour components are more evident. Since concentrations of some of the putative bioactive phytochemicals in coffee are affected by the brewing method, there may be limitations when extrapolating epidemiological evidence on coffee consumption from North European or US populations to Mediterranean populations.

Coffee is rich in antioxidants and was by found to be the major contributor of antioxidants from beverages in the Spanish diet (64%, compared with 19% from red wine) [56]. Although over a thousand compounds have been detected in coffee, the major compounds both quantitatively and in terms of putative health effects are phenolics, especially chlorogenic acid, the alkaloid caffeine, and the diterpene alcohols cafestol and kahweol.

Chlorogenic acid

'Chlorogenic acid' is actually a group of compounds consisting of esters formed between quinic acid and hydroxycinnamates. By far the most abundant chlorogenic acid in coffee is 5-O-caffeoylquinic acid (an ester between quinic acid and caffeic acid). Chlorogenic acid has antioxidant activity *in vitro*, and not only is coffee the main source of chlorogenic acid in the Mediterranean diet, but chlorogenic acid was found in one study to be the phenolic compound that contributed most to the overall antioxidant activity of the Spanish diet [57]. However, chlorogenic acid is extensively metabolised *in vivo* to metabolites with lower antioxidant activity, and the significance of chlorogenic acid *in vivo* is unclear.

Caffeine

A general estimate is that a cup of coffee contains about 100 mg of the alkaloid caffeine. Although espresso contains approximately two to three times the caffeine concentration of filter coffee, it is generally consumed in far smaller amounts Caffeine is rapidly and almost completely absorbed in the stomach and small intestine, and distributes to all tissues including the brain. Caffeine is an antagonist of A_{2A} subtypes of the adenosine receptor, and this may be associated with protection against Parkinson's disease (see Chapter 13).

Diterpenes

The diterpenes cafestol and kahweol are extracted from ground coffee during brewing, and are present at relatively high levels in Turkish coffee (6–12 mg per cup) and at about 4 mg per cup in espresso (due to the smaller serving size). However, they are largely removed from coffee by filtration and during the production of instant coffee. These diterpenes raise LDL cholesterol levels [58]. However, in relation to cancer, cell culture and animal studies have shown these diterpenes to have a broad range of anti-carcinogenic effects [59].

Other compounds

Many compounds are produced during the process of roasting green coffee beans, due to a series of complex reactions, mainly between sugars and amino acids (the Maillard reaction, see Chapter 4). Many of these Maillard reaction products are associated with the increase in the antioxidant capacity of coffee that occurs during roasting, but their biological significance is unclear [60].

References

1. Jackson, R.S. *Wine science: principles and applications*. 3rd ed. 2008, London: Academic.
2. Cordova, A.C. et al. The cardiovascular protective effect of red wine. *J Am Coll Surg*, 2005. **200**(3): 428–39.
3. German, J.B., Walzem, R.L. The health benefits of wine. *Annu Rev Nutr*, 2000. **20**: 561–93.
4. Crozier, A. et al. Secondary metabolites in fruits, vegetables, beverages and other plant-based dietary components. In: *Plant secondary metabolites: occurrence, structure and role in the human diet*, ed. A. Crozier, M.N. Clifford and H. Ashihara. 2006, Oxford: Blackwell.
5. Stervbo, U., Vang, O., Bonnesen, C. A review of the content of the putative chemopreventative phytoalexin resveratrol in red wine. *Food Chemistry*, 2006. **101**: 449–457.

6. Guerrero, R.F. et al. Wine, resveratrol and health: a review. *Nat Prod Commun*, 2009. **4**(5): 635–58.
7. Schroder, H. et al. Alcohol consumption is associated with high concentrations of urinary hydroxytyrosol. *Am J Clin Nutr*, 2009. **90**(5): 1329–35.
8. de Andres-de Prado, R. et al. Effect of soil type on wines produced from Vitis vinifera L. cv. Grenache in commercial vineyards. *J Agric Food Chem*, 2007. **55**(3): 779–86.
9. Seitz, H.K., Becker, P. Alcohol metabolism and cancer risk. *Alcohol Res Health*, 2007. **30**(1): 38–41, 44–7.
10. Covas, M.I. et al. Wine and oxidative stress: up-to-date evidence of the effects of moderate wine consumption on oxidative damage in humans. *Atherosclerosis*, 2010. **208**(2): 297–304.
11. Goldberg, D.M.,Yan, J., Soleas, G.J. Absorption of three wine-related polyphenols in three different matrices by healthy subjects. *Clin Biochem*, 2003. **36**(1): 79–87.
12. Dragoni, S. et al. Red wine alcohol promotes quercetin absorption and directs its metabolism towards isorhamnetin and tamarixetin in rat intestine in vitro. *Br J Pharmacol*, 2006. **147**(7): 765–71.
13. O'Keefe, J.H., Bybee, K.A., Lavie, C.J. Alcohol and cardiovascular health: the razor-sharp double-edged sword. *J Am Coll Cardiol*, 2007. **50**(11): 009–14.
14. Klatsky, A.L. Alcohol and cardiovascular health. *Integr Comp Biol*, 2004. **44**: 324–328.
15. Baglietto, L. et al. Average volume of alcohol consumed, type of beverage, drinking pattern and the risk of death from all causes. *Alcohol Alcohol*, 2006. **41**(6): 664–71.
16. Della Valle, E. et al. Drinking habits and health in Northern Italian and American men. *Nutr Metab Cardiovasc Dis*, 2009. **19**(2): 115–22.
17. Rimm, E., Moats, C. Alcohol and coronary heart disease: drinking patterns and mediators of effect. *Ann Epidemiol*, 2007. **17**(S1): S3–S7.
18. Ellison, R. Closing remarks. *Ann Epidemiol*, 2007. **17**(5 Supplement 1): S114–S115.
19. Sieri, S. et al. Patterns of alcohol consumption in 10 European countries participating in the European Prospective Investigation into Cancer and Nutrition (EPIC) project. *Public Health Nutr*, 2002. **5**(6B): 1287–96.
20. Smith, D.E. Cultural convergence: consumer behavioral changes in the European wine market. *J Wine Research*, 2007. **18**(2): 107–112.
21. Zamora-Ros, R. et al. Resveratrol metabolites in urine as a biomarker of wine intake in free-living subjects: The PREDIMED Study. *Free Radic Biol Med*, 2009. **46**(12): 562–6.
22. Trevisan, M. et al. Drinking pattern and mortality: the Italian Risk Factor and Life Expectancy pooling project. *Ann Epidemiol*, 2001. **11**(5): 312–9.
23. Dorn, J.M. et al. Alcohol drinking pattern and non-fatal myocardial infarction in women. *Addiction*, 2007. **102**(5): 730–9.
24. Stranges, S. et al. Relationship of alcohol drinking pattern to risk of hypertension: a population-based study. *Hypertension*, 2004. **44**(6): 813–9.
25. Fan, A.Z. et al. Lifetime alcohol drinking pattern is related to the prevalence of metabolic syndrome. The Western New York Health Study (WNYHS). *Eur J Epidemiol*, 2006. **21**(2): 129–38.
26. Kalant, H. Effects of food and body composition on blood alcohol levels. In: *Comprehensive handbook of alcohol related pathology*, ed. V.R. Preedy and R.R. Watson. 2005, Amsterdam; London: Elsevier Academic.
27. Franke, A. et al. Effect of ethanol and some alcoholic beverages on gastric emptying in humans. *Scand J Gastroenterol*, 2004. **39**(7): 638–44.
28. Weisse, M.E., Eberly, B., Person, D.A. Wine as a digestive aid: comparative antimicrobial effects of bismuth salicylate and red and white wine. *BMJ*, 1995. **311**(7021): 1657–60.
29. Johansen, D. et al. Food buying habits of people who buy wine or beer: cross sectional study. *BMJ*, 2006. **332**(7540): 519–22.
30. Alcacera, M.A. et al. Alcoholic beverage preference and dietary pattern in Spanish university graduates: the SUN cohort study. *Eur J Clin Nutr*, 2008. **62**(10): 1178–86.
31. Carmona-Torre, F. et al. Relationship of alcoholic beverage consumption to food habits in a Mediterranean population. *Am J Health Promotion*, 2008. **23**(1): 27–30.
32. Walzem, R.L. Wine and health: state of proofs and research needs. *Inflammopharmacology*, 2008. **16**(6): 265–71.
33. Iacopini, P. et al. Catechin, epicatechin, quercetin, rutin and resveratrol in red grape: Content, in vitro antioxidant activity and interactions. *Journal of Food Composition and Analysis*, 2008. **21**: 589–598.

34. Baur, J.A. et al. Resveratrol improves health and survival of mice on a high-calorie diet. *Nature*, 2006. **444**(7117): 337–42.
35. Baur, J.A., Sinclair, D.A. Therapeutic potential of resveratrol: the in vivo evidence. *Nat Rev Drug Discov*, 2006. **5**(6): 493–506.
36. Barreiro-Hurle, J., Colombo, S., Cantos-Villar, E. Is there a market for functional wines? Consumer preferences and willingness to pay for resveratrol-enriched red wine. *Food Quality and Preference*, 2008. **19**: 360–371.
37. Knutson, M.D., Leeuwenburgh, C. Resveratrol and novel potent activators of SIRT1: effects on aging and age-related diseases. *Nutr Rev*, 2008. **66**(10): 591–6.
38. Zamora-Ros, R. et al. Concentrations of resveratrol and derivatives in foods and estimation of dietary intake in a Spanish population: European Prospective Investigation into Cancer and Nutrition (EPIC)-Spain cohort. *Br J Nutr*, 2008. **100**(1): 188–96.
39. Boocock, D.J. et al. Phase I dose escalation pharmacokinetic study in healthy volunteers of resveratrol, a potential cancer chemopreventive agent. *Cancer Epidemiol Biomarkers Prev*, 2007. **16**(6): 1246–52.
40. Vitaglione, P. et al. Bioavailability of trans-resveratrol from red wine in humans. *Mol Nutr Food Res*, 2005. **49**(5): 495–504.
41. Opie, L.H., Lecour, S. The red wine hypothesis: from concepts to protective signalling molecules. *Eur Heart J*, 2007. **28**(14): 1683–93.
42. Miksits, M. et al. Expression of sulfotransferases and sulfatases in human breast cancer: impact on resveratrol metabolism. *Cancer Lett*, 2010. **289**(2): 237–45.
43. Pasqualini, J.R. The selective estrogen enzyme modulators in breast cancer: a review. *Biochim Biophys Acta*, 2004. **1654**(2): 123–43.
44. Bertelli, A.A. Wine, research and cardiovascular disease: instructions for use. *Atherosclerosis*, 2007. **195**(2): 242–7.
45. Russo, G.L. Ins and outs of dietary phytochemicals in cancer chemoprevention. *Biochem Pharmacol*, 2007. **74**(4): 533–44.
46. Brereton, P. et al. Analytical methods for the determination of spirit drinks. *Trends Anal Chem*, 2003. **22**(1): 19–25.
47. Anand, P. et al. Cancer is a preventable disease that requires major lifestyle changes. *Pharm Res*, 2008. **25**(9): 2097–116.
48. Somjen, D. et al. Estrogenic activity of glabridin and glabrene from licorice roots on human osteoblasts and prepubertal rat skeletal tissues. *J Steroid Biochem Mol Biol*, 2004. **91**(4–5): 241–6.
49. Lairon, D. *pers. comm.*
50. Dimitrios, B. Sources of natural phenolic antioxidants. *Trends in Food Science & Technology*, 2006. **17**: 505–512.
51. Peterson, J. et al. Major flavonoids in dry tea. *Journal of Food Composition and Analysis*, 2005. **18**: 487–501.
52. Labbe, D., Tremblay, D.A., Bazinet L. Effect of brewing temperature and duration on green tea catechin solubilization: Basis for production of EGC and EGCG-enriched fractions. *Separ Purif Technol*, 2006. **49**: 1–9.
53. Popkin, B.M. et al. A new proposed guidance system for beverage consumption in the United States. *Am J Clin Nutr*, 2006. **83**(3): 529–42.
54. Gardner, E.J., Ruxton, C.H., Leeds, A.R. Black tea – helpful or harmful? A review of the evidence. *Eur J Clin Nutr*, 2007. **61**(1): 3–18.
55. Yang, C.S. et al. Bioavailability issues in studying the health effects of plant polyphenolic compounds. *Mol Nutr Food Res*, 2008. **52 Suppl 1**: S139–51.
56. Pulido, R., Hernandez-Garcia, M., Saura-Calixto, F. Contribution of beverages to the intake of lipophilic and hydrophilic antioxidants in the Spanish diet. *Eur J Clin Nutr*, 2003. **57**(10): 1275–82.
57. Saura-Calixto, F., Goni, I. Definition of the Mediterranean diet based on bioactive compounds. *Crit Rev Food Sci Nutr*, 2009. **49**(2): 145–52.
58. Bonita, J.S. et al. Coffee and cardiovascular disease: in vitro, cellular, animal, and human studies. *Pharmacol Res*, 2007. **55**(3): 187–98.
59. Cavin, C. et al. Cafestol and kahweol, two coffee specific diterpenes with anticarcinogenic activity. *Food Chem Toxicol*, 2002. **40**(8): 1155–63.
60. Dorea, J.G., da Costa, T.H. Is coffee a functional food? *Br J Nutr*, 2005. **93**(6): 773–82.

Section 2
HEALTH EFFECTS

8 Epidemiological Methods

Summary

- A correct understanding of epidemiological methods and interpretation of epidemiological results is of paramount importance for understanding the place of public health in the prevention of chronic degenerative diseases (CDDs); and no more so than in relation to the MedDiet, since this diet and its effect on CDDs has been the subject of many epidemiological studies.
- Epidemiological methods have evolved from simple descriptions of the prevalence or incidence of a disease, to the search for a causal relationship between a factor (environmental or genetic) and the incidence of, or death from, a disease.
- Absolute evidence supporting an aetiological relationship between the considered factor and disease is difficult to establish from epidemiological methods. Rather, an hierarchy for increasing strength of evidence can be established from ecological studies (weakest) to analytical prospective studies and intervention studies (strongest).
- Even for the strongest evidence, a single study cannot by itself establish with certainty a causal relationship. Rather, a portfolio, or mosaic, of different studies, including experimental studies supporting biological plausibility of the relationship, is necessary in order to either establish the level of evidence as convincing or probable, or to refute any relationship.

8.1 Introduction

Chapters 10–13 examine epidemiological evidence for the health benefits of a MedDiet. Several methods are used in epidemiology which, although all of some value, differ in their capacity to establish a causal relationship between an observed effect and a supposed cause. This chapter discusses the strengths and limitations of various epidemiological methods for establishing a causal relationship between cause and effect. Also discussed are the criteria and requirements for assessing the validity of epidemiological studies and for estimating the level of evidence.

The Mediterranean Diet: Health and Science, First Edition. Richard Hoffman and Mariette Gerber.
© 2012 Richard Hoffman and Mariette Gerber. Published 2012 by Blackwell Publishing Ltd.

8.2   Study designs

8.2.1   Descriptive epidemiology

A description of a pathological event (incidence or mortality) or distribution of a risk factor in various populations is the basis for the first approach of epidemiology, known as descriptive epidemiology. Acquiring these data is necessary in order to support further studies, but they are insufficient in themselves to identify a causal factor.

Comparing different end-points observed among the populations under study generates hypotheses about which factors could be responsible for the observed differences, namely genes or the environment (climate, food, lifestyle). For example, in his first report, the 'Seven countries study', Ancel Keys showed that there were significant differences in cardiovascular and all causes of mortality among the 16 cohorts of men from Japan, the US, Northern Europe (Finland, the Netherlands), Southern Europe (Italy, Yugoslavia) and Crete, Greece (Figure 8.1) [1]. These populations were differentiated by many factors, including genetic polymorphisms, and consequently further research was needed in order to comprehend the rationale for these strong differences.

The Monica study (Figure 8.2) also showed strong differences in coronary heart disease among European populations, and even among samples from regions within the specific country under study (as shown for France) [2]. These were characterised by different dietary patterns, and this supports the hypothesis of diet-related factors.

Migrant studies add time to space and show if the suspected factor needs time and adaptation of the subject to the new environment in order to produce an effect. This is illustrated by the change in breast cancer incidence observed among migrant Japanese women as adults in Hawaii, and daughters of these migrant women, compared with

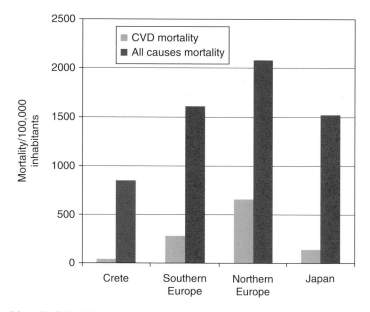

Figure 8.1   Mortality/100,000 inhabitants of selected countries of 'The seven countries study' over a 15 years follow-up [1].

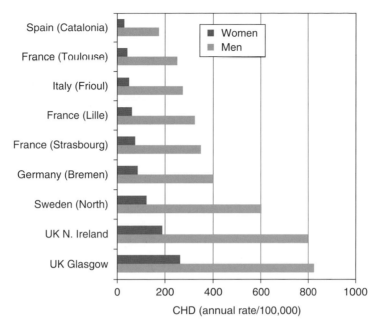

Figure 8.2 Coronary heart disease incidence (annual rate per 100,000) in selected countries of the Monica study (1990s) (from data from [2]).

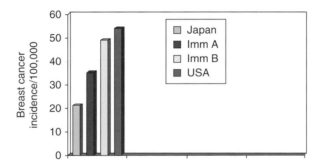

Figure 8.3 Variation of incidence of breast cancer/100,000, by birth place and age at immigration (adjusted for age) adapted from [3]. Imm A: immigrants as adults; Imm B: immigrants born in US.

Japanese women in Japan and American women in Hawaii (Figure 8.3) [3]. Thus, diet may be a factor influencing the incidence and mortality of chronic diseases in human populations.

Prevalence and incidence

Prevalence: The proportion of individuals in a population having a disease. Prevalence is a statistical concept referring to the number of cases of a disease that are present in a particular population at a given time.

Incidence: The frequency with which something, such as a disease, appears in a particular population or area. In disease epidemiology, the incidence is the number of newly diagnosed cases during a specific time period. The incidence is distinct from the prevalence which refers to the number of cases alive on a certain date.

8.2.2 Ecological studies

Ecological studies, or international comparative correlation studies, calculate the correlation coefficient between a nutrient and the incidence of, or mortality from, a disease among several populations in the world, e.g. fat consumption and breast cancer incidence. This type of study is based on aggregated data (food disappearance for the whole population) and cannot avoid confounding with other factors that could also be related to the disease. For example, fat might be found in certain types of meat, which may also contain mutagenic heterocyclic amines. The ecological study cannot distinguish between these two potential risk factors. Therefore, ecological studies reinforce the hypothesis of diet as a factor for chronic diseases, but require studies based on individual data to eliminate, as much as is possible, confounding factors and to get closer to establishing a level of evidence.

8.3 Analytical epidemiology

Analytical epidemiology refers to studies that are based on collecting data on an individual basis. This is usually through a questionnaire, and elicits information on demographics, anthropometrics, education variables, socio-economic status, characteristics of reproductive life (e.g. age at menarche and menopause, age at first pregnancy, number of pregnancies and children), life-style factors, physical activity and diet. All of these factors could either be potential risk factors or confounding factors. Statistical techniques (adjustment, multivariate analysis, logistic regression) enable identification, as much as is possible, of the specific risk factor(s) implicated in the disease.

Nutritional epidemiology is a special field of epidemiology because specific epidemiological techniques needed to be devised in relation to nutrition [4]. These include food composition tables and *ad hoc* software that transform food intake into corresponding nutrients, and also a variety of food questionnaires including dietary recall, food records and food-frequency questionnaires (FFQ). This last questionnaire is the one used most often in studies on the relationship between food and disease because the usual diet over a certain period is quite well captured by this method. Important criteria to ensure the validity and the strength of a study include: (1) using a sizeable number of items (≥ 100) to ensure good coverage of food and energy intake; (2) the judicious constitution of food groups (e.g. potatoes should not be included in the group 'vegetables' when analysing the association with disease risk because of the difference in micronutrients between potatoes and other vegetables).

Food records have been shown to be less prone to measurement error, but their use is more cumbersome for large samples [5]. A questionnaire must be validated on a sub-sample of the study population by another nutritional epidemiology technique in order to detect measurement errors [6]. These errors are never completely avoidable, but they should be identified as much as is possible and minimised. Validation can lead to the correction of errors in nutritional assessment.

Another way to assess nutritional intake is to measure nutritional markers either shortly after intake or in the previous days, weeks or months. A nutritional marker must reflect variations in intake of a nutrient, and the choice of time will depend on the tissue source of the biomarker. For example, fatty acids in plasma reflect intake over the previous day, in erythrocytes intake over the previous week, and in adipose tissue intake over the previous month.

For nutritional epidemiology, specific statistical techniques were developed because of the correlation between nutrient intake, especially macronutrients, with energy intake [4]. Thus, controlling for energy in analytical nutritional epidemiology is a criterion of validity of the study.

8.3.1   Case-control and prospective studies

Analytical epidemiology is applied in two designs: case-control and prospective studies. Case-control studies compare a sample of subjects presenting with the disease under study (the 'cases') with a sample of subjects not affected by the disease (the 'controls'). The variables suspected of playing a role in the disease, as well as those susceptible to confound these risk factors, are assessed through a questionnaire (and/or biomarkers for nutrients). Correct diagnosis of the disease must be confirmed in the cases. The controls are recruited either in the general population or among patients suffering from a condition not related to the one under study, e.g. trauma surgery. Controls from the general population may appear to be less biased than those recruited from hospitalised patients. However, it can be argued that the latter are more disposed to give the same time and attention to the questionnaire as the cases, whereas controls in the general population might be less inclined to answer questionnaires. Case-control studies might be biased by memory faults, given that the investigated factors may have happened years before the disease. This is especially true in nutritional epidemiology because the effects of nutrients upon the disease often depend upon food consumption years before disease diagnosis. Also, cases might be inclined to emphasise some characteristics that they think might be related to their disease. In case-control studies, results obtained from nutritional assessment by biomarkers should be regarded with caution, especially if they are short-term markers, and also because these markers can be modified by the concurrent disease.

The memory biases are absent in the *prospective study* of a cohort of subjects, since they answer the questionnaires before the disease. This also ensures the correct temporal relationship between exposure to the factor and diagnosis of the disease. In this design, nutritional biomarkers that are relevant to the nutritional assessment are also collected at entry into the study. The main difficulty is that a large number of subjects need to be recruited in order to achieve a sufficient number of cases in the follow-up. This particularly applies when looking for risk factors for diseases characterised by a low incidence. This explains why there are many studies on cardiovascular diseases and some cancers (e.g. lung, breast, colon), but less on some other less common cancers (e.g. ovary, rectum, bile duct). After a follow-up of several years, certified cases are registered, and exposure of the ill and non-ill subjects in the cohort to the risk factors under consideration is compared.

Although it avoids memory bias, a prospective study is not completely exempt from bias. The subjects recruited for the cohort are usually volunteers or part of a community (e.g. nurses, members of a professional insurance company), and are therefore not exactly representative of the general population. Hence, results from these studies cannot always be extrapolated. The European multi-centre EPIC study obviates this pitfall by including cohorts from different countries, thus combining the advantages of both prospective and ecological studies.

8.4   Intervention studies

Intervention studies are designed to establish whether or not there is a causal relationship between a factor and a disease. They reproduce scientific experimental studies, i.e. an experimental group of subjects is exposed to the factor (a nutrient or a chemical or a specified diet postulated to be beneficial) and this group is compared to a group exposed to a placebo. Both groups are subjects at risk for a disease, and they are recruited based on precise criteria such as being smokers, hypercholesterol-aemic, overweight or obese. Results cannot be as clear-cut as those obtained from experimental studies in animal models since individual variability is not controlled for (such as genetic polymorphisms, and lifestyle and environmental factors). This design generally tests one nutrient or plant constituent as opposed to whole diets, thus emphasising the potential importance of a single molecule, and it might also show other effects within the context of a dietary pattern.

8.5   Expression and interpretation of data from epidemiological studies

Using analytical epidemiology, it is possible to calculate the probability of the risk for a subject becoming ill when exposed to the risk factor under consideration. In a prospective study, the relative risk is expressed by the hazard ratio (HR) or relative risk (RR). These measure the actual probability for the disease to appear in a population. By contrast, in a case-control study, the risk is an estimated relative risk, and this is expressed as the odds ratio (OR) between predetermined exposed and non-exposed populations. The use of OR is only valid if the incidence of the disease is low. In both cases, the risk is evaluated against a reference category, most often the subjects the least exposed to the risk factor, for which the HR/RR or OR = 1. For each category of exposure, a relative risk may then be calculated. When the factor is increasing the risk, HR or OR >1. When the factor is decreasing the risk, HR or OR <1. Confidence intervals (CI) are calculated. These are most often 95% CI and in this book CI values are 95% CI unless otherwise stated. If the value for the HR/RR or OR = 1, this would indicate no effect. When the exposure can be expressed as a continuous value, the HR or OR is calculated for a given increment of exposure. OR are also used to express the results of intervention studies.

From this basic technique, other statistical approaches have been developed:

- A *population attributable risk (PAR)* is the proportion of the incidence of a disease in the population (exposed and nonexposed) that is increased (negative exposure) or decreased (favourable exposure) following the exposure. It is the incidence of a disease *in the population* that would be eliminated if exposure were eliminated (negative exposure) or generalised to all the population (favourable exposure). It is necessary to know the number of subjects exposed in the population and the risk probability of the disease. If there is a high level of exposure in the population, then even if the risk probability is low the PAR might still be rather large, and this is the case for many nutritional factors.
- A *trend* in increasing or decreasing risk might be observed through the various categories of exposure. Significance of this trend is calculated, and when significant it assumes a linear relationship between exposure and the observed effect.

- The *meta-analysis* technique has been developed to increase the statistical power of a study, as this might be insufficient from a single study due to there being too few subjects in each individual study. This technique was considered to mark a major improvement in epidemiological analysis. However, the validity of the result depends upon the validity of each study included in the meta-analysis. Thus, criteria for selecting the studies must always be carefully described and studies with comparable methods and design should be included. A test to estimate the validity of the meta-analysis is the heterogeneity test, which evaluates the degree of heterogeneity among the selected studies. If this is large, it casts some doubt on the final result.

8.6   Dietary patterns

Nutritional data are analysed either by food or by nutrient, for which the HR or OR expresses the relationship with the disease under consideration. However, a holistic approach of *dietary patterns* may also be used based on either *a priori* or *a posteriori* dietary patterns. In *a priori* dietary patterns, a score or index groups several nutritional values characteristic of a dietary pattern fixed *a priori*, i.e. from prior knowledge. The composite index is then statistically treated as a single variable. The *a posteriori* dietary pattern uses data obtained from the population under study and analyses them by specific statistical techniques (multiple correspondence or principal component analysis) to reveal groups of foods that describe the food patterns of the population under study. Dietary patterns have the ability to integrate the complex and subtle interactive effects of many dietary exposures and bypass problems generated by testing multiple variables and the high correlations that may exist among these exposures.

8.6.1   *A priori* dietary patterns

A first method using an *a priori* dietary pattern to comprehensively understand diet was the construction of the diet quality index (DQI). A selection of foods or nutrients assumed to represent diet quality, either by their presence in high amounts or in low amounts, receive a score, which results in a quality index. Patterson et al. designed the first DQI in 1994 based on US nutritional guidelines [7]. It cannot be applied to the MedDiet because, except for SFA, there was no mention of other FAs. Subsequently, Trichopoulou et al. built a first Mediterranean diet score (MDS) as a reference for the MedDiet based on the consumption by a population of elderly Greeks of greens, legumes, fruit and nuts, cereals, MUFA/SFA ratio, meats and dairy products [8]. Another MDQI was published in 2000 by Gerber et al., which introduced foods such as olive oil and fish [9]. The construction of the index is shown in Table 8.1. The amount of food is based on the amount that has been shown to be protective or deleterious in epidemiological studies. Each food or nutrient is scored accordingly. The MDQI ranges from 0, which is the closest to an idealised MedDiet, to 14, which is the furthest from a MedDiet. Because of the use of olive oil, this score can only be used to characterise the maintenance of a MedDiet in populations in Mediterranean areas [10].

Later, Trichopoulou et al. improved their first score by adding fish, and applied it to the Greek component of the European Prospective Investigation into Cancer and Nutrition (EPIC) which included a total of 28,572 participants aged 20 to 86 years

Table 8.1 Construction of a MedDiet score based on daily intake [9]. With permission from Elsevier.

Score/ nutrient or food	SFA (% TEI[1])	Cholesterol (mg)	Red meat and dairy foods (g)	Olive oil (ml)	Fish (g)	Cereals[2] (g)	Fruit + Vegetables (g)
0	<10	<300	<200	>15	>60	>300	>700
1	10–13	300–400	200–400	15–5	60–30	300–100	700–400
2	>13	>400	>400	<5	<30	<100	<400

[1]Total energy intake.
[2]Not including fast foods and pastries.

Table 8.2 Scores attributed to each food or nutrient, and the median intake by elderly Greeks (g/day) [11].

	Vegeta- bles	Legumes	Fruits + nuts	Dairy produce	Cereals	Meat	Alcohol	MUFA/ SFA	Fish
Men	550	9	363	197	178	121	10–50	1.7	24
Women	500	7	356	191	140	90	5–25	1.7	19
Score	>:1[1]	>:1	>:1	>:0	>:1	>:0	<c>:1[3]	>:1	>:1
	<:0[2]	<:0	<:0	<:1	<:0	<:1	< >:0[4]	<:0	<:0

[1]>:1 – assigned a value of 1 if consumption > median.
[2]<:0 – assigned a value of 0 if consumption < median.
[3]<c>:1 – assigned a value of 1 if consumption is between the two values.
[4]< >:0 – assigned a value of 0 if consumption is outside the two values.

old [11]. The MDS was constructed by assigning a value of 0 or 1 to each of nine indicated components with the use of the sex-specific median as the cut-off. For beneficial components (vegetables, legumes, fruits and nuts, cereal, and fish), persons whose consumption was below the median were assigned a value of 0, and persons whose consumption was at or above the median were assigned a value of 1. For components presumed to be detrimental (meat, poultry, and dairy products – which are rarely non-fat or low-fat in Greece), persons whose consumption was below the median were assigned a value of 1, and persons whose consumption was at or above the median were assigned a value of 0. For ethanol, a value of 1 was assigned to men who consumed between 10 and 50 g per day and to women who consumed between 5 and 25 g per day (Table 8.2). Thus, the total MDS ranged from 0 (minimal adherence to the traditional MedDiet) to 9 (maximal adherence).

The MDS had to be modified (M-MDS) when applied to other European elderly cohorts of the EPIC study [12]. The MUFA/SFA ratio in the context of the MDS represents the ratio of oleic acid – which is mainly from olive oil – and SFA – which is mainly from animal fat (meat and dairy products). However, in other European countries, especially in North European countries, a large part of MUFA intake is provided by meat, whereas the use of vegetable oils provides mainly PUFAs. Therefore the MUFA/SFA ratio became MUFA+PUFA/SFA. In addition, the values of the score cut-offs change when they are applied to different populations since they are the medians of the population that is being analysed. For example, the median consumption of vegetables for all the EPIC cohorts was 157 g whereas in the Greek cohort it was 500 g, which also had one-third more dairy product intake. Another pitfall might be that this *a priori* dietary pattern described by the MDS correlates with other nutritional or lifestyle factors that also have a potential role in risk reduction in Mediterranean countries, and these may not necessarily be present in non-Mediterranean countries. For example, in a comparative study on the maintenance of a MedDiet in Malta and Sardinia, it was shown that a timely organisation of meals through the day, their structure, and the conviviality at the meals, were important characteristics of this MedDiet [13]. In another report, from the HALE project, it was shown that when other lifestyle factors (non-smoking, physical activity and moderate use of alcohol) were combined with the MDS (without wine) the HR was 0.35 (CI 0.28–0.44), whereas it was 0.77 (CI 0.68–0.88) for the MDS alone [14]. Another lifestyle factor which might be correlated with the variables of the MDS is taking a siesta [15].

The MDS was further modified in later studies. For studies conducted in the US, Fung and colleagues (2006) excluded potato products from the vegetable group, separated fruits and nuts into two groups, eliminated the dairy group, included whole-grain products only, included only red and processed meats in the meat group, and allocated 1 point for alcohol intake between 5 and 15 g/d [16]. It was called the alternate MDS (aMDS). In 2010, another modification was developed [17]. Each component (apart from alcohol) was calculated as a function of energy density (g/1000 Kcal/d) and was then divided into tertiles of intake. A score of 0 to 2 was assigned to the first, second and third tertiles of intake for the five components presumed to fit the MedDiet, namely fruit (including nuts and seeds), vegetables (excluding potatoes), legumes, fish (fresh or frozen, excluding fish products and preserved fish), and cereals. The scoring was inverted for the two components presumed not to fit the MedDiet, namely total meat and dairy products. The scoring for olive oil was modified because of the relatively large number of non-consumers. Therefore, 0 was assigned to non-consumers, 1 for subjects below the median (calculated only within olive oil consumers), and 2 for subjects equal or above this median. Alcohol was assigned either 2 for moderate consumers (range: 5–25 g/d for women and 10–50 g/d for men) or 0 for subjects outside (above or below) the sex-specific range. This modification was called the relative-MDS (rMDS). The rMDS were then grouped into low (0–6), medium (7–10), and high (11–18).

Another index, called the Mediterranean Adequacy Index (MAI), was proposed in 2004 [18]. It was computed by dividing the sum of the percentage of total energy from typical Mediterranean food groups by the sum of the percentage of total energy from non-typical Mediterranean food groups. The reference Italian-Mediterranean diet that was used was that of subjects from Nicotera (Southern Italy) in 1960.

8.6.2   *A posteriori* dietary patterns

A posteriori refers to knowledge gained from experience or empirical evidence. *A posteriori* techniques in nutrition collect nutritional data from a population sample, and then use these data to identify the dietary patterns present in this population. The nutritional data collected in the population under study are analysed by 'multiple correspondences' or 'principal component analysis' (PCA). Multiple correspondences analyse one variable with respect to a series of variables (disease yes or no, with respect to nutritional variables). Principal component analysis forms linear combinations of the original food groups, thereby grouping together variables that correlate with each other. These linear combinations are specific food items or food groups aggregated together on the basis of the degree to which the food items in the dataset are correlated with one another. A summary score for each pattern is then derived and can be used in either correlation or regression analysis to examine relationships between various eating patterns and the outcome of interest, such as nutrient intake, cardiovascular risk factors and other biochemical indicators of health [19]. 'Cluster analysis' identifies clusters of individuals with the same dietary pattern using similar principles discussed above. *A posteriori* dietary patterns, identified primarily based on the correlations between the food groups as observed in a population sample, have been analysed by principal component analysis.

The *a posteriori* approach has been used mainly in non-Mediterranean countries and identified essentially two patterns: a 'prudent' or 'plant based' pattern and a 'Western' pattern. The consistent features of the prudent diet are a high intake of vegetables, fruit, legumes fish/seafood and whole grains, whereas the Western diet is characterised by a high intake of red and processed meat, butter, potatoes, refined grains and high-fat dairy products [19]. Depending on the population and the study, other food groups that can be found in the prudent diet include poultry, low-fat dairy products, salad dressings, fruit juices and wine, whereas in the Western diet sweets, French fries, high sugar drinks, pizzas, mayonnaise and margarine may occur.

A 'plant-based diet' was defined as the first component of the PCA of the EPIC cohorts; that is, it is a diet rich in plant foods such as vegetables and vegetable oils, fruit, pasta/rice/other grains and legumes, but poor in potatoes, margarine and non-alcoholic beverages [20].

8.7 Criteria for judging epidemiological data

As discussed above, it is an absolute requirement when considering the results of an epidemiological study to have used validated cases, to have validated food questionnaires with sufficient and pertinent items, and to have detected and controlled for confounding factors. Another criterion is the sample size. Large confidence intervals reflect an insufficient number of subjects. A satisfactory sample size for questionnaire-based case-control studies is about 500, whereas it might be reduced to 100 in prospective studies, mainly when nutritional assessment is based on biomarkers.

Despite maximising validity, one epidemiological study cannot by itself be considered sufficient to establish a causal relationship between a factor and a disease. Hill in 1965 was the first to propose a series of criteria to characterise a causal inference from epidemiological data [21]. These were: (1) consistency among the studies devoted to a factor and a disease; (2) strength of the association (that is to say, the value of the HR/OR); (3) dose-response relationship; (4) temporality (the exposure to the factor must precede the diagnosis by a relevant time); (5) biological plausibility; (6) congruent experimental studies.

Temporality between cause and effect is sometimes difficult to assess and this consideration gave rise to the concept of *reverse causality*. Reverse causality describes the situation where the effect precedes the cause. The problem arises when the assumption is that A causes B when the truth may actually be that B causes A: an example that can be given is loss of appetite and weight in Alzheimer's disease.

An *hierarchy* among studies has been proposed to help to establish a causal inference [22]. Top of the hierarchy are data from prospective studies, which then might be supported by intervention studies, when they exist. Case-control studies are judged by these authors to be in third position, followed by experimental studies. Another way to look at various types of studies is the *portfolio* (or mosaic) approach. In this case, all the criteria should be considered together, each providing a piece of the puzzle [23]. However, each study might be weighted, and in this perspective, it is acknowledged that prospective studies have the highest weighting. Finally, the World Cancer Research Fund/American Institute for Cancer Research in 2007 proposed criteria for grading evidence [24]:

- *Convincing* (unlikely to be modified by further studies): evidence from more than one type of study and from at least two prospective cohort studies; no substantial unexplained heterogeneity within or between studies types or in different populations; valid studies (as defined above); dose response effect, not necessarily linear as long as the explanation is biologically plausible; strong experimental evidence (human or animal) that exposure to the factor can lead to the disease.
- *Probable*: the same as the points above except for the first one – evidence from at least two prospective cohort studies or at least five case-control studies;
- *Limited-suggestive*: not enough studies, or studies with methodological flaws, but show generally consistent direction of effect, in spite of some unexplained heterogeneity.
- *Limited-no conclusion*: evidence so limited that no firm conclusion can be made.
- *Substantial effect on risk unlikely*: the same as convincing but with studies showing absence of effect.

When the level of evidence is judged convincing or probable, preventive recommendations should be made in the perspective of public health.

References

1. Keys, A. et al. Epidemiological studies related to coronary heart disease: characteristics of men aged 40–59 in seven countries. *Acta Med Scand Suppl*, 1966. **460**: 1–392.
2. Tunstall-Pedoe, H. et al. Contribution of trends in survival and coronary-event rates to changes in coronary heart disease mortality: 10-year results from 37 WHO MONICA project populations. Monitoring trends and determinants in cardiovascular disease. *Lancet*, 1999. **353**(9164): 1547–57.
3. Ziegler, R.G. et al. Migration patterns and breast cancer risk in Asian-American women. *J Natl Cancer Inst*, 1993. **85**(22): 1819–27.
4. Willett, W. *Nutritional epidemiology*. 2nd ed. 1998, New York; Oxford: Oxford University Press.
5. Bingham, S.A. et al. Are imprecise methods obscuring a relation between fat and breast cancer? *Lancet*, 2003. **362**(9379): 212–4.
6. Daures, J.P. et al. Validation of a food-frequency questionnaire using multiple-day records and biochemical markers: application of the triads method. *J Epidemiol Biostat*, 2000. **5**(2): 109–15.
7. Patterson, R.E., Haines, P.S., Popkin, B.M. Diet quality index: capturing a multidimensional behavior. *J Am Diet Assoc*, 1994. **94**(1): 57–64.
8. Trichopoulou, A. et al. Diet and overall survival in elderly people. *BMJ*, 1995. **311**(7018): 1457–60.
9. Gerber, M.J. et al. Profiles of a healthful diet and its relationship to biomarkers in a population sample from Mediterranean southern France. *J Am Diet Assoc*, 2000. **100**(10): 1164–71.
10. Scali, J., Richard, A., Gerber, M. Diet profiles in a population sample from Mediterranean southern France. *Public Health Nutr*, 2001. **4**(2): 173–82.

11. Trichopoulou, A. et al. Adherence to a Mediterranean diet and survival in a Greek population. *N Engl J Med*, 2003. **348**(26): 2599–608.
12. Trichopoulou, A. et al. Modified Mediterranean diet and survival: EPIC-elderly prospective cohort study. *BMJ*, 2005. **330**(7498): 991.
13. Tessier, S., Gerber, M. Comparison between Sardinia and Malta: the Mediterranean diet revisited. *Appetite*, 2005. **45**(2): 121–6.
14. Knoops, K.T. et al. Mediterranean diet, lifestyle factors, and 10-year mortality in elderly European men and women: the HALE project. *Jama*, 2004. **292**(12): 1433–9.
15. Naska, A. et al. Siesta in healthy adults and coronary mortality in the general population. *Arch Intern Med*, 2007. **167**(3): 296–301.
16. Fung, T.T. et al. Diet quality is associated with the risk of estrogen receptor-negative breast cancer in postmenopausal women. *J Nutr*, 2006. **136**(2): 466–72.
17. Buckland, G. et al. Adherence to a Mediterranean diet and risk of gastric adenocarcinoma within the European Prospective Investigation into Cancer and Nutrition (EPIC) cohort study. *Am J Clin Nutr*, 2010. **91**(2): 381–90.
18. Alberti-Fidanza, A., Fidanza, F. Mediterranean Adequacy Index of Italian diets. *Public Health Nutr*, 2004. **7**(7): 937–41.
19. Hu, F.B. Dietary pattern analysis: a new direction in nutritional epidemiology. *Curr Opin Lipidol*, 2002. **13**(1): 3–9.
20. Bamia, C. et al. Dietary patterns and survival of older Europeans: the EPIC-Elderly Study (European Prospective Investigation into Cancer and Nutrition). *Public Health Nutr*, 2007. **10**(6): 590–8.
21. Hill, A.B. The environment and disease: association or causation? *Proc R Soc Med*, 1965. **58**: 295–300.
22. Smit, L.A., Mozaffarian, D., Willett, W. Review of fat and fatty acid requirements and criteria for developing dietary guidelines. *Ann Nutr Metab*, 2009. **55**(1–3): 44–55.
23. Gerber, M. Fiber and breast cancer: another piece of the puzzle–but still an incomplete picture. *J Natl Cancer Inst*, 1996. **88**(13): 857–8.
24. WCRF/AICR, *World Cancer Research Fund / American Institute for Cancer Research. Food, Nutrition, Physical Activity, and the Prevention of Cancer: a Global Perspective.* 2007, AICR: Washington DC.

9 General Mechanisms for Disease Prevention

Summary

- Experimental systems used to evaluate the effects of nutrients on disease mechanisms include *in vitro* models (biochemical assays, cell organelle preparations, cell lines, tissue slices), animal models and human intervention studies.
- Many chronic degenerative diseases (CDDs) are thought to be associated with an accumulation of oxidative damage to DNA, proteins and lipids.
- The MedDiet is an excellent source of antioxidant vitamins, minerals and phytochemicals, and these come from a wide range of sources including fruit and vegetables, nuts, extra virgin olive oil, legumes, and drinks such as coffee and wine. However, the role of dietary antioxidants *in vivo* in disease prevention has not been clearly established.
- A wide range of CDDs is associated with an inflammatory response and anti-inflammatory components in Mediterranean foods include *n*-3 fatty acids in fish, various phenolics found in olive oil (such as oleocanthal), flavonoids and other phenolics in fruits and vegetables.
- *n*-3 fatty acids (EPA and DHA) are the starting material for the production of various anti-inflammatory eicosanoids, and also induce the production of anti-inflammatory cytokines, whereas phenolics may exert anti-inflammatory effects by acting as antioxidants and by inhibiting pro-inflammatory enzymes such as COX-2.
- Flavonoids may exert anti-proliferative effects by inhibiting protein kinases involved in signalling pathways for cell proliferation.
- Nutrigenetics (how the genetic make-up of an individual influences their response to dietary components) and nutrigenomics (how dietary components alter the expression of genes affecting health) are having a major impact on understanding how dietary factors such as phenolics and PUFAs influence health.
- Some of the beneficial effects of dietary phenolics may be mediated via inhibition of the pro-inflammatory transcription factor NFκB or via activation of the transcription factor Nrf2 that induces a "cytoprotective" effect in cells. Dietary PUFAs can act via activation of transcription factors known as PPARs.
- Hormesis is an adaptive beneficial response to a low dose of a nutrient which at higher doses is harmful, and hormesis offers a new conceptual framework for understanding the roles of phytochemicals in the MedDiet.
- Benefits of the Mediterranean dietary pattern over the use of supplements or single foods include minimising potentially toxic spikes in plasma nutrient concentrations, and benefits from synergistic interactions between nutrients.

9.1   Introduction

About 75% of people over 65 in the UK and other western countries die from either cancer or CVD. Other chronic degenerative diseases (CDDs) such as diabetes and dementias cause fewer deaths but contribute to considerable suffering for many older people. Most CDDs are the result of complex interactions between lifestyle factors and predisposing genes and hence these disorders are said to be "multifactorial".

Many CDDs such as cancer, CVD and diabetes have common aetiological (causal) factors, a point that was highlighted when the American Cancer Society, the American Diabetes Association, and the American Heart Association issued a "common agenda" in 2004 for action against these disorders [1]. Diabetes and dementia – two apparently quite distinct disorders – can be used to illustrate common underlying causes [2]. Both disorders are associated with poor diet and inadequate physical exercise, and these factors increase the risk for abdominal obesity which, in turn, is associated with inflammation of the vasculature and dysregulation of fat and glucose metabolism (Figure 9.1). Specific inherited predisposing genes may contribute to how these physiological changes progress pathogenically, such as by influencing the development of insulin resistance (the failure of normal concentrations of insulin to exert its normal effects) or of mild cognitive impairment (MCI). For example, the APOE ε4 allele is associated with an increased risk of Alzheimer's disease (AD). Individuals with the APOE ε4 allele together with a critical number of other contributory factors (sometimes referred to as "liabilities") will go on to develop AD. However, not all individuals with the APOE ε4 allele will develop AD: the APOE ε4 allele is present in 15% of the general

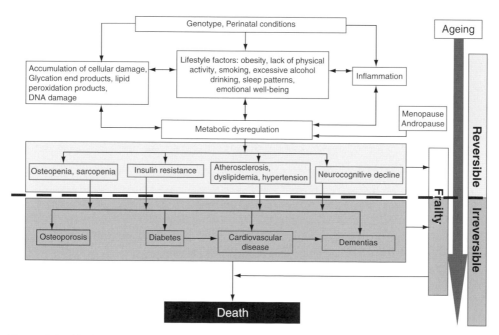

Figure 9.1   Mechanisms leading to age-related disorders [2]. With permission from Elsevier.

population, but not all individuals in this sub-set with the APOE ε4 allele will develop AD. Also, many people who develop AD do not have the APOE ε4 allele. (About 40% of individuals with AD have the APOE ε4 allele.)

Insulin resistance and MCI can be thought of as "pre-disease" states, and untreated these pre-disease states may lead to diabetes and dementia, respectively. There is strong epidemiological evidence that many pre-disease states are potentially reversible by dietary intervention or other means (e.g. drugs). By contrast, the full-blown clinical diseases – diabetes and dementia in this case – are far more difficult to reverse since they are the consequence of complex disease processes.

Common biochemical changes in pre-disease states, such as oxidative stress and inflammation, are of great interest since they help explain why the same dietary factors can help prevent a diverse range of diseases. A few types of nutrients, such as antioxidants, anti-inflammatory agents and *n*-3 fatty acids, crop up again and again as constituents that help reverse early pathological changes. The favourable combination of these beneficial nutrients in the MedDiet probably goes a long way to explaining how this diet helps protect against a diverse range of diseases.

9.2 Methods for studying the effects of nutrients on disease mechanisms

9.2.1 General considerations

Chapters 10–13 consider not only the epidemiological evidence for beneficial effects of the MedDiet, but also experimental evidence from laboratory and clinical studies. When interpreting data from these studies of the effects of nutrients on diseases, it is important to recognise their limitations, just as it is for epidemiological studies. When evaluating experimental data, one consideration is when, and for how long, the study is conducted. Food is consumed at (more-or-less) regular intervals throughout our lives. By contrast, most laboratory-based scientific studies in nutrition take place over a relatively short period (days or weeks) and do not attempt to mimic the way our bodies are normally exposed to nutrients; instead, short-term (acute) biochemical changes are usually measured rather than long-term (chronic) effects. Secondly, it is now recognised that the postprandial state may be an important aspect of disease risk, but this is difficult to study in the laboratory. For example, hyperlipidaemia resulting from the consumption of a high-fat meal is associated with oxidative stress and this might contribute to increased cardiovascular risk. Another consideration is the type of nutrient under investigation, such as whether it is a purified substance, and if so its dose, or whether the substance constitutes part of a more complex food matrix (Table 9.1).

Experimental systems that evaluate the effects of nutrients on disease mechanisms range from simple biochemical assays, to cell culture models, animal models and studies in humans (Table 9.1) [3]. Many cell culture, animal or human studies with isolated phytochemicals use far higher doses than those commensurate with consumption of a MedDiet. Also, of course, the use of isolated phytochemicals does not allow for possible interactions with other dietary substances.

Table 9.1 Types of nutritional studies.

Nutritional approach	Experimental system
• purified nutrient • food extract (e.g. fruit juice) • single food • dietary pattern	• biochemical assay (e.g. enzyme, antioxidant) • cell system • animal model (acute or chronic dosing) • human intervention trials (acute or chronic)

It is worth considering some of the limitations of using purified phytochemicals in acute experimental models (such as a biochemical assay or in cell culture) when attempting to extrapolate these observations to a consumer of the MedDiet.

1. Usually the aglycone form of the phytochemical is tested experimentally whereas many phytochemicals (particularly flavonoids) occur naturally in the diet as glycosides (sugar conjugates). *In vitro* models do not take into account absorption across the gut which can be highly variable (see Chapter 4).
2. Enantiomeric forms may differ between test substance and the dietary form.
3. Many phytochemicals are extensively metabolised in the body and little parent phytochemical may be present in the blood stream (see Chapter 4). For example, many flavonoids are rapidly metabolised in the body, whereas most *in vitro* studies use the parent molecule.

9.2.2   *In vitro* models

The increasing order of complexity of *in vitro* models is:

biochemical assay
cell organelle preparation
cell lines
tissue slices

Biochemical assays are one of the simplest *in vitro* models, and may test the effect of a nutrient on an enzyme activity or be used to determine antioxidant activity (see below). The next level of complexity includes microsomes, which are a cell organelle preparation consisting of ribosomes and fragments of the endoplasmic reticulum. Microsomes, and in particular those derived from the liver, are used to study the phase I and phase II metabolism of xenobiotics such as phytochemicals. More complex again are cell lines, i.e. cells of animal or human origin that can be grown in cell culture; many have been cultured over many years. A widely-used human cell line is Caco-2, which was originally established from a colorectal cancer. It retains many of the characteristics of human intestinal enterocytes and can be used to examine the intestinal absorption of phytochemicals. A second example is the human hepatoma (liver-derived) cell line HepG2 which is used to evaluate the metabolism of nutritional factors. Primary cell lines are cells that are used soon after isolation from their tissue of origin (either freshly obtained or from cryopreserved specimens), and these are increasingly being used since they have undergone far fewer changes than most cell lines. Tissue slices retain 3-dimensional interactions between neighbouring cell populations, and these so-called paracrine interactions are now recognised as important influences on cell function. Tissue slices can be used to study the effects of nutrients on cell signalling, anti-cancer effects and metabolic effects. However, tissue slices can usually only be maintained for a short period in culture.

9.2.3   Animal models

Animal models aim to bridge the gap between *in vitro* studies and human studies. Although animals mimic the human situation in as much as they encompass the complete metabolic pathway from absorption to excretion, there are often significant differences between these processes in animals and humans, and so ultimately human studies must still be undertaken. Animal models can be used to study effects either on normal body functioning or effects on a disease process.

Animal models are important in cancer research. Apc^{Min} mice are a model for human adenomatous polyposis coli, a pre-malignant condition that leads to colon cancer. Apc^{Min} mice carry a genetic defect that gives rise to this condition, and it is passed on to subsequent generations. Tumours can also be induced chemically in animals or by genetic manipulation (either by introducing a gene that confers an increased likelihood of cancer – a transgenic animal – or by eliminating a gene that protects against cancer – so-called knockouts) and the effects of nutrients on the disease process can be studied.

Animals are also important in CVD research. One of the most widely-used models is the apolipoprotein E-deficient (ApoE -/-) mouse. These mice have an impaired ability to remove lipoproteins and this results in the spontaneous development of atherosclerotic lesions resembling those observed in humans.

There are several limitations associated with animal models. Dosages (usually of pure compound) administered to the animals are often far higher than would occur as part of the normal diet. For example, resveratrol has been tested in a wide range of experimental systems, but far higher doses are administered to animals than will be obtained from moderate consumption of red wine. Administration is usually acute rather than chronic and this is important when considering the relevance of short-term findings in relation to disease processes that may take many years to develop. For example, the prevention of LDL oxidation by antioxidant phytochemicals is used as an assay for CVD. However, atherosclerotic plaques develop slowly over many years and oxidative stress may be involved at several stages during the formation of the lesions.

9.2.4   Human intervention studies

These studies may examine the effects of a nutrient or diet on a marker for a disease process (biomarker) such as oxidative stress (see Section 9.3) or, more rarely, the disease itself. Increasingly, the effects of nutrients on gene expression are being examined, either of single genes or simultaneously of multiple genes using a nutrigenomics approach (see Section 9.6). Dietary substances being evaluated for their specific activity may need many years in order for an overall health benefit to be demonstrable, and it has been suggested that prematurely terminating trials with antioxidants may be one explanation for the failure of some of these trials to demonstrate a therapeutic benefit [4].

9.3   Oxidative stress

Many CDDs are thought to be associated with an accumulation of oxidative damage to DNA, proteins and lipids, and much has been made of the putative health benefits of antioxidants and their ability to neutralise the harmful effects of free radicals. However, there is now good evidence that most antioxidant supplements do not have the once hoped-for health benefits [5]. The MedDiet contains a high level of antioxidants and consumption of a MedDiet is associated with a reduction in markers for oxidative stress [6]. This section considers the possible significance of antioxidants in the MedDiet.

9.3.1   What are free radicals?

Atoms consist of a nucleus around which electrons revolve in "orbitals". Each orbital normally contains a pair of electrons. Atoms or molecules that contain an unpaired electron in one or more orbitals are known as free radicals. Most free radicals are highly reactive since they try to restore an electron pair by taking electrons from proteins, lipids or nucleic acids. Loss of electrons (e.g. from a protein) is referred to as oxidation, and hence free radicals act as oxidising agents. The unpaired electron is usually denoted by a dot or minus sign, or both. For example, the superoxide radical is denoted as $O_2^{\bullet}$ or O_2^{-} or $O_2^{\bullet-}$.

Aide memoire: OIL RIG

OIL – Oxidiation Is Loss of electrons
RIG – Reduction Is Gain of electrons

Free radicals derived from oxygen are examples of reactive oxygen species (ROS). The reactivity of oxygen-derived free radicals varies considerably, the most reactive being the hydroxyl radical. Some other species of oxygen are reactive without being free radicals, and these are also referred to as ROS, a good example being hydrogen peroxide (Table 9.2). Various reactive nitrogen species (RNS) also have important physiological and pathological effects and include both free radicals such as nitric oxide, and non-radicals such as peroxynitrite (Table 9.2). ROS and RNS are sometimes grouped together under the name "reactive species".

9.3.2   Production of reactive species

Reactive species are formed on exposure to various external factors such as atmospheric pollution and chemicals in cigarette smoke, and during normal metabolic processes in the cell. The electron transport chain in mitochondria is a major source of superoxide in most cells. "Leakage" of electrons from the mitochondria reduces molecular oxygen (which is itself a free radical and has two unpaired electrons) to superoxide (which has one unpaired electron) [7]. (Remember: reduction is gain of an electron.) O_2 is the terminal electron acceptor in the electron transport chain, and normally forms water, but it is thought that about 1–3% of O_2 is partially reduced by electron leakage and forms superoxide, $O_2^{\bullet-}$. Hydrogen peroxide is generated by the enzyme superoxide dismutase acting on superoxide. Nitric oxide (NO) is another

Table 9.2   Some physiologically occurring reactive species.

Reactive oxygen species (ROS)		Reactive nitrogen species (RNS)	
Free radicals	Non radicals	Free radicals	Non radicals
superoxide $O_2^{\cdot-}$ hydroxyl OH$^{\cdot}$ peroxyl $RO_2^{\cdot}$	hydrogen peroxide H_2O_2 hypochlorous acid HOCl singlet oxygen $^1O_2$	nitric oxide NO* nitrogen dioxide $NO_2^{\cdot}$	peroxynitrite ONOO$^-$

*Usually just written as NO

Table 9.3   Sources of some reactive species. See [8] for further information.

Reactive species	Production	Possible consequence/ disease association
superoxide radical	• electron transport chain • cytochrome P450 enzymes • white blood cells (respiratory burst)	relatively non toxic
hydrogen peroxide	• superoxide dismutase • oxidation of long chain FAs in peroxisomes • reactions in ischaemic tissue	conversion to hydroxyl radical
hydroxyl radical	• free iron (Fenton reaction) or free copper • reaction between hydrogen peroxide and superoxide	lipid peroxidation
singlet oxygen	• photochemical reaction • respiratory burst	may contribute to age-related macular degeneration
nitric oxide	• nitric oxide synthase	• vasorelaxant • can generate peroxynitrite
peroxynitrite	• reaction between nitric oxide and superoxide	nitrates lipids and amino acids

important reactive species, and it is produced enzymically by nitric oxide synthase. NO reduces the risk of CVD by acting as a vasorelaxant, but it can also react with superoxide to form peroxynitrite, a damaging RNS. Some sources of reactive species are shown in Table 9.3.

Most transition metals (such as iron and copper) contain an unpaired electron and thus qualify as free radicals. The majority of iron in the body is present in haemoglobin, and either free iron or haem generated from the degradation of haemoglobin can act as free radicals causing lipid peroxidation (see below). Fe^{2+} can also react with hydrogen peroxide to generate the hydroxyl radical by the so-called Fenton reaction.

9.3.3   Effects of reactive species

Free radicals are often thought of as damaging agents. However, it is now recognised that a cell must maintain the correct "redox" status in order to function optimally, and redox reactions regulate normal cellular functions. This delicate balancing act is called "redox homeostasis". It is an important concept in relation to nutrition since overwhelming the normal redox status of a cell with antioxidants could explain some of the adverse effects of antioxidant supplements.

Adverse effects

Reactive species such as free radicals can damage a wide range of cell components. Polyunsaturated fatty acids are particularly susceptible to attack by free radicals. Free radicals such as the hydroxyl radical oxidise a methylene group situated between two double bonds:

$$-CH=CH-CH_2-CH=CH-$$

$$\downarrow \cdot OH$$

$$-CH=CH-\cdot CH-CH=CH-$$

This initiation reaction is followed by "propagation" reactions in which the products of one reaction serve as reactants in another reaction generating lipid peroxides. This process sets up a chain reaction which can be terminated by antioxidants (see below). The major products of lipid peroxidation are malondialdehyde (MDA) and 4-hydroxy-2-nonenal (HNE), and these, along with other related products such as oxidised isoprostanes, are useful biomarkers for lipid peroxidation reactions *in vivo* (see Table 9.5).

Reactive species can also damage DNA, either directly or via lipid peroxidation products. The major damage is caused by the hydroxyl radical which oxidises bases, especially guanine, to form 8-hydroxy deoxyguanosine, which can be used as a marker for DNA damage. Oxygen-derived free radicals such as the hydroxyl radical will react almost instantaneously at their site of production, whereas non-radicals such as hydrogen peroxide can pass through cell membranes and so act at a greater distance.

For neurological and cardiovascular disorders and others, it is unclear whether reactive species are the main factor that *initiates* the disease. But there is more evidence that reactive species are important for the *progression* of these diseases. In the case of cancer, it is clear that reactive species can damage DNA and so result in a mutation that *initiates* cancer. However, reactive species are more commonly associated with events in tumour promotion and tumour progression such as angiogenesis, carcinogen metabolism and metastasis, and most cancers are initiated by mutagens (i.e. carcinogens) other than reactive species [8]. Reactive species are also involved in inducing an inflammatory response, which is an important component in many chronic diseases, although again the inflammatory response may not necessarily have initiated the disease process.

Beneficial effects

It is now established that reactive species at low to moderate concentrations have many beneficial effects [9]. One well-established beneficial effect is defence against infectious agents resulting from ROS generation by phagocytic cells during the respiratory burst. Nitric oxide has a diverse range of beneficial physiological effects, including regulating blood pressure and immune function. Maintaining the correct

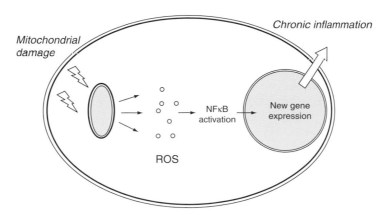

Figure 9.2 Chronic inflammation resulting from the continual production of ROS.

redox status in the cell is also important for regulating a number of intracellular signalling pathways in cells that regulate many basic cell functions such as growth, differentiation and death.

Oxidative stress

An imbalance of ROS in favour of too much pro-oxidant activity is called oxidative stress. Oxidative stress can initiate various pathological events such as cell death (e.g. of neurones) or possibly lead to the continual activation of transcription factors involved in inflammatory responses resulting in chronic inflammation (Figure 9.2).

Different degrees of oxidative stress can result in quite different outcomes for a cell. These variable effects are nicely illustrated by considering the effects of oxidative stress on tumour development: low levels of oxidative stress promote the growth of tumour cells (e.g. via activation of signalling pathways), moderate levels can cause DNA damage (mutagenesis), whereas high levels will trigger cell death (apoptosis or necrosis) (Figure 9.3).

9.3.4   Antioxidant defences

An antioxidant has been defined as "any substance that delays, prevents or removes oxidative damage to a target molecule" [8]. The potentially harmful effects of reactive species are normally kept in check by various antioxidant defences that are either produced physiologically or obtained from the diet. Hydrophilic defences tend to act in aqueous solutions such as the blood or cytoplasm, whereas hydrophobic antioxidants are more active in cell membranes (Table 9.4).

Physiologically produced antioxidants include enzymes such as superoxide dismutase (SOD), glutathione peroxidase and catalase. SOD helps eliminate superoxide, and the importance of SOD is clearly demonstrated in knock-out mice which lack SOD since they have an increased rate of cancer development. SOD exists in extracellular, cytoplasmic and mitochondrial forms. The extracellular and cytoplasmic forms require zinc and copper as cofactors whereas the mitochondrial form uses manganese. Hence, these metals are required in sufficient amounts from the diet in order for SODs to work. Another very important metal involved in antioxidant

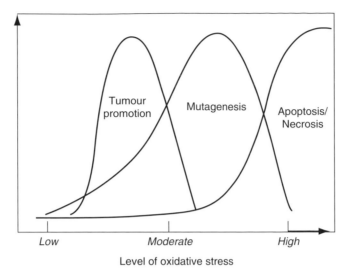

Level of oxidative stress

Figure 9.3 The dose-dependent effects of oxidative stress on tumour development [9]. With permission from Elsevier.

Table 9.4 Antioxidant defences and their cellular locations.

Reactive species	Antioxidant defences	Location
superoxide	vitamin C	blood, cytoplasm
	CuZn SOD*	blood (especially arterial blood), cytoplasm
	Mn SOD	mitochondria
hydrogen peroxide	vitamin C	blood, cytoplasm
	glutathione peroxidase (Se)	cytoplasm, mitochondria, blood
	catalase	peroxisomes
hydroxyl radical	vitamin C, uric acid, glutathione, dihydrolipoic acid, metallothionein	aqueous solutions
singlet oxygen	carotenoids	membrane
	vitamin C	blood, cytoplasm
lipid peroxides	vitamin E, carotenoids	membranes
	vitamin C	
	glutathione	

*SOD: superoxide dismutase.

mechanisms is selenium. Selenium is a cofactor for glutathione peroxidase which removes hydrogen peroxide. Glutathione peroxidase also requires glutathione (a peptide consisting of three amino acids) in its reduced form (GSH) as a reducing agent. GSH becomes oxidised during the reaction to glutathione disulphide (GSSG):

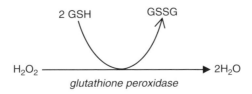

$glutathione\ peroxidase$

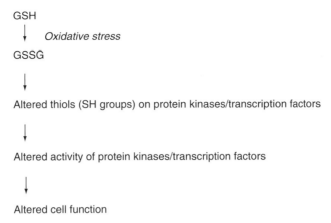

Figure 9.4   Role of GSSG as a redox sensor to alter cell function.

Non-enzymic antioxidants can act directly to scavenge free radicals. In addition to acting as a cofactor for glutathione peroxidase, glutathione performs many other protective roles in the cell. Glutathione is present in cells in millimolar concentrations and is a pivotal non-enzymic antioxidant in the cell. Glutathione (GSH) becomes oxidised to GSSG during redox reactions, and the ratio of GSSG:GSH is a good measure of oxidative stress in a cell or organism; i.e. the higher the GSSG:GSH ratio, the higher the degree of oxidative stress. GSSG is a sensor for the cell of its redox status, enabling the cell to make appropriate functional modifications. GSSG acts by modifying thiol groups on signalling molecules, such as protein kinases and some transcription factors, and this affects their activity and hence in turn causes changes in cell function (Figure 9.4).

The MedDiet is a rich source of directly-acting antioxidants, including vitamins C and E, and various phytochemicals such as carotenoids and possibly phenolics. These are discussed in Section 9.2.6.

Direct antioxidants are consumed or oxidised in the process of their antioxidant activity, and they in turn become pro-oxidants with varying degrees of activity. For example, vitamin C reacts with the hydroxyl radical to generate the fairly non-reactive semidehydroascorbate radical. Glutathione reacts with the hydroxyl radical generating a glutathione radical that typically reacts with another glutathione radical to form GSSG. Other scavengers of hydroxyl radicals include uric acid and coenzyme Q.

Some antioxidants become potentially damaging pro-oxidants after reacting with free radicals. Hence, these newly formed pro-oxidants need to be returned to their antioxidant status. This can be achieved by antioxidants interacting in networks as can be illustrated by considering vitamin E. Being lipid soluble, vitamin E is an important antioxidant that terminates many chain reactions propagated by lipid peroxides present in cell membranes. During this process vitamin E is itself oxidised, forming the potentially toxic vitamin E radical. Various antioxidants, including glutathione and vitamin C, can regenerate vitamin E, which requires the vitamin E radical to migrate to the membrane surface so that it can react with these water-soluble antioxidants (Figure 9.5). Vitamin E may play a role in preventing the oxidation of lipids present in LDL (see Section 9.2.6).

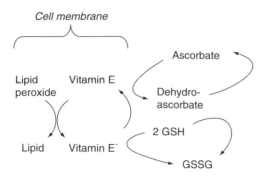

Figure 9.5   Part of an antioxidant network regenerating vitamin E.

9.3.5   Measuring antioxidant activity

The "total antioxidant capacity" (TAC) is a commonly-used method that avoids measuring individual antioxidants, and is often used to measure the antioxidant capacity of a foodstuff. The TAC of foods can be measured by preparing water-soluble and lipid-soluble extracts and measuring the ability of the extract to delay oxidation generated by a free radical-initiating substance such as AAPH (2,2'-azobis-(2-amidino-propane)dihydrochloride) or ABTS (2,2'azinobis-(3-ethylbenzothiazoline 6-sulphonate) [8]. The delay in oxidation is often expressed as the "lag time": the higher the lag time of oxidation the greater the antioxidant capacity of the test substance. Alternatively, the ability of foodstuffs to act as reductants can be measured by assaying for the reduction of Fe^{3+} to Fe^{2+} by the foodstuff extract or of plasma (the FRAP assay, ferric antioxidant power of plasma). These biochemical assays measure only one aspect of oxidation, and since antioxidants work in a variety of ways, this type of assay only gives a crude estimate of overall antioxidant action. Using these assays, various "league tables" of the TAC of foods have been compiled [10–12]. For some foods it has been possible to correlate antioxidant activity with the level of a particular nutrient or group of nutrients. For example, there was found to be a good correlation between TAC as measured by the ABTS assay in 26 herbs and spices with their total phenolic content, suggesting that phenolic compounds contribute significantly to the TAC (Figure. 9.6) [13].

The TAC does not give an overall measure of antioxidant capacity in plasma since the antioxidant status of people is due to both directly-acting antioxidants – which are measured in these assays – and antioxidant enzymes, which are not. A more commonly-used approach in human subjects is to assay for various biomarkers of oxidative stress in plasma. Some biomarkers are associated with oxidative damage in a wide range of diseases, whereas others are more disease-specific. For example, 8-hydroxy deoxyguanosine is indicative of oxidative damage to DNA damage and can be used as a biomarker for cancer risk, whereas advanced glycation end products have been used as a biomarker for Alzheimer's disease [9]. Measuring the ratio of reduced glutathione (GSH) to glutathione disulphide (GSSG) is used as a biomarker for oxidative stress in cancer risk, CVD, Alzheimer's disease and Parkinson's disease [9]. F_2-isoprostanes are lipid peroxidation products formed from arachidonic acid, and are used both as an index of lipid peroxidation and oxidative DNA damage to white blood cells, and have been used as a biomarker for CVD and Alzheimer's disease.

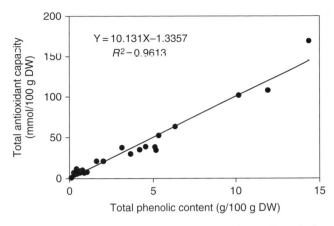

Figure 9.6 Relationship between total antioxidant capacity and total phenolic content of methanolic extracts from 26 spices [13]. With permission from American Chemical Society.

Assaying for F_2-isoprostanes is considered by many authorities to be the best method currently available for measuring lipid peroxidation *in vivo* and is preferred to MDA measurements that were previously used [14].

Oxidation of LDL particles is a commonly-used method for assessing oxidative stress, particularly in relation to CVD. LDL particles are rich in cholesterol, cholesterol esters (i.e. cholesterol linked to a fatty acid) and triglycerides packaged in an outer coat of more polar phospholipids and protein. The fatty acids (particularly PUFAs) and protein are prone to oxidation, and oxidised LDL particles (ox-LDL) are associated with the pathology of CVD (see Chapter 11). Oxidised LDL particles can be measured directly in serum samples using an enzyme-linked immunosorbent assay kit (ELISA). Alternatively, LDL particles can be isolated from plasma and incubated with Cu^{2+} to induce peroxidation. The longer the time taken for lipid peroxidation to accelerate (measured by the "lag-time"), the more resistant the particles are to oxidation.

Antioxidant assays have been used in order to help assess the possible impact of antioxidants on specific diseases. For example, the effect of antioxidants on copper-induced oxidation of LDL was used in a study to identify Mediterranean-style dishes with high antioxidant capacity [15]. Total lipids were extracted from the dishes and the inhibitory effects of the extracts on Cu-induced LDL oxidation were measured. The dishes with the highest antioxidant activities were then given over a four-week period to type 2 diabetic patients (who are at high risk of developing CVD). It was subsequently found that the plasma from patients given these dishes had a higher antioxidant capacity in an experimental assay against lipid oxidation than the plasma from patients who maintained their normal diet [15].

9.3.6   Antioxidant activity in the Mediterranean diet

"Lifetime consumption of the complex mixture of antioxidants in foods is more effective than large doses of a single antioxidant given for a finite period. The latter might deplete the endogenous antioxidant pool, thus turning an antioxidant into a prooxidant in vivo." [16]

Table 9.5 Sources of foods in the Spanish diet with *in vitro* antioxidant activity [6]. With permission from Taylor & Francis Group.

Source	Daily antioxidant capacity[1]
Nuts	176
Fruits	342
Vegetables	272
Legumes	135
Cereals	33
Beverages	
∘ Coffee	1582
∘ Wine	617
∘ Others	378
Vegetable oils	
∘ Olive	13
∘ Others	2
Total antioxidant capacity	3549

[1]Measured by ABTS method (μmol trolox equivalents).

The many antioxidants in the MedDiet come from a wide range of sources, including fruit and vegetables, nuts, extra virgin olive oil, legumes, and drinks such as coffee and wine [17]. Wild greens are also an important source of antioxidants in a more traditional MedDiet consumed in some Mediterranean countries [18]. This diversity of sources increases the likelihood of consuming antioxidants that act in different ways and may interact in beneficial ways as discussed above. An estimation of the daily contribution of antioxidant activity from various foodstuffs in the Spanish diet is shown in Table 9.5. It is interesting to note that the largest contributor in the Spanish diet (as measured by the ABTS assay) was found to be coffee.

A number of studies have examined the relationship between a MedDiet and TAC, or markers of oxidative stress, in human subjects. The PREDIMED is a randomised controlled trial assessing the effects of a traditional MedDiet on the primary prevention of CVD. The effects of a traditional MedDiet were already apparent three months into the intervention since 372 participants at high risk for CVD consuming a traditional MedDiet enriched with olive oil had significantly decreased levels of circulating ox-LDL compared to participants on a low-fat diet ($p = 0.02$) even after this relatively short period of time [16]. After three years of follow-up in the PREDIMED study, 187 subjects were randomly selected to analyse the influence of an olive oil- or nut-enriched MedDiet on plasma TAC (using the ABTS assay). Subjects in the intervention group had a significantly higher plasma TAC than control subjects. The correlation between the plasma TAC and the intervention diet was significant and independent from age and sex [19].

In a cross-sectional study from the Attica region of Greece (the ATTICA study), greater adherence to a MedDiet was correlated with higher serum TAC (coefficient of adjusted multivariate regression, R^2 29%, $p < 0.001$) and lower ox-LDL cholesterol (R^2 26%) [20]. The Twins Heart Study (THS) is a US study that allows genetic factors to be considered as possible confounding factors. Oxidative stress was measured by assaying for GSH and GSSG. A one-unit increment in the diet score was associated with a 7% higher GSH/GSSG ratio ($p = 0.03$) after adjustment for energy intake, other nutritional factors, CVD risk factors, and medication use. These results are also independent of genetic factors since the interaction test for zygosity was non-significant [21].

F_2-isoprostanes have not been measured in many of the large-scale epidemiological studies of the MedDiet despite their value as a marker for lipid peroxidation. A small study (12 subjects) did find a significant increase in vitamin C and a reduction in F2-isprostanes following consumption of *gazpacho* (a Spanish soup containing tomato, cucumber and peppers) for 14 days [22].

Antioxidant activity of phytochemicals

Although the MedDiet is an excellent source of antioxidant vitamins, minerals and phytochemicals, their roles *in vivo* as antioxidants in disease prevention have not been clearly established. This section will highlight some of the issues, particularly in relation to phytochemicals, since much of the controversy lies here.

Carotenoids

Carotenoids are important antioxidants for plants since they protect the plant against singlet oxygen that is formed during photosynthesis. Singlet oxygen is an electronically "excited" form of oxygen in which an electron has been excited into a higher orbit. This electron can be "quenched" by carotenoids due to the conjugated double bond system absorbing the excess energy.

Carotenoids may also be important for protecting humans against singlet oxygen. Singlet oxygen causes the peroxidation of lipids, particularly of vulnerable PUFAs in the lipid bilayer of cell membranes and in LDL particles. Carotenoids can prevent these actions in experimental systems. However, although carotenoids are readily absorbed by the gut, the relevance of the antioxidant activity of carotenoids in human health is unclear [8]. Two conditions in which the antioxidant activities of carotenoids are implicated are protection against LDL-oxidation (a risk factor for CVD) and reducing the risk of age-related eye disorders.

LDL -oxidation   Subjects at high risk of CVD who adopted a MedDiet were found to have reduced circulating levels of ox-LDL [16]. Antioxidants present in the MedDiet which are associated with LDL particles – and so could in principle reduce LDL oxidation – include vitamin E (α-tocopherol and γ-tocopherol) and carotenoids. Different carotenoids vary in their efficacy as inhibitors of LDL oxidation in *in vitro* assays, some commentators promoting the merits of the xanthophyl class such as astaxanthin, although there is at present no consensus on the overall merits of various carotenoids [23]. The antioxidant efficacy of carotenoids is also influenced by the presence of other antioxidants. The oleic acid content of olive oil may also contribute to a reduction in ox-LDL in subjects consuming a MedDiet since oleic acid present in LDL particles will be relatively resistant to oxidation. Hence, the relative contribution of dietary carotenoids or vitamin E to the prevention of LDL-oxidation is unclear. It is also worth noting that carotenoids can act as pro-oxidants under some circumstances, although there is no indication that this is a concern for carotenoids which are consumed as part of a MedDiet. (However, pure carotenoids are not very stable and can generate potentially toxic products, hence care is needed when taking carotenoids supplements.)

Age-related eye disorders   The potential for oxidative reactions in the eye is high since it is exposed to several sources of oxidation such as the double dangers of atmospheric oxygen and sunlight, and hence to the risk of photo-oxidation. The eye also has the highest rate of uptake of oxygen in the body due to its intense energy demands. Light triggers the formation of singlet oxygen in the eye and this can lead to lipid peroxidation. The lipids in the membranes of cells in the retina are particularly susceptible to oxidation since they are very rich in the PUFA docosahexaenoic acid (DHA). DHA is required for the correct functioning of photoreceptors. A history of exposure to sunlight (blue light) has been associated with an increased risk of age-related macular degeneration (AMD) in some studies, especially when the antioxidant status of the individual is low [24]. AMD is the most common cause of untreatable blindness in the western world with an incidence of 12% in people aged 80 years.

Not surprisingly, the eye has evolved a complex arsenal of antioxidant defences. The macular region of the retina, which surrounds the fovea and has the highest level of visual acuity, is yellow because of a high concentration of the antioxidant carotenoids lutein and zeaxanthin (also present as meso-zeaxanthin)[1]. In fact, the full name for the macular region is macula lutea which translates from the Latin as "yellow spot". It is thought that lutein and zeaxanthin protect the eye by helping prevent peroxidation of DHA in the retina caused by oxidation products such as superoxide [24]. There is a good deal of interest in determining if lutein and zeaxanthin can help prevent AMD and this is discussed in Section 13.7.

Polyphenols

Mediterranean foods contain a huge variety of phenolic compounds (see Section 2.7.3 and Chapter 5) and many of these have antioxidant activity in *in vitro* assays, in particular polyphenols, i.e. phenolics with at least two phenolic rings [27]. Two mechanisms have been postulated to explain how polyphenols act as antioxidants in *in vitro* conditions. Firstly, the hydroxyl groups on polyphenols such as flavonoids can donate an electron and scavenge a wide variety of free radicals such as superoxide, hydroxyl radical and peroxyl radicals. Secondly, many polyphenols chelate metal ions such as iron and copper that can have pro-oxidant activity in the body.

Establishing that these polyphenols are responsible for any antioxidant activity observed *in vivo* is complicated by the fact that foods may also contain non-phenolic antioxidants. Extra virgin olive oil (EVOO) contains a range of well-characterised antioxidant polyphenols. The concentrations of polyphenols varies quite widely between olive oils, so these various oils can be examined to see if there is a correlation between polyphenol content and antioxidant activity *in vivo*. Consumption of extra virgin olive oil (EVOO) was found to increase the TAC of serum in a small intervention study (12 subjects) [28]. In the so-called EUROLIVE study there was a correlation between the polyphenol content of olive oils and a reduction in markers of lipid oxidation, thus suggesting that the polyphenols in the olive oil may be responsible for the reduction in lipid oxidation seen in the subjects (reviewed in [29]).

---

[1] The retina contains specific binding proteins for zeaxanthin (glutathione-S-transferase P1) and lutein which can explain how the retina concentrates these carotenoids to concentrations that are several orders of magnitude greater than those found in the plasma [25, 26].

Although polyphenols have good *in vitro* antioxidant activity, the relevance of these observations to the situation *in vivo* is unclear. Studies found no reduction in F_2-isoprostane production – considered to be one of the best markers of oxidative stress – in subjects given a flavonoid-rich diet versus a flavonoid-poor diet and, similarly, there was no reduction in F_2-isoprostane levels in the EUROLIVE study [14]. The relevance of polyphenols *in vivo* can be questioned based on what is known about their metabolism: as discussed in Chapter 4, the concentrations of the ingested forms of most polyphenols in the plasma are very low due to rapid conjugation with glucuronate or sulphate groups. These conjugation reactions occur on the hydroxyl groups of the flavonoids, and these are the very sites that are responsible for scavenging free radicals. Studies have found that most of these conjugates have reduced antioxidant activity compared to the unconjugated forms. Based on these considerations, it is now thought that dietary polyphenols do not have good antioxidant activity in the systemic circulation, and that this is not their main mechanism of action.

There is no consensus on whether or not the antioxidant capacity of wine correlates simply with the total polyphenol content of wine or whether certain polyphenols contribute disproportionately to the antioxidant capacity [30]. Wine producers are developing wines with high polyphenol content, and there is consumer interest in purchasing these wines [31]. Health claims have been made for red wines with high polyphenol content, although an EU Food Law effective from 1 July 2007 makes it illegal to make any health claims on alcoholic beverages containing more than 1.2% alcohol.

Despite these conclusions, there are some situations where polyphenols may act as antioxidants. Although few polyphenols are in their native form by the time they reach the systemic circulation, there may still be time whilst they are in the gut for them to exert an antioxidant effect. Quite high levels of intact and unmetabolised polyphenols can occur in the stomach and many polyphenols remain unabsorbed in the small intestine, raising the possibility for antioxidant activity [14]. Although flavonoids and other polyphenols are extensively metabolised by bacteria in the colon to more simple phenolics, these metabolites may still retain some antioxidant activity, particularly by scavenging metal ions.

Based on reservations about the bioavailability of wine polyphenols and the likelihood that they retain antioxidant activity in the plasma, it has been suggested that wine polyphenols may be most active in the GI tract. i.e. before they are metabolised by the liver and elsewhere. One way that polyphenols may act in the stomach and small intestine is by reducing the formation and/or the absorption of toxic lipid oxidation products called advanced lipoxidation end-products (ALEs). ALEs are produced during digestion and it is thought that they may affect gut health or enter the circulation and promote inflammatory disorders including CVD [32].[2] One interesting study found that red wine consumed with fatty food was able to prevent the generation and absorption of cytotoxic ALEs, and this was ascribed to the polyphenols in the red wine [34]. The authors of this study suggested that in their view the main site of action of polyphenols could be in the digestive system *before* absorption, and that systemic effects are not the main sites of action. The affinity

---

[2] It should be noted however that at present the significance of ALEs in disease processes remains a controversial point [33].

beween red wine and fatty foods has long been appreciated by food lovers, and it remains to be seen if this combination may also prevent deleterious effects.

Far lower levels of intact flavonoids will be needed if they interact synergistically with other antioxidants rather than acting on their own. This provides another framework to explain how only low levels of unconjugated flavonoids may still be active as antioxidants. It is clear from *in vitro* observations that antioxidants can act in interlocking networks to recharge each other. Indications that antioxidants from foods interact after consumption is derived from observations that the antioxidant activity of extracts from fruits and vegetables is often higher than can be accounted for by individual antioxidants [35]. For example, drinking orange juice resulted in the white blood cells of the subjects having greater protection against oxidative DNA damage than could be accounted for by the vitamin C content alone, and this could be due to the vitamin C interacting with flavanones (or possibly other antioxidant phytochemicals) in the orange juice [36]. In a study with hamsters, it was found that flavonoids from almond skin acted synergistically with vitamins C and E [37]. The many antioxidant nutrients present in the MedDiet mean that there are many possibilities for synergistic interactions to occur.

A third scenario is if polyphenols are acting as antioxidants in microdomains in the body rather than having any major effects on systemic markers. For example, it has been suggested that olive oil phenolics act in the artery walls (intima) by directly preventing the oxidation of lipids in LDL and this explains why there was no effect on systemic markers such as F_2 isoprostanes [29].

Although the balance of current evidence suggests that most individual polyphenols probably do not act systemically as *direct* antioxidants, diets rich in polyphenols have often been shown to reduce markers of oxidation such as ox-LDL in blood. How can this be? One possible explanation is that flavonoids and other polyphenols act *indirectly* as antioxidants by inducing the expression of genes encoding antioxidant enzymes. This is discussed in Section 9.6.2.

9.3.7   Limitations of the dietary antioxidant theory

It is evident from the previous discussion that a role for the antioxidant properties of phytochemicals is far from resolved. Some of the issues are summarised here:

1. If oxidative stress is an important aspect of the pathology of various chronic disorders then it would be expected that antioxidant therapy would show clear benefits. However, several major trials with antioxidants have failed to show any benefits, and indeed some supplements have had harmful effects [38].
2. Only micromolar or nanomolar concentrations of dietary antioxidants are usually present in plasma or some organs of the body, and these concentrations are significantly lower (by an order of magnitude) than some endogenous antioxidants such as glutathione, and are thought to be too low to protect against hydroxyl radicals [39]. This is particularly evident for flavonoids, where the low plasma concentrations are due to poor absorption by the gut and extensive metabolism.
3. Metabolism of flavonoids to various conjugates significantly alters their redox potential.
4. It has been argued that the increase in antioxidant capacity of plasma observed after consuming a meal rich in flavonoids is due not to an increase in plasma

flavonoid levels, but instead to an increase in urate levels [40]. Fruits, and some vegetables, contain relatively high levels of sugars such as fructose and sorbitol, which can increase the production of urate in the body.

5. There is now good evidence that ROS play an important role in cell signalling by normal, healthy cells. This is supported by the fact that the redox status in the body is under strict homeostatic control. Hence, it is possible that high doses of antioxidants could have a detrimental effect by inhibiting cell signalling pathways that are necessary for health.

6. A number of other plausible cellular mechanisms that can explain the health benefits of antioxidant phytochemicals have now been identified (e.g. see Section 9.5).

It is worth ending this section by quoting this cautionary statement by one of the most eminent researchers in the field of antioxidants, Professor Halliwell: "Despite decades of research, it is currently impossible to state what, if any, contribution is made to the health-promoting effects of fruits and vegetables by the antioxidants present" [41].

9.4   Inflammation

Diseases associated with an inflammatory response include rheumatoid arthritis, diabetes, neurodegenerative diseases, atherosclerosis and cancer. It is also now thought that inflammation is important in obesity. The specific role of inflammation in the pathology of these diseases is discussed more fully in Chapters 10–13, and this chapter discusses more general aspects of inflammation.

9.4.1   The inflammatory response

The body responds to infection or injury by initiating an inflammatory response (Figure 9.7). This includes an increase in blood flow, and an increase in the permeability of capillaries which allows white blood cells and large molecules, such as complement, antibodies and cytokines, to leave the blood stream and cross the endothelial wall. The inflammatory response initiates an immunological response to eliminate invading pathogens and toxins. These responses are carefully regulated. Adhesion molecules (such as intercellular adhesion molecule 1 (ICAM-1), vascular cell adhesion molecule 1 (VCAM-1) and E-selection) are up-regulated on endothelial cells, and this allows white blood cells, such as granulocytes, monocytes and lymphocytes, to bind. These then pass across endothelial cells, and in the underlying tissue they are stimulated to produce various cytokines (including tumour necrosis factor α (TNFα), interleukin-1 (IL-1), IL-6 and IL-8), some eicosanoids[3], nitric oxide (NO) and enzymes known as matrix metalloproteinases (MMPs). These factors act locally to regulate the inflammatory and immunological responses. Some cytokines also act systemically by causing fever or by stimulating the liver to produce so-called acute phase proteins, e.g. IL-6 induces the liver to produce C-reactive protein (CRP).

---

[3] A family of signalling molecules including prostaglandins (PGs), prostacyclins (PCs), thromboxanes (TXs), and leukotrienes (LTs).

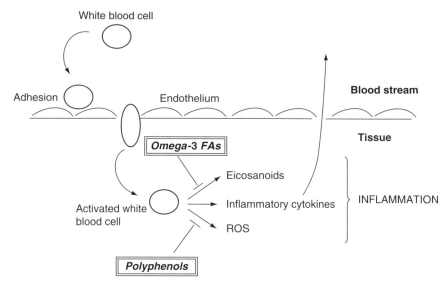

Figure 9.7   Steps in an inflammatory response.
⊣ = inhibits.

Mediators in the systemic circulation such as TNFα, IL-1, IL-6 and CRP are useful inflammatory markers that are readily measured in blood samples. Although inflammation is a normal response to injury, it can become uncontrolled in chronic conditions and this can result in tissue damage.

9.4.2   The MedDiet and inflammation

A number of epidemiological studies have examined the relationship between consumption of a MedDiet and inflammatory markers. The effect of a MedDiet on circulating markers of inflammation was assessed in a large cohort of subjects asymptomatic, but at high risk, for CVD (participants in the PREDIMED study). The consumption of certain components of the MedDiet, namely fruits, cereals, virgin olive oil and nuts, was associated with lower serum concentrations of inflammatory markers, especially those related to endothelial function, although this was only statistically significant for fruit or cereal consumption for IL-6 (p=0.005 for both), nut consumption for ICAM-1 (p=0.003) and virgin olive oil consumption for VCAM-1 (p=0.02) [42]. There was no statistically significant relationship between overall adherence to a MedDiet and inflammatory markers in this study. By contrast, adherence to a MedDiet was associated with reduced levels of IL-6 (p<0.001) (but not CRP) in a group of middle-aged American men asymptomatic for CVD [43].

In a randomised controlled trial of German patients with coronary artery disease, there was no effect of a MedDiet on inflammatory biomarkers related to vascular injury and also on metabolic plasma molecules [44]. It has been argued that this negative finding could have been due to failure of the intervention group to adhere to virgin olive oil consumption, a potentially important food for the anti-inflammatory effects of the MedDiet, or that the control group may also have changed their diet [45]. A small study (12 subjects) that looked at the effects of olive oil found that

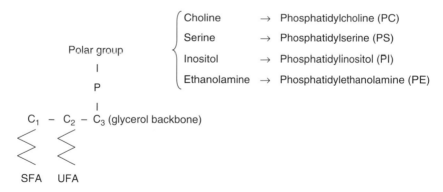

Figure 9.8 Typical structure of a phospholipid. P: phosphate group; SFA: saturated fatty acid; UFA: unsaturated fatty acid.

post-prandial levels of the eicosanoids TXB2 and LTB4 were lower in subjects consuming EVOO compared to control subjects consuming OO or corn oil [28]. There was no effect of non-virgin olive oil (or corn oil), suggesting that polyphenols in the EVOO may have been responsible for these effects. A cross-sectional study on 1514 subjects asymptomatic for CVD from the ATTICA region of Greece showed that fish consumers (>300 g per week) had significantly lower markers of various inflammatory markers, including IL-6, CRP and TNFα (all $p < 0.05$), than non-fish eaters [46].

In summary, a number of foods present in the MedDiet, including EVOO, nuts, fish, fruits and vegetables, have been demonstrated to have anti-inflammatory properties. In addition, the MedDiet is typically low in foods thought to promote inflammation, including meats, processed foods and dairy products. Components in the MedDiet with possible anti-inflammatory activity include n-3 FAs from fish, and various phenolics found in olive oil (such as oleocanthal) and fruits and vegetables (especially flavonoids). Possible mechanisms for the anti-inflammatory actions of these constituents will now be discussed.

9.4.3   *n-3* Fatty acids

n-3 fatty acids are the starting material for the production of various anti-inflammatory eicosanoids, and to understand how a diet rich in *n-3* FAs is associated with a reduction in some inflammatory disorders it is necessary to consider:

1. how dietary FAs are incorporated into the membranes of inflammatory cells
2. how these fats are used for the production of eicosanoids with anti-inflammatory actions

Dietary FAs and cell membranes

Phospholipids are the principal components of cell membranes. Phospholipids consist of a 3 carbon glycerol backbone bound to two fatty acids and to a phosphate group which is in turn joined to another small polar group (Figure 9.8).

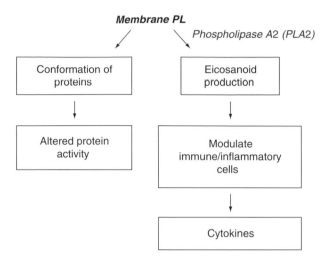

Figure 9.9 Effects of membrane phospholipids on cellular processes.

The fatty acid at C_1 (sn-1) is usually saturated whereas the fatty acid at C_2 (sn-2) is usually unsaturated. Two major factors affecting the fatty acid composition of membrane PLs are:

1. location – e.g. PLs in the membranes of retinal cells are rich in docosahexaenoic acid (DHA)
2. diet – e.g. dietary oily fish increases the EPA content of membrane PLs

The FA composition of PLs has two major influences (Figure 9.9). Firstly, it affects the conformation of proteins embedded in the membrane and this in turn will affect their activity, e.g. DHA influences the conformation of rhodopsin in the retina. Secondly, some PUFAs are used to generate eicosanoids. Eicosanoids are factors that act locally and influence immune and inflammatory cells e.g. by regulating the production of cytokines (some of which can then act systemically).

Production of anti-inflammatory eicosanoids

Eicosanoids are principally generated from the 20-carbon PUFAs arachidonic acid (AA) and eicosapentaenoic acid (EPA), and also from the 22-carbon PUFA DHA. Inflammatory cells contain a high proportion of AA, so this is usually the main substrate for eicosanoid synthesis. AA is cleaved from PLs (mostly PC) by phospholipase A_2. AA is then converted into various prostaglandins (PGs) and thromboxanes (TXs) by the enzyme cyclooxygenase (COX), and to leukotrienes (LTs) by lipoxygenase (LOX) (Figure 9.10). These are sometimes referred to as 2-series PGs and 4-series LTs. The specific eicosanoids that are generated depend on the cell type and specific enzymes present in these cells. Although the precise roles of these various eicosanoids are complicated, the general effect is pro-inflammatory. Hence, a diet that leads to high levels of AA in the membranes of inflammatory cells (such as a diet high in red meat) will tend to have a pro-inflammatory effect since increased consumption of AA seems to be associated with an increased production of inflammatory eicosanoids, although not necessarily of inflammatory

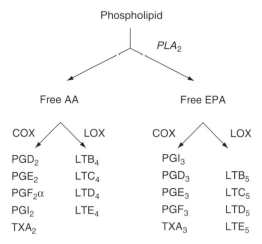

Figure 9.10   Synthesis of eicosanoids from AA and EPA [48].

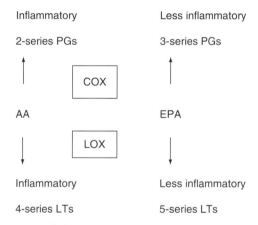

Figure 9.11   Relative potency of eicosanoids derived from AA and EPA.

cytokines [47]. AA is also produced in the body from LA, but the precise relationship between intake of LA and an increase in AA has not been fully established.

Consumption of fish oils increases the amount of EPA and DHA in membrane PLs and decreases the amount of AA. This has been found to reduce the production of pro-inflammatory eicosanoids from AA. Importantly, like AA, EPA and DHA are substrates for COX and LOX and fish oil consumption results in the production of relatively more eicosanoids derived from these PUFAs. Eicosanoids from EPA, referred to as 3-series PGs and 5-series LTs, are different to those derived from AA and tend to be less inflammatory (Figure 9.11). Recently, a new family of eicosanoids derived from either EPA or DHA has been identified. These so-called resolvins are potent anti-inflammatory eicosanoids and may be responsible for many of the anti-inflammatory effects of consuming EPA and DHA [49]. Although there is some conversion of dietary ALA into EPA, the role of dietary ALA intake on the subsequent production of anti-inflammatory eicosanoids derived from EPA has not been fully established [47].

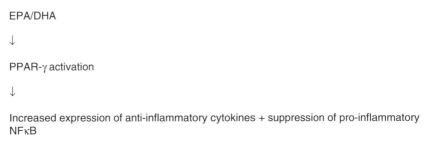

Less important pathway?	More important pathway?
EPA/DHA	EPA/DHA
↓	↓
Anti-inflammatory eicosanoids	Immune cell
↓	↓
Immune cells	Altered gene expression
↓	↓
Reduced pro-inflammatory cytokine production	Altered cytokine production

Figure 9.12   Two possible mechanisms by which EPA and DHA can affect cytokine production.

EPA/DHA

↓

PPAR-γ activation

↓

Increased expression of anti-inflammatory cytokines + suppression of pro-inflammatory NFκB

Figure 9.13   PPAR-γ mediated anti-inflammatory effects of EPA/DHA.

Cytokine production

As well as reducing the production of eicosanoids, fish oil consumption also decreases the production of inflammatory cytokines such as TNFα, IL-1 and IL-6. Although some of these effects may be via modulation of eicosanoid production, it appears that alterations in gene expression may be more important [49] (Figure 9.12).

One target for EPA and DHA which results in altered cytokine gene expression is the transcription factor PPAR-γ (Figure 9.13). Activation of PPAR-γ may directly result in the production of anti-inflammatory cytokines, and also suppress activation of the pro-inflammatory transcription factor NFκB.

9.4.4   Phenolics

Two ways by which phenolics can potentially exert anti-inflammatory effects are: (1) by acting as antioxidants; and (2) by inhibiting pro-inflammatory enzymes.

ROS can induce the production of pro-inflammatory cytokines via activation of the transcription factor NFκB, one the most important transcription factors for cytokine gene expression (see below). Hence, by neutralising ROS, the antioxidant activity of polyphenols can potentially exert an anti-inflammatory effect. Extracts from a number of wild food plants from the Calabria region of Italy with *in vitro* antioxidant activity were found to inhibit croton oil-induced ear oedema in mice,

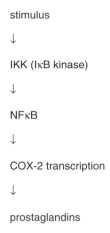

stimulus

↓

IKK (IκB kinase)

↓

NFκB

↓

COX-2 transcription

↓

prostaglandins

Figure 9.14   Induction of COX-2.

an animal model for inflammation, although it was not established which of the plant constituents, such as flavonoids and plant sterols, may have been responsible for this effect [50].

Phenolics inhibit many enzymes associated with inflammation [51]. For example, some flavonoids inhibit PLA_2, but generally quite high concentrations are required. Perhaps of greater interest are the effects on LOX and COX enzymes. COX exists in two forms (isoenzymes). COX-1 is generally considered to be a "house-keeping" enzyme in most tissues since it catalyses the production of various eicosanoids that are required for normal cell function, it is constitutively present in cells and its levels do not change in response to stimuli. By contrast, COX-2 is rapidly induced during inflammation by various stimuli such as growth factors and cytokines via activation of the transcription factor NFκB (Figure 9.14). Overexpression of COX-2 is associated with a number of pathological conditions such as colorectal cancer, and there is a good deal of interest in specifically targeting COX-2 to prevent this cancer.

Phytochemicals in the MedDiet can act by either (1) directly inhibiting the enzyme activity of COX-2, or (2) by *indirectly* inhibiting COX-2 by inhibiting the pathway that leads to its production, i.e. inhibiting COX-2 transcription. For example, both flavonoids and flavonoid metabolites inhibit COX-2 transcription, and since most flavonoids exist in the body as metabolites and not as the parent molecule, this is potentially an important mechanism by which flavonoids could be exerting beneficial effects in the body [52–54]. In addition, some flavonoids directly inhibit the activity of COX-2. Phenolics in extra virgin olive oil (EVOO) may also have anti-inflammatory activity due to inhibition of COX enzymes. Consumption of EVOO was found to reduce the levels of the pro-inflammatory cytokines TXB_2 and LTB_4 in 12 human subjects after consuming an EVOO-rich meal compared to either an OO- or corn oil-rich meal [28]. This effect was not seen after consuming more processed olive oil, suggesting that it is the phenolic fraction in EVOO that is responsible for this effect. EVOO contains a phenolic called oleocanthal that inhibits the activities of COX 1 and 2 enzymes, and this could be contributing to the anti-inflammatory effect of EVOO [55].

9.4.5   Pro-inflammatory foods

A number of nutrients that enhance inflammation, such as trans fatty acids (TFAs) and foods with a high glycaemic index, are consumed in only low amounts in a traditional MedDiet. Technologically-produced TFAs were absent from traditional Med-Diets and their consumption is still low in modern MedDiets [56]. TFAs have been found to raise serum levels of various inflammatory markers such as CRP. Lowering the glycaemic index of a meal is also associated with a reduction in CRP levels [57].

9.5   Modulation of cell signalling pathways by phenolics

The realisation that the beneficial effects of flavonoids probably cannot be explained simply by their antioxidant activity stimulated scientists to look for alternative mechanisms of action for these, and similar, compounds. Many flavonoids have been shown to inhibit intracellular signalling pathways. Flavonoids and other phenolics have a bewildering range of effects on cell signalling pathways: pathways may be inhibited or stimulated and the same phenolic may have opposite effects on different cell types, and opposite effects at different concentrations. However, the evidence that the anti-proliferative effects of some flavonoids on cancer cells is due, at least in part, to inhibition of cell signalling is generally considered to be quite strong.

9.5.1   Cell signalling pathways in disease

Signalling pathways control fundamental aspects of a cell such as death, survival and proliferation [58]. Signalling pathways are initiated by a signal such as a growth factor or cytokine that then results in activation of a series of components resulting in a cell response. The signal passing down these components is referred to as signal transduction. Many of these molecules are proteins and a key change that they undergo when registering a signal is by becoming phosphorylated. Protein phosphorylation is cata-lysed by protein kinases, and these can act both to phosphorylate a protein substrate and to be substrates themselves for other protein kinases (Figure 9.15). Protein kinases are enzymes that use ATP as a source of phosphate for phosphorylating proteins.

Flavonoids have been shown to inhibit a number of protein kinases involved in signalling pathways (see Figure 9.15). The flavonoids usually inhibit protein kinases by binding to the site on the protein kinase that normally binds ATP, thus preventing ATP from binding (in enzymological parlance, the flavonoid is acting as a competitive inhibitor), and hence the protein kinase no longer has a source of phosphate with which to phosphorylate its target. A flavonoid may inhibit many protein kinases and so inhibit many signalling pathways. The overall outcome generally seems to be favourable, and it has been suggested that the anti-tumour activity of flavonoids in animal models of cancer may, at least in part, be due to inhibition of signalling pathways associated with cell proliferation [58]. Flavonoids can also inhibit signalling pathways associated with cell survival and this promotes cell death (apoptosis) – another important mechanism for arresting the growth of a tumour (Figure 9.15). Flavonoids also specifically *activate* signalling pathways that increase apoptosis.

As discussed above, a major criticism levelled against the hypothesis that flavonoids act as antioxidants in the systemic circulation is that most flavonoids are present in the body as metabolites, and these metabolites have greatly reduced antioxidant

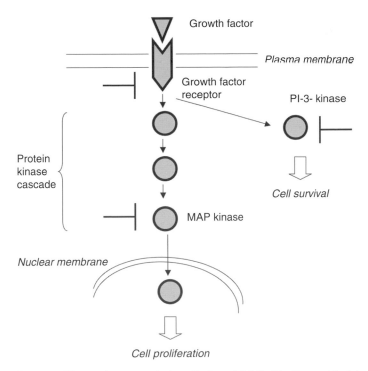

Figure 9.15   Cell signalling pathways and steps that are inhibited by flavonoids (shown by ⊣).

activity. By contrast, there is some limited evidence that flavonoid metabolites retain inhibitory effects against signalling molecules and also that the parent flavonoid molecules can, in some cases, be active at quite low concentrations [58]. However, it is clear that more work needs to be done in this area in order to clarify the precise role of phenolics as inhibitors of signalling pathways.

9.6   Gene interactions

> *"Nutrition can no longer be viewed as simply epidemiological studies whose aims are to identify relationships between nutrition and chronic disease in genetically uncharacterized populations; rather, complex cell and molecular biology coupled with biochemistry and genetics are required if the ambitious goals of nutrigenomics are to be realized."* [59]

Increased understanding of the relationship between genes and diet is revolutionising nutrition. The science of nutrigenetics is used to study how the genetic make-up (genotype) of an individual influences their response to dietary components, and their risk of developing diet-related diseases. Nutrigenomics is used to study how dietary components alter the expression of genes affecting health. These relationships are shown in Figure 9.16.

9.6.1   Genetic predisposition to diet – nutrigenetics

The genome of an individual is an important determinant of that person's response to diet (see box below). The human genome consists of about 20,000–25,000 genes,

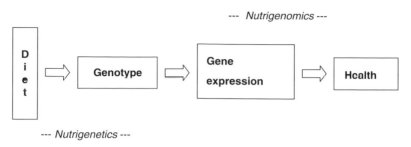

Figure 9.16   Nutrigenomics and nutrigenetics.

but not all of these genes are of equal importance in relation to diet and disease. Those of particular importance are referred to as "candidate" genes or "susceptibility" genes. Candidate genes will usually have an important role in a disease process and may be responsive to changes in diet. Genetic heterogeneity between populations is now thought to be one of the main reasons for the variability seen between epidemiological studies examining the link between diet and health.

A short primer on human genetics

The human genome comprises approximately 3.2×10^9 nucleotides organised into 23 pairs of chromosomes. It includes about 20,000–25,000 genes that encode cellular proteins and RNA. However, only about 2% of the genome encodes genes, and most DNA is termed non-coding and has structural or regulatory roles or is of unknown function. A single gene can encode more than one RNA or protein due to changes that occur after transcription: these are termed post- transcriptional and post-translational changes. These changes involve modifications such as alternative splicing of RNA or differential methylation. The consequence of these processes is that there are over 100, 000 proteins with distinct primary sequences (ie sequences of amino acids) in human cells.

The primary sequence of nucleotides varies by approximately 0.2%–0.4% between individuals. These variations are referred to as polymorphisms and are a molecular reason for phenotypic variations between people. Variations in single nucleotides between individuals, known as SNPs (single nucleotide polymorphisms), are a major source of variation in human DNA. These variations are due to substitution of one base pair for another (A, T, G or C) or, less frequently, to insertions or deletions of bases.

Genetic heterogeneity between people results from polymorphisms in genes. Polymorphic genes are those that occur in a population in two or more forms. A particular polymorphism that confers an advantage can become enriched in a population by natural selection. One widely-studied example is lactose tolerance that displays positive selection in certain geographical regions where there are nutritional benefits for drinking milk. It has also been hypothesised that there may have been positive selection for beneficial polymorphisms associated with diet in the Mediterranean region.

Evolutionary aspects of polymorphisms

It is possible that enrichment of particular polymorphisms may have occurred during evolution in the Mediterranean region. The type of food supply and its relative abundance influences the expansion of polymorphisms, and hence polymorphisms are not evenly distributed throughout populations. The consumption of wild greens in the Mediterranean may represent an example of positive selection. Man has consumed wild greens over many thousands of years, and well before agriculture was invented, and so there has been a long time for adaption to occur to enable positive selection of detoxification mechanisms that will enable potentially toxic plants to be consumed. Hence, it has been postulated that certain benefits of a MedDiet could be more likely in Mediterranean people than others since Mediterranean people may have evolved the best genetic make-up to most benefit from components in the MedDiet [60].

The most common genetic polymorphisms are due to single nucleotide polymorphisms (SNPs). These are single base pair differences between two or more forms of the same gene. SNPs are not the same thing as mutations: the most common form of an SNP must, by definition, occur at a prevalence of no more than 90% in the population, and SNPs occur in the germline and so are heritable whereas most mutations occur in somatic (i.e. non-germ) cells. It is estimated that there are more than 10 million SNPs in the human genome [61, 62]. Many candidate genes are polymorphic within a population.

The importance of polymorphisms in genes in relation to disease can be illustrated by considering CVD. Low fat diets are generally considered to be associated with a reduced risk of CVD. However, there is considerable variability between individuals in their responses to this type of diet, and some individuals in fact exhibit a response associated with an increased risk of atherogenesis, rather than a decreased risk as might be expected from a low fat diet. Genetic differences, for example in SNPs, are a main reason for this variability of response between individuals. An epidemiological study carried out to examine susceptibility to heart attack in a Greek population analysed as part of the EPIC programme included analysis of polymorphisms. Composite analysis of 11 genetic polymorphisms indicated that together they accounted for a significant proportion (approx. 22%) of the risk of having a heart attack in this Greek population [63]. However, most epidemiological studies do not take genetic background into account, thus highlighting the limitations of these studies.

Evidence for the importance of interactions between SNPs and metabolic responses to a MedDiet has come from the Medi-RIVAGE study. In this study, participants with a habitual western-type diet and moderate cardiovascular risks (hypercholesterolaemia, hypertriglyceridaemia, elevated BMI or hypertension) were advised to eat either a low-fat diet or a Mediterranean type-diet for three months. Correlations analysed in the whole study sample were observed between cardiovascular risk factors (such as total plasma cholesterol) and SNPs in genes associated with regulating cholesterol secretion and uptake such as apo B (the main apoprotein of LDL and VLDL) and apo E (an apoprotein in LDL, VLDL and chylomicrons) [64]. SNPs have also been shown to influence the response of individuals to putative anti-cancer phytochemicals such as sulforaphane and folate (see Section 4.3.7).

9.6.2   Effects of diet on gene expression

The effect of diet on the expression of proteins is traditionally studied by examining changes in single biomarkers, i.e. well characterised factors related to a disease state, such as cholesterol or CRP in the case of CVD. A limitation of these biomarkers is that they are single changes, and they are based on a presumed understanding of the disease process. Hence, novel mechanisms of action of dietary factors will be missed.

There is now good evidence that many substances in the MedDiet modulate gene expression, and this is likely to contribute to its protective effects. A normal diet will be associated with multiple changes in genes and biochemical pathways, and many of these have the potential to influence a disease process. Important new technological advances, particularly using microarray technology, now enable the simultaneous analysis of the expression of many genes and proteins in response to a dietary component or to a complete diet. The names of the various sciences that simultaneously analyse many different components use the suffix "ome" which means "complete" or "all". Several of these omic sciences are being applied to nutrition research. The study of multiple gene changes is referred to as genomics – or, more specifically, as nutrigenomics when it relates to changes in multiple genes in response to diet. The study of changes to multiple proteins is referred to as proteomics (although the corresponding term "nutriproteomics" is not yet widely used). Other omics of relevance to nutrition are transcriptomics which analyses mRNA, and metabolomics which analyses metabolites. Omics are beginning to have a profound effect on epidemiological studies, particularly nutrigenomics, since the technology is currently the most advanced in this area. Not only can omic approaches simultaneously examine multiple changes, but no *a priori* assumptions about disease processes are made, hence opening up the possibility of identifying novel mechanisms of action for dietary components.

Two important constituents in the MedDiet that influence gene expression are phytochemicals and fatty acids. These changes are being studied using both conventional single gene approaches and by nutrigenomics.

Phytochemicals

Phytochemicals have been shown to modulate the activity of a number of transcription factors. Transcription factors are proteins that induce new gene expression, and most bind onto the promotor regions of genes. Several genes may share the same promotor region, and genes encoding several proteins can be co-induced by the same transcription factor.

Phytochemicals can modulate the activity of transcription factors in both normal cells and pathologically altered cells (see Figure 9.17):

- In normal cells, phytochemicals can activate transcription factors that then induce the expression of genes encoding various defence proteins. Examples of defence proteins are those that increase the resistance of cells to potentially damaging insults such as oxidants and electrophiles: this has been dubbed a "cytoprotective" response.
- In "activated" or "abnormal" cells, such as activated inflammatory cells or cells that are in the early stages of forming a tumour (i.e. the early stages of carcinogenesis), phytochemicals can suppress over-active transcription factors and so return a cell to a baseline or normal function.

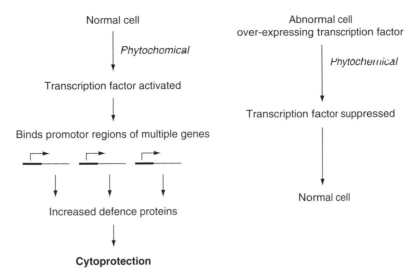

Figure 9.17 Modulation of gene expression by phytochemicals in normal and abnormal cells.

Table 9.6 Cytoprotective proteins induced by Nrf2.

Metabolic process	Protein involved	Role
Phase 2 metabolism	glutathione transferases (GSTs)	conjugates molecules with glutathione
	UDP-glucuronosyltrans-ferases (UGTs)	conjugates molecules with glucuronate
	quinone reductase (NAD(P)H: quinone oxidoreductase)	reduces quinones
Antioxidant proteins	haem oxygenase	degrades haem
	γ-glutamylcysteine synthase	synthesises glutathione
	glutathione reductase	regenerates reduced glutathione
	glutathione peroxidase	removes hydrogen peroxide using reduced glutathione
	catalase	removes hydrogen peroxide
	ferritin	stores iron
	thioredoxin	quenches free radicals

Phytochemicals modulate a number of transcription factors, either by increasing or decreasing their activity, and the next section considers some which may play a role in the protective effects of a MedDiet.

Cytoprotection of normal cells
One of the most important transcription factors induced by phytochemicals is called Nrf2. Nrf2 binds to a promotor region on genes known as the anti-oxidant response element (ARE). Many different genes contain the ARE and can be co-ordinately expressed following activation of Nrf2. Examples of genes induced by Nrf2 are those that encode phase 2 detoxifying enzymes and antioxidant proteins (Table 9.6).

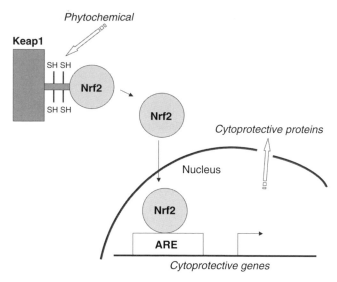

Figure 9.18   Induction of cytoprotective proteins by phytochemicals.

Increased expression of phase 2 enzymes and antioxidant proteins reduces the likelihood of tumours developing (see Chapter 12), and this may be an important mechanism by which some phytochemicals may help prevent cancer. For example, sulforaphane protects against carcinogen-induced tumours in animal models and this protective effect is lost in animals lacking Nrf2 (Nrf2 knockouts), elegantly demonstrating the essential role of Nrf2 for this protection [65]. Resveratrol protects endothelial cells against oxidative stress *in vitro* and in animal models in an Nrf2-dependent manner [66]. Other phytochemicals consumed as part of a MedDiet that have been shown to act in an Nrf2-dependent way include isoliquiritigenein found in shallots, caffeic acid phenethyl ester present in honey, carnosol in rosemary, diallyl sulphide in garlic and quercetin in onions [67]. It should be noted that it has not been established if consuming a MedDiet results in plasma concentrations of these phytochemicals sufficient to activate Nrf2.

Although a diverse range of phytochemicals can activate Nrf2, they all act via a common mechanism, namely by reacting with sulphydryl (i.e. thiol or SH) groups on a protein called Keap1 (Figure 9.18). Normally Nrf2 is kept in an inactive form in the cell by binding to Keap1. This binding requires the presence of the sulphydryl groups on Keap1. Phytochemicals that interact with the SH groups cause the dissociation of Keap1 from Nrf2. Nrf2 is then free to bind to the anti-oxidant response element (ARE) and activate the transcription of cytoprotective genes.

Restoration of normal function
Many disease processes, including cancer, neurological disorders and CVD, are associated with chronic inflammation. Transcription factors are activated in inflammatory cells and may be over-expressed in abnormal cells, such as premalignant

cells. Hence, suppressing the activation of these transcription factors can help revert these cells back to a base-line function. Inflammatory stimuli produced at sites of inflammation can up-regulate a transcription factor known as NFκB (NF kappa B) in peripheral blood cells and other target cells. NFκB in turn increases the expression of genes associated with inflammation, and this can help perpetuate a chronic inflammatory state via a positive feedback mechanism. For example, various inflammatory cytokines and oxidised-LDL are implicated in the development of atherosclerosis, and these activate NFκB in cells that in turn causes the transcription of inflammatory genes.

Several studies have evaluated the ability of a MedDiet rich in VOO to suppress the activation of NFκB and of other genes associated with a pro-atherogenic state. A MedDiet rich in VOO was found to decrease NFκB activation in mononuclear cells in 16 healthy men compared to the level of NFκB activation resulting from a Western diet [68]. However, this study did not establish whether or not it was constituents in the VOO or in some other foodstuffs in the MedDiet that were responsible for this effect. A second study used a nutrigenomics approach to analyse the effect of a MedDiet on the expression of a number of pro-atherogenic genes in the monocytes of 49 subjects within the PREDIMED study with one or two cardiovascular risk factors such as overweight, diabetes or elevated blood pressure. A traditional MedDiet enriched in VOO prevented an increase in various pro-inflammatory genes compared to participants on a control diet or a traditional MedDiet enriched in nuts [69]. Hence, this study suggested that constituents in virgin olive oil may be responsible for reducing the expression of pro-atherogenic genes. Although this study did not determine whether the polyphenols or the MUFA content of the virgin olive oil were responsible, this can be evaluated by using oils with different polyphenol contents. One such randomised control trial in healthy volunteers (n = 90), used a nutrigenomics approach to study the effect of a traditional MedDiet supplemented with a polyphenol-rich olive oil on pro-oxidative and pro-inflammatory genes. The traditional MedDiet resulted in a significantly greater decrease in pro-atherogenic genes, and the polyphenol-rich olive oil supplemented diet was also shown to induce a significantly higher decrease in the expression of most of these genes compared with the results observed in the group of participants consuming their usual diet. This decrease was higher than the decrease observed with a similar diet supplemented with a low polyphenol olive oil although the difference was not significant, but a significant trend was observed comparing the decrease in expression of atherosclerosis-related genes associated with consumption of the usual diet, the diet supplemented with a low polyphenol olive oil and the polyphenol-rich olive oil supplemented diet. This suggests that polyphenols in the olive oil are making a significant contribution to the overall effect of the traditional MedDiet [70].

A similar conclusion was reached from a double-blinded, randomised, crossover designed study in 20 patients with metabolic syndrome. Microarray analysis identified 98 differentially expressed genes (79 under-expressed and 19 over-expressed) when comparing the intake of a phenol-rich olive oil with a low-phenol olive oil [71]. In the 26 genes related with a high probability to "inflammatory diseases", two genes showed a decreased expression, namely IL1B (p = 0.006) and PTGS2 (p = 0.118), as compared to low-phenol olive oil intake. These effects could contribute to reduced inflammation during the postprandial period. In addition, EGR2, over-expressed in type 2 diabetes, was also found to be significantly repressed (p = 0.014) [71].

Genes mediated by NFκB as well as genes associated with obesity, dyslipidaemia and type 2 diabetes could also be decreased by phenol-rich olive oil. Although these studies demonstrate the important role that polyphenols in virgin olive oil have on genes associated with CVD and metabolic syndrome, the relative contribution of these observations to the overall protective effect of virgin olive oil, or indeed of the overall MedDiet, is not known. Several other dietary phytochemicals found in the MedDiet, such as metabolites from red wine, have also been shown to suppress the expression of multiple genes, including NFκB [72].

One of the advantages mentioned earlier of omics over conventional approaches is the ability to examine multiple changes in genes or proteins without any *a priori* knowledge of the mechanism involved. An illustration of the benefits of this approach was a transcriptomic analysis (i.e. examining mRNA expression) that studied how the polyphenol catechin reduces the development of atherosclerotic lesions in apo E-deficient mice. Gene expression was examined in samples from the aortas of the mice and the expression of 450 genes was found to be altered in the catechin-treated mice. These mice showed no changes in other parameters frequently implicated in the benefits of catechin such as antioxidant and anti-inflammatory effects, and the transcriptomic approach allowed an empirical analysis of a wide range of changes without making any *a priori* assumptions about how catechin may be working [73].

Epigenetic regulation
Epigenetics refers to the regulation of gene activity and expression by changes in DNA methylation, and by modifications to histones such as the addition of acetyl and methyl groups. Modifying the activity of enzymes that add these methyl or acetyl groups can thus influence gene expression. Epigenetic changes are involved in many disease processes, including cancer, CVD and neurological diseases. Hence phytochemicals that modify epigenetic changes may also modify these disease processes.

An enzyme causing epigenetic changes that has attracted a good deal of attention is sirtuin 1 (Sirt1). Changes in Sirt1 activity are associated with an increase in longevity in various organisms. Sirt1 is a deacetylase enzyme that removes acetyl groups from histones and from a variety of transcription factors that mediate cellular responses to fasting, insulin, and inflammation [74]. Resveratrol, a polyphenol found in red wine, is an activator of the Sirt1 deacetylase, and resveratrol fed to animals has a range of positive health effects (see Chapter 7). However, the role of dietary resveratrol in human health is controversial (see Chapter 7).

Fatty acids

Since a MedDiet is associated with a high consumption of olive oil, nuts, fish and some oil-rich plant foods, it is particularly rich in a variety of monounsaturated and polyunsaturated fatty acids (OA, EPA, DHA, ALA). Increasing evidence suggests that these fatty acids can influence disease processes by modulating gene expression. Although much of this information currently comes from *in vitro* and animal studies, human studies are now taking place. Since fatty acid consumption influences many chronic diseases including cancer, CVD, neurological diseases, obesity, arthritis, osteoporosis and diabetes, it is of great interest to understand how these dietary factors may influence gene expression.

Table 9.7 Distribution and function of PPARs.

PPAR	Main tissue (other tissues)	Main functions
PPAR-α	liver (heart, muscle)	fatty acid oxidation
PPAR-γ	adipose tissue	fat cell (adipocyte) formation, lipid storage
PPAR-β/δ	throughout body, but low in liver	fatty acid oxidation, energy homeostasis

PPARs – transcription factors that bind fatty acids

Long chain monounsaturated fatty acids and long chain polyunsaturated fatty acids (LC-PUFAs) and some of their metabolites (such as prostaglandins and leukotrienes) are particularly important in regulating gene expression. One of the most important families of transcription factors that bind LC-PUFAs are known as the PPARs. PPAR is the abbreviation for peroxisome proliferator-activated receptor. This somewhat obscure-sounding name derives from the observation that PPARs act as receptors for substances that activate the proliferation of peroxisomes – organelles that contribute to the oxidation of fatty acids. However, it is now known that the roles of PPARs extend well beyond regulating fatty acid oxidation, and include effects on lipid storage and many other aspects of cell metabolism such as carbohydrate metabolism, immune modulation, inflammation and the proliferation, differentiation and survival of cells. These diverse effects are possible since there are several sub-types of PPARs that differ in their tissue distribution and effects on cell metabolism (see Table 9.7). The diverse functions of PPARs are implicated in many pathological processes ranging from obesity to CVD, diabetes, cancer and others.

PUFAS, PPARs and obesity

Many of the effects of dietary PUFAs on the concentrations of fat in tissues and in the circulation are mediated by dietary PUFAs affecting gene transcription [75]. A few hours after feeding animals a diet rich in PUFAs, there is a rapid and sustained activation of genes that result in lipid oxidation and a decrease in genes that result in lipid synthesis [76]. The suppression of lipogenic genes by PUFAs in the liver, the central organ that regulates whole body lipid metabolism, even overrides the pro-lipogenic effects of insulin and carbohydrates which is high after a meal [76].

The effects of PUFAs on gene transcription are mediated by PUFAs binding to (i.e. acting as ligands for) various nuclear receptors and transcription factors. These include PPARs, liver X receptor (LXR), hepatocyte nuclear factor-4 alpha (HNF-4α) and sterol regulatory element binding protein (SREBP). These various factors act as fat sensors and have major metabolic effects in the body. To take one example, PUFAs function as activator ligands for PPARα in the liver. PPARα induces genes involved in lipid oxidation, and hence reduces the fatty acid load in the liver [75]. EPA is a particularly potent activator of PPARα, and hence of lipid oxidation, whereas *n*-6 fatty acids, such as arachidonic acid, are significantly less potent activators [75]. Whilst induction of PPARα by PUFAs promotes fatty acid oxidation in the liver, PUFAs inhibit hepatic fatty acid synthesis by suppressing SREBP. SREBP regulates several aspects of fatty acid synthesis [77]. These observations mainly come from animal studies and it is not known if PUFAs may have "anti-obesity" effects in humans.

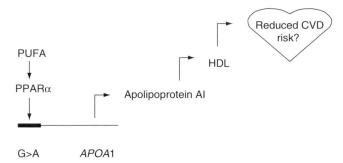

Figure 9.19   How binding of PUFAs to PPARα influences HDL expression.

Many of the promotor regions of genes that bind PPARs are polymorphic and this can have a significant impact on the response of an individual to dietary fats. PPARα binds PUFAs and this resulted in increased levels of HDL (Figure 9.19), but only in a sub-population of people studied. People showing a favourably elevated HDL response to PUFAs carried a SNP in the promotor region of the gene for apolipoprotein A-I (*APOA1*) (G to A change, which is written as G>A). This G>A increases the binding of PPARα that results in increased apolipoprotein A-I (apo AI) production. Apo AI is the major protein component in HDL. Hence high induction of *APOA1* results in high levels of beneficial HDL and hence possibly in a reduced risk of CVD.

9.7   Increased stress resistance

There is a good deal of interest in the concept that various environmental factors can increase stress resistance in normal cells and that this is associated with increased disease resistance. Many of these environmental factors are associated with the MedDiet, although it is currently not known to what extent this concept may directly apply to the MedDiet.

9.7.1   The general concept

Most normal cells and tissues need to operate within a fairly narrow range of function and so maintain a steady state, i.e. homeostasis. However, pathologists have long recognised that cells exposed to mild stressors can adapt and achieve a new but altered steady state within which the cell is still able to function. This cell adaption is associated with biochemical or morphological changes. For example, increased demand on cells in the heart results in increased cell size (hypertrophy). The adapted cells are then better able to respond to the new conditions.

Experimental evidence indicates that low doses of some phytochemicals can activate cellular pathways that adapt cells to increased stress. These biochemically-adapted cells may then be better able to resist a more severe stress, one that in non-adapted cells and tissues could increase risk for a chronic disease such as cancer. Besides phytochemicals, a variety of lifestyle factors – many of which are characteristic of a Mediterranean lifestyle such as exercise and moderate alcohol – may, it has been suggested, act through this mechanism to provide protection against a range of

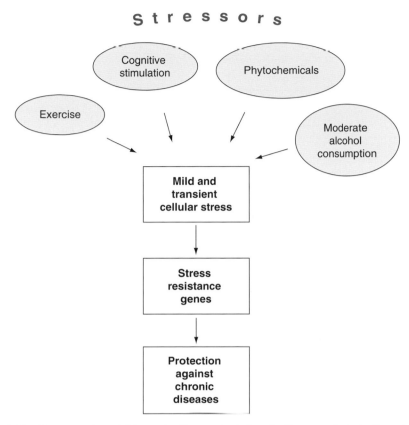

Figure 9.20 Conceptual model for protection against chronic diseases via induction of a stress response.

chronic disorders (Figure 9.20) [78]. For example, dietary restriction, exercise and cognitive stimulation may act as mild stressors on nerve cells and increase resistance to neurodegenerative diseases [79].

Only low doses of the stressor are considered to be beneficial, and higher doses are toxic. This is analogous to the increasing evidence that there is an upper threshold for many vitamins and minerals (such as folic acid, iron, copper, iodide, and selenium), above which there can be adverse effects [80]. As has been succinctly stated in relation to micronutrients and cancer prevention: "the notion that some is good and therefore more is better has been proven wrong; it is more likely that for any given micronutrient, there is an optimal range of intake" [81].

This biphasic response – i.e. benefit at low dose and toxicity at high dose – has been described by the memorable phrase "that which does not kill makes us stronger" [82]. This concept is now referred to as hormesis and agents that can induce this type of response are called hormetins. Hormesis has been defined as "a process in which exposure to a low dose of a chemical agent or environmental factor that is damaging at higher doses induces an adaptive beneficial effect on the cell or organism" [79].

A typical dose-response curve for this effect is shown in Figure 9.21. A minimum dose is required for an effect, there is then a dose range where a beneficial effect is seen and this can be regulated by normal homeostatic mechanisms, and beyond this dose range there is toxicity.

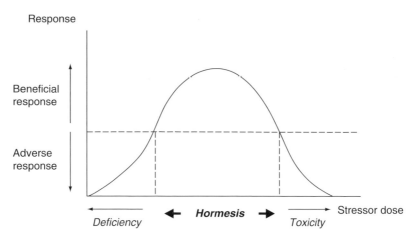

Figure 9.21   Hormetic dose response.

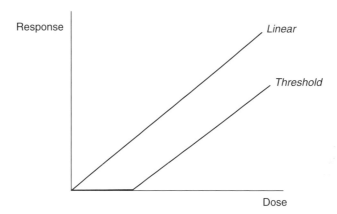

Figure 9.22   Linear and threshold dose-response curves.

This type of dose response contrasts with the more familiar concept in which there is a single direct relationship between dose and response: either a threshold model (no effect until a threshold dose, above which the response is linear) or a linear non-threshold (response directly proportional to dose without any threshold) (Figure 9.22). The hormesis dose response is the only one that offers a simple explanation of why high doses of vitamin and mineral supplements can be harmful.

Phytochemicals are considered by some scientists to be good examples of hormetins. Phytochemicals are recognised by the body as foreign chemicals or "xenobiotics". As such, the body responds by inducing a plethora of protective mechanisms to minimise any potential damage, and this cytoprotective response is associated with increased protection against various disease processes (see the section on Phytochemicals above) [65]. Phytochemicals that have been reported to have protective effects at low doses but that are toxic at higher doses include quercetin, resveratrol and sulforaphane [79, 83].

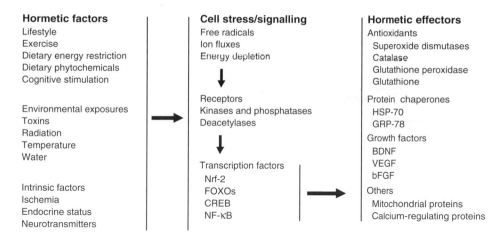

Figure 9.23 Proposed mechanism for hormetic effects [79]. With permission from Elsevier.
Extrinsic factors or intrinsic changes to cells result in mild cell stress that induces an adaptive response.

Alcohol and hormesis

In some respects, alcohol could also be considered as a hormetin, since low concentrations produce favourable increases in HDL-cholesterol which is associated with cardiovascular protection, whereas high concentrations of alcohol lead to a wide variety of adverse effects such as cirrhosis of the liver, increased blood pressure and increased cancer risk.

9.7.2   Mechanistic basis of hormesis

The cellular and molecular mechanisms underlying hormesis are very active areas of research. Hormetins activate a variety of signalling pathways that can activate transcription factors. These transcription factors in turn result in the production of effector proteins that protect cells against more severe stress (Figure 9.23). Some of these general effectors, such as antioxidant proteins, have already been discussed previously. More specialised effectors include brain-derived neurotrophic factor (BDNF) which affords neurological protection. Other hormetic changes include decreased inflammation, increased insulin sensitivity and increased stress resistance.

Xenohormesis hypothesis

The hormesis hypothesis has been extended to explain how the physiology of early humans adapted to stressful environments. Production of many polyphenols in plants increases when the environment in which the plant is growing is stressful to the plant (e.g. the plant is being exposed to excess UV light, drought, or attack by herbivores). It has been suggested that the "polyphenol content provides a chemical signature of the state of the environment" [84]. The xenohormesis hypothesis proposes that the human body has evolved to recognise these chemical signals from the environment (plants) and adapt accordingly [84].

These adaptations include changes to many signalling pathways, such as those that decrease inflammation, increase insulin sensitivity and increase stress resistance. Adapting to a stressful environment would increase the chances of survival during difficult times.

In the case of the MedDiet, this may have been particularly relevant in relation to the consumption of wild greens. Wild greens were collected as "famine food" during periods of famine. The growth and production of polyphenols by wild greens is directly influenced by natural environmental conditions, unlike cultivated crops whose growth and polyphenol content are modified by agricultural practices. Consumption of wild greens with a high phytochemical content could trigger a xenohormetic response, with increased stress resistance in the consumer.

This xenohormesis hypothesis has also been used to explain why the majority of phytochemicals are surprisingly safe with no side-effects and indeed often with multiple beneficial effects. For example, resveratrol found in red wine interacts with over 20 molecular targets but the vast majority of these targets increase resistance against cancer, cardiovascular disease and others and by generally increasing the stress resistance by the body.

In summary, phytochemicals and various lifestyle factors may afford protection against CDDs through a hormetic mechanism. This conceptual framework is increasingly being evaluated in the context of the MedDiet, but is currently at an early stage.

9.8 Nutrient interactions and the Mediterranean dietary pattern

"It seems a good assumption that the vast majority of components of plant and animal-based food is functional, that it has some kind of biological activity." [85]

From an extensive examination of the epidemiological evidence, there is now good evidence that no single food group, such as fruit or fish, has the same health benefits as the overall MedDiet (see Chapters 10–13) [86]. These studies thus indicate that understanding the complex interactions between food components in the MedDiet will lead to a greater understanding of its protective effects. This new holistic approach, referred to as a "dietary pattern" approach, is a departure from the current more reductionist approach, and represents an important challenge for future nutrition research [87].

The importance of analysing the overall dietary pattern can be illustrated by considering factors that affect cancer risk. A study compared three dietary patterns for risk of colon cancer: a Western diet (high intake of processed and red meats, fast food, refined grain, added sugar and high fat dairy food and a low intake of yogurt), a "prudent" diet (high intake of fish, fresh fruit, legumes, crucifers, carrots, tomatoes and other vegetables) and a "drinker" diet (high intake of fish, liquor and wine). Both the Western diet and the "drinker" diet showed an increased risk of colon cancer, but importantly *both* had a high consumption of fish [88]. This demonstrates that considering a single food, in this case fish, can lead to a misinterpretation of the data.

This prompted the development of tools that can evaluate cancer risk with multiple components of the MedDiet such as the Mediterranean Dietary Quality Index (MDQI) [89], and this has been discussed in Chapter 8.

In contrast to the dietary pattern approach, nutritional supplements epitomise a reductionist approach to nutrition. Although supplements can be appropriate for people who are deficient in certain nutrients, studies have found that some supplements are of no benefit when given to people with adequate nutritional status, and indeed in some cases they may increase disease risk.

Supplements

Why not simply substitute multivitamin pills for the MedDiet? Although epidemiological studies have highlighted various antioxidants in fruits and vegetables as potential reasons for their protection against cancer, CVD and other diseases, most randomised trials with antioxidant supplements have failed to fulfil their initial promise. One of the most unexpected outcomes came from studies that examined whether β-carotene could reduce the incidence of lung cancer in smokers. Contrary to expectations, these studies showed that the incidence of lung cancer actually increased in the people taking supplements. The specific reason for this effect is not fully understood but it could be that β-carotene is toxic at high concentrations or it may have blocked the uptake from the diet of more protective factors [8]. Also, many carotenoids including β-carotene are not stable in their pure form and can generate toxic products when they break down [8]. Another large-scale study, looking at the cancer preventative effects of supplementation with selenium and vitamin E (the SELECT study), has also reported negative results [90].

A review of 68 trials with anti-oxidant supplements such as β-carotene and vitamins A, C or E showed that overall mortality was higher in people taking the supplements [91]. It was suggested by the authors that most of these deaths were probably due to increased rates of cancer and CVD. This is of public health concern since it is estimated that 10–20% of the population (80–160 million) of N. America and Europe take these types of supplements.

Various potential benefits of taking nutrients as part of an overall dietary pattern, rather than as pure supplements, have been enumerated, and these include:

- Minimising spikes in plasma concentrations of nutrients
- Synergistic interactions

9.8.1   Minimising spikes in plasma concentrations

Although it has long been recognised that an insufficient intake of vitamins and minerals results in deficiency disorders, it is now recognised that too high an intake of many vitamins and minerals is associated with toxicity [92]. Hence, the optimal beneficial effects are only obtained within a certain range of concentrations ie neither too low nor too high. (This is comparable to the hormetic dose response shown in Figure 9.21.) The designation of some vitamins and minerals as GRAS (generally recognised as safe) therefore needs to be qualified by specifying intake ranges.

Table 9.8 Estimated relative risk of breast cancer according to selected combined dietary intake [89].

Food intake – test	Food intake – reference for comparison	OR (CI)
Highest β-carotene and Se, lowest PUFA	Lowest β-carotene and Se, highest PUFA	1.00 (0.47–2.13)
Lowest total lipids	Highest total lipids	0.57 (0.36–0.90)
Highest fibre, fermented milk	Lowest fibre, fermented milk	0.62 (0.35–1.09)
Highest fibre, fermented milk, lowest total lipids	Lowest fibre, fermented milk, highest total lipids	0.33 (0.15–0.73)

Most vitamin and mineral supplements are taken orally as a single pill and rapid absorption can lead to a plasma concentration "spike" that swamps normal homeostatic mechanisms for regulating plasma concentrations. This can result in adverse effects, particularly in people who do not have a prior deficiency of the nutrient in question. By contrast, many vitamins, minerals and phytochemicals consumed in foods are absorbed more slowly due to a buffering effect of the food matrix, and this generally[4] results in a lower peak plasma concentrations. For this reason, it is sometimes recommended that nutrient supplements are taken with a meal in order to slow absorption, and so mitigate against the "bolus" effect [94] Many nutrients are present in more than one meal of the day when consuming a MedDiet, and this will also minimise a "bolus effect" whilst still achieving the recommended daily intake (RDI).

9.8.2 Synergistic interactions

A central argument used to support claims for the superiority of dietary patterns over supplements is that beneficial interactions and synergies can occur between dietary components, both of known compounds and between compounds that have yet to be discovered. The benefits of combining various foods can be illustrated by considering breast cancer. Increased risk of breast cancer is known to be associated with high exposure to oestrogens. Many nutritional factors influence oestrogen levels in the body: a high fat diet increases oestrogen levels in the body, whereas fibre and fermented milk products may decrease oestrogen levels by increasing the rate of excretion of oestrogen metabolites (fibre and fermented milk products are thought to promote a favourable bacterial population in the colon which metabolises oestrogens). In a study to examine the role of various food combinations in breast cancer risk, the combination of a low intake of fat with a high intake of fibre and fermented milk products achieved the greatest decrease in breast cancer risk (Table 9.8), thus illustrating how a specific combination of foods can achieve the best overall benefit [89].

Unravelling significant interactions in the MedDiet is a complex issue when one considers that there are thousands of different compounds, especially a wide variety of phytochemicals. Interactions may occur both between components in different

---

[4] However this is not necessarily the case for all phytochemicals. For example, quercetin glycosides were found to be absorbed at similar rates whether they were given in isolated form or as part of the food matrix in onions [93].

Table 9.9 Examples of beneficial interactions and synergies between foods that are part of the MedDiet.

Stage	Food effector	Acts on	Effect
Food preparation	red wine marinade	fried food	Inhibition of Maillard reaction products
Digestion	red wine (or other polyphenol-rich food)	fatty foods	Inhibition of the production or absorption of ALEs in the gi tract
Metabolic effects	quercetin	inhibits sulphotransferase	Decreased sulphation of polyphenols
	olive oil	fat-soluble nutrients	Increased uptake
Cellular effects	mixture of antioxidants	mixture of antioxidants	Increased antioxidant effects

ALEs: advanced lipid oxidation end-products.

foods, and between components present in a single food, and these interactions can act during food preparation, digestion, metabolism or at cellular targets. Some examples that are discussed elsewhere in this book are summarised in Table 9.9.

Synergistic interactions can also occur between different constituents within a single foodstuff. Some nutrients are packaged together in Nature for specific reasons. For example, unsaturated fats in nuts are protected from oxidation by vitamin E, and by antioxidant phenolics that form a protective barrier in the nut's skin that surrounds the fatty region. Thus, eating whole nuts results in the fats being consumed simultaneously with protective antioxidants which may help reduce oxidation of the fats in the body. By contrast, there is an increased likelihood of purified unsaturated fats (e.g. in refined vegetable oils) becoming oxidised during storage, or in the body of the consumer if the person's antioxidant status is low.

There are several examples of whole extracts of fruits or vegetables having greater beneficial effects against cancer and other diseases than individual components from these extracts. For example, polyphenols from pomegranate juice exhibit synergistic inhibition of cancer cell proliferation (see Chapter 12). Some of the beneficial interactions between phytochemicals in fruits and vegetables may be due to the way in which antioxidant phytochemicals and vitamins interact mechanistically (Section 9.3.4). Not all interactions between food components are necessarily beneficial, however. Examples of compounds with possible anti-nutrient effects include some polyphenols (e.g. tannins in tea), oxalic acid (found in spinach) and phytate (inositol hexaphosphate) (in grains and legumes), all of which can inhibit the absorption of certain minerals. Modelling these complex interactions between nutrients, especially between micronutrients, is now being developed in the new area of biological networks [95].

References

1. Eyre, H. et al. Preventing cancer, cardiovascular disease, and diabetes: a common agenda for the American Cancer Society, the American Diabetes Association, and the American Heart Association. *Stroke*, 2004. **35**(8): 1999–2010.
2. Franco, O.H. et al. Changing course in ageing research: The healthy ageing phenotype. *Maturitas*, 2009. **63**(1): 13–19.

3. Mortensen, A. et al. Biological models for phytochemical research: from cell to human organism. *Br J Nutr*, 2008. **99 E Suppl 1**: ES118–26.
4. Steinhubl, S.R. Why have antioxidants failed in clinical trials? *Am J Cardiol*, 2008. **101**(10A): 14D–19D.
5. McCormick, D.B. Vitamin/mineral supplements: of questionable benefit for the general population. *Nutr Rev*, 2010. **68**(4): 207–13.
6. Saura-Calixto, F., Goni, I. Definition of the Mediterranean diet based on bioactive compounds. *Crit Rev Food Sci Nutr*, 2009. **49**(2): 145–52.
7. Lindsay, D.G., Astley, S.B. European research on the functional effects of dietary antioxidants – EUROFEDA. *Mol Aspects Med*, 2002. **23**(1–3): 1–38.
8. Halliwell, B., Gutteridge, J.M.C. *Free radicals in biology and medicine*, 4th ed. 2007: Oxford University Press.
9. Valko, M. et al. Free radicals and antioxidants in normal physiological functions and human disease. *Int J Biochem Cell Biol*, 2007. **39**(1): 44–84.
10. Halvorsen, B.L. et al. Content of redox-active compounds (ie, antioxidants) in foods consumed in the United States. *Am J Clin Nutr*, 2006. **84**(1): 95–135.
11. Halvorsen, B.L. et al. A systematic screening of total antioxidants in dietary plants. *J Nutr*, 2002. **132**(3): 461–71.
12. Carlsen, M.H. et al. The total antioxidant content of more than 3100 foods, beverages, spices, herbs and supplements used worldwide. *Nutr J*, 2010. **9**: 3.
13. Shan, B. et al. Antioxidant capacity of 26 spice extracts and characterization of their phenolic constituents. *J Agric Food Chem*, 2005. **53**(20): 7749–59.
14. Halliwell, B., Rafter, J., Jenner, A. Health promotion by flavonoids, tocopherols, tocotrienols, and other phenols: direct or indirect effects? Antioxidant or not? *Am J Clin Nutr*, 2005. **81**(1 Suppl): 268S–276S.
15. Aronis, P. et al. Effect of fast-food Mediterranean-type diet on human plasma oxidation. *J Med Food*, 2007. **10**(3): 511–20.
16. Fito, M. et al. Effect of a traditional Mediterranean diet on lipoprotein oxidation: a randomized controlled trial. *Arch Intern Med*, 2007. **167**(11): 1195–203.
17. Bogani, P., Visioli, F. Antioxidants in the Mediterranean diets: an update. *World Rev Nutr Diet*, 2007. **97**: 162–79.
18. Vardavas, C.E.A. The antioxidant and phylloquinone content of wildly grown greens in Crete. *Food Chem*, 2006. **99**: 813–821.
19. Razquin, C. et al. A 3 years follow-up of a Mediterranean diet rich in virgin olive oil is associated with high plasma antioxidant capacity and reduced body weight gain. *Eur J Clin Nutr*, 2009. **63**(12): 1387–93.
20. Pitsavos, C. et al. Adherence to the Mediterranean diet is associated with total antioxidant capacity in healthy adults: the ATTICA study. *Am J Clin Nutr*, 2005. **82**(3): 694–9.
21. Dai, J. et al. Association between adherence to the Mediterranean diet and oxidative stress. *Am J Clin Nutr*, 2008. **88**(5): 1364–70.
22. Sanchez-Moreno, C. et al. Mediterranean vegetable soup consumption increases plasma vitamin C and decreases F2-isoprostanes, prostaglandin E2 and monocyte chemotactic protein-1 in healthy humans. *J Nutr Biochem*, 2006. **17**(3): 183–9.
23. Krinsky, N.I., Johnson, E.J. Carotenoid actions and their relation to health and disease. *Mol Aspects Med*, 2005. **26**(6): 459–516.
24. Thurnham, D.I. Macular zeaxanthins and lutein – a review of dietary sources and bioavailability and some relationships with macular pigment optical density and age-related macular disease. *Nutr Res Rev*, 2007. **20**(2): 163–79.
25. Bhosale, P. et al. Identification and characterization of a Pi isoform of glutathione S-transferase (GSTP1) as a zeaxanthin-binding protein in the macula of the human eye. *J Biol Chem*, 2004. **279**(47): 49447–54.
26. Bhosale, P. et al. Purification and partial characterization of a lutein-binding protein from human retina. *Biochemistry*, 2009. **48**(22): 4798–807.
27. Dimitrios, B. Sources of natural phenolic antioxidants. *Trends in Food Science & Technology*, 2006. **17**: 505–512.
28. Bogani, P. et al. Postprandial anti-inflammatory and antioxidant effects of extra virgin olive oil. *Atherosclerosis*, 2007. **190**(1): 181–6.

29. Fito, M., de la Torre, R., Covas, M.I. Olive oil and oxidative stress. *Mol Nutr Food Res*, 2007. **51**(10): 1215–24.
30. Di Majo, D. et al. The antioxidant capacity of red wine in relationship with its polyphenolic constituents. *Food Chemistry*, 2008. **111**: 45–49.
31. Barreiro-Hurle, J., Colombo, S., Cantos-Villar, E. Is there a market for functional wines? Consumer preferences and willingness to pay for resveratrol-enriched red wine. *Food Quality and Preference*, 2008. **19**: 360–371.
32. Kanner, J. Dietary advanced lipid oxidation endproducts are risk factors to human health. *Mol Nutr Food Res*, 2007. **51**(9): 1094–101.
33. Baynes, J.W. Dietary ALEs are a risk to human health–NOT! *Mol Nutr Food Res*, 2007. **51**(9): 1102–6.
34. Gorelik, S. et al. A novel function of red wine polyphenols in humans: prevention of absorption of cytotoxic lipid peroxidation products. *Faseb J*, 2008. **22**(1): 41–6.
35. Liu, R.H. Health benefits of fruit and vegetables are from additive and synergistic combinations of phytochemicals. *Am J Clin Nutr*, 2003. **78**(3 Suppl): 517S–520S.
36. Guarnieri, S., Riso, P., Porrini, M. Orange juice vs vitamin C: effect on hydrogen peroxide-induced DNA damage in mononuclear blood cells. *Br J Nutr*, 2007. **97**(4): 639–43.
37. Chen, C.Y. et al. Flavonoids from almond skins are bioavailable and act synergistically with vitamins C and E to enhance hamster and human LDL resistance to oxidation. *J Nutr*, 2005. **135**(6): 1366–73.
38. Bardia, A. et al. Efficacy of antioxidant supplementation in reducing primary cancer incidence and mortality: systematic review and meta-analysis. *Mayo Clin Proc*, 2008. **83**(1): 23–34.
39. Holst, B., Williamson, G. Nutrients and phytochemicals: from bioavailability to bioefficacy beyond antioxidants. *Curr Opin Biotechnol*, 2008. **19**(2): 73–82.
40. Lotito, S.B., Frei, B. Consumption of flavonoid-rich foods and increased plasma antioxidant capacity in humans: cause, consequence, or epiphenomenon? *Free Radic Biol Med*, 2006. **41**(12): 1727–46.
41. Halliwell, B. The wanderings of a free radical. *Free Radic Biol Med*, 2009. **46**(5): 531–42.
42. Salas-Salvado, J. et al. Components of the Mediterranean-type food pattern and serum inflammatory markers among patients at high risk for cardiovascular disease. *Eur J Clin Nutr*, 2008. **62**(5): 651–9.
43. Dai, J. et al. Adherence to the Mediterranean diet is inversely associated with circulating interleukin-6 among middle-aged men: a twin study. *Circulation*, 2008. **117**(2): 69–75.
44. Michalsen, A. et al. Mediterranean diet has no effect on markers of inflammation and metabolic risk factors in patients with coronary artery disease. *Eur J Clin Nutr*, 2006. **60**(4): 478–85.
45. Serrano-Martinez, M., Martinez-Gonzalez, M.A. Effects of Mediterranean diets on plasma biomarkers of inflammation. *Eur J Clin Nutr*, 2007. **61**(8): 1035–6; author reply: 1036.
46. Zampelas, A. et al. Fish consumption among healthy adults is associated with decreased levels of inflammatory markers related to cardiovascular disease: the ATTICA study. *J Am Coll Cardiol*, 2005. **46**(1): 120–4.
47. Calder, P.C. n-3 polyunsaturated fatty acids, inflammation, and inflammatory diseases. *Am J Clin Nutr*, 2006. **83**(6 Suppl): 1505S–1519S.
48. Yaqoob, P., Calder, P. The immune and inflammatory systems. In: *Nutrition and metabolism*, ed. M. Gibney, I.A. McDonald. H. Roche. 2003: Blackwell Publishing.
49. Calder, P.C. Polyunsaturated fatty acids and inflammatory processes: New twists in an old tale. *Biochimie*, 2009. **91**(6): 791–5.
50. Conforti, F. et al. In vivo anti-inflammatory and in vitro antioxidant activities of Mediterranean dietary plants. *J Ethnopharmacol*, 2008. **116**(1): 144–51.
51. Middleton, E., Jr., Kandaswami, C., Theoharides, T.C. The effects of plant flavonoids on mammalian cells: implications for inflammation, heart disease, and cancer. *Pharmacol Rev*, 2000. **52**(4): 673–751.
52. Williamson, G. et al. In vitro biological properties of flavonoid conjugates found in vivo. *Free Radic Res*, 2005. **39**(5): 457–69.
53. O'Leary, K.A. et al. Effect of flavonoids and vitamin E on cyclooxygenase-2 (COX-2) transcription. *Mutat Res*, 2004. **551**(1–2): 245–54.
54. Rahman, I., Biswas, S.K., Kirkham, P.A. Regulation of inflammation and redox signaling by dietary polyphenols. *Biochem Pharmacol*, 2006. **72**(11): 1439–52.

55. Beauchamp, G.K. et al. Phytochemistry: ibuprofen-like activity in extra-virgin olive oil. *Nature*, 2005. **437**(7055): 45–6.
56. Saadatian-Elahi, M. et al. Plasma phospholipid fatty acid profiles and their association with food intakes: results from a cross-sectional study within the European Prospective Investigation into Cancer and Nutrition. *Am J Clin Nutr*, 2009. **89**(1): 331–46.
57. Esfahani, A. et al. The glycemic index: physiological significance. *J Am Coll Nutr*, 2009. **28 Suppl**: 439S–445S.
58. Williams, R.J., Spencer, J.P., Rice-Evans, C. Flavonoids: antioxidants or signalling molecules? *Free Radic Biol Med*, 2004. **36**(7): 838–49.
59. Mutch, D.M., Wahli, W., Williamson, G. Nutrigenomics and nutrigenetics: the emerging faces of nutrition. *Faseb J*, 2005. **19**(12): 1602–16.
60. Ordovas, J.M., Kaput, J., Corella, D. Nutrition in the genomics era: cardiovascular disease risk and the Mediterranean diet. *Mol Nutr Food Res*, 2007. **51**(10): 1293–9.
61. Stover, P.J., Caudill, M.A. Genetic and epigenetic contributions to human nutrition and health: managing genome-diet interactions. *J Am Diet Assoc*, 2008. **108**(9): 1480–7.
62. Stover, P.J. Human nutrition and genetic variation. *Food Nutr Bull*, 2007. **28**(1 Suppl International): S101–15.
63. Yiannakouris, N. et al. A direct assessment of genetic contribution to the incidence of coronary infarct in the general population Greek EPIC cohort. *Eur J Epidemiol*, 2006. **21**(12): 859–67.
64. Lairon, D. et al. Nutrigenetics: links between genetic background and response to Mediterranean-type diets. *Public Health Nutr*, 2009. **12**(9A): 1601–6.
65. Dinkova-Kostova, A.T., Talalay, P. Direct and indirect antioxidant properties of inducers of cytoprotective proteins. *Mol Nutr Food Res*, 2008. **52 Suppl 1**: S128–38.
66. Ungvari, Z. et al. Resveratrol confers endothelial protection via activation of the antioxidant transcription factor Nrf2. *Am J Physiol Heart Circ Physiol*, 2010. **299**(1): H18–24.
67. Eggler, A.L., Gay, K.A., Mesecar, A.D. Molecular mechanisms of natural products in chemoprevention: induction of cytoprotective enzymes by Nrf2. *Mol Nutr Food Res*, 2008. **52 Suppl 1**: S84–94.
68. Perez-Martinez, P. et al. The chronic intake of a Mediterranean diet enriched in virgin olive oil, decreases nuclear transcription factor kappaB activation in peripheral blood mononuclear cells from healthy men. *Atherosclerosis*, 2007. **194**(2): e141–6.
69. Llorente-Cortes, V. et al. Effect of Mediterranean diet on the expression of pro-atherogenic genes in a population at high cardiovascular risk. *Atherosclerosis*, 208(2): 442–50.
70. Konstantinidou, V. et al. In vivo nutrigenomic effects of virgin olive oil polyphenols within the frame of the Mediterranean diet: a randomized controlled trial. *Faseb J*, 2010. **24**(7): 2546–57.
71. Camargo, A. et al. Gene expression changes in mononuclear cells in patients with metabolic syndrome after acute intake of phenol-rich virgin olive oil. *BMC Genomics*, 2010. **11**: 253.
72. Virgili, F., Marino, M. Regulation of cellular signals from nutritional molecules: a specific role for phytochemicals, beyond antioxidant activity. *Free Radic Biol Med*, 2008. **45**(8): 1205–16.
73. Auclair, S. et al. Catechin reduces atherosclerotic lesion development in apo E-deficient mice: a transcriptomic study. *Atherosclerosis*, 2009. **204**(2): e21–7.
74. Knutson, M.D., Leeuwenburgh, C. Resveratrol and novel potent activators of SIRT1: effects on aging and age-related diseases. *Nutr Rev*, 2008. **66**(10): 591–6.
75. Minihane, A.M. Nutrient gene interactions in lipid metabolism. *Curr Opin Clin Nutr Metab Care*, 2009. **12**(4): 357–63.
76. Sampath, H., Ntambi, J.M. Polyunsaturated fatty acid regulation of genes of lipid metabolism. *Annu Rev Nutr*, 2005. **25**: 317–40.
77. Jump, D.B. et al. Fatty acid regulation of hepatic gene transcription. *J Nutr*, 2005. **135**(11): 2503–6.
78. Hayes, D.P. Nutritional hormesis. *Eur J Clin Nutr*, 2007. **61**(2): 147–59.
79. Mattson, M.P. Hormesis defined. *Ageing Res Rev*, 2008. **7**(1): 1–7.
80. Langman, M.E.A. *Safe upper levels for vitamins and minerals*. 2003, Expert Group on Vitamins and Minerals.
81. Kristal, A.R., Lippman, S.M. Nutritional prevention of cancer: new directions for an increasingly complex challenge. *J Natl Cancer Inst*, 2009. **101**(6): 363–5.
82. Gems, D., Partridge, L. Stress-response hormesis and aging: "that which does not kill us makes us stronger". *Cell Metab*, 2008. **7**(3): 200–3.

83. Vargas, A.J., Burd, R. Hormesis and synergy: pathways and mechanisms of quercetin in cancer prevention and management. *Nutr Rev*, 2010. **68**(7): 418–28.
84. Howitz, K.T., Sinclair, D.A. Xenohormesis: sensing the chemical cues of other species. *Cell*, 2008. **133**(3): 387–91.
85. Jacobs, D.R., Jr., Tapsell, L.C. Food, not nutrients, is the fundamental unit in nutrition. *Nutr Rev*, 2007. **65**(10): 439–50.
86. Benetou, V. et al. Conformity to traditional Mediterranean diet and cancer incidence: the Greek EPIC cohort. *Br J Cancer*, 2008. **99**(1): 191–5.
87. Katan, M.B. et al. Which are the greatest recent discoveries and the greatest future challenges in nutrition? *Eur J Clin Nutr*, 2009. **63**(1): 2–10.
88. Slattery, M.L. et al. Eating patterns and risk of colon cancer. *Am J Epidemiol*, 1998. **148**(1): 4–16.
89. Gerber, M. The comprehensive approach to diet: a critical review. *J Nutr*, 2001. **131**(11 Suppl): 3051S–5S.
90. Klein, E.A. Selenium and vitamin E: interesting biology and dashed hope. *J Natl Cancer Inst*, 2009. **101**(5): 283–5.
91. Bjelakovic, G. et al. Mortality in randomized trials of antioxidant supplements for primary and secondary prevention: systematic review and meta-analysis. *Jama*, 2007. **297**(8): 842–57.
92. Mulholland, C.A., Benford, D.J. What is known about the safety of multivitamin-multimineral supplements for the generally healthy population? Theoretical basis for harm. *Am J Clin Nutr*, 2007. **85**(1): 318S–322S.
93. Graefe, E.U. et al. Pharmacokinetics and bioavailability of quercetin glycosides in humans. *J Clin Pharmacol*, 2001. **41**(5): 492–9.
94. Jacobs, D.R., Jr. et al. Food synergy: an operational concept for understanding nutrition. *Am J Clin Nutr*, 2009.
95. van Ommen, B. et al. A network biology model of micronutrient related health. *Br J Nutr*, 2008. **99 Suppl 3**: S72–80.

10 Metabolic Disorders

Summary

- Obesity, metabolic syndrome and diabetes are closely inter-related disorders.
- Epidemiological evidence linking a MedDiet with a reduction in obesity is inconclusive, although experimental studies suggest that favourable features of the MedDiet that may limit weight gain include its typical fatty acid composition (relatively high in medium chain fatty acids and oleic acid and low in long chain SFAs) and high dietary fibre intake.
- Diagnosis of metabolic syndrome is based on three or more of the following symptoms: abdominal obesity, elevated blood pressure, elevated triglycerides, reduced HDL cholesterol, elevated fasting glucose; physiologically, metabolic syndrome is associated with an increase in the resistance of the body to the effects of insulin.
- Epidemiological studies have found that decreasing SFA and increasing MUFA improves insulin sensitivity when total fat intake is moderate; fibre intake and moderate alcohol consumption also improve markers for metabolic syndrome.
- A number of studies indicate that an overall Mediterranean-style dietary pattern might be effective in reducing the prevalence of the metabolic syndrome and the associated risk of CVD.
- The MedDiet may reduce metabolic syndrome risk by reducing adiposity and inflammation; olive oil, wine cinnamon and green tea have been shown to improve insulin sensitivity.
- A few studies have shown that Mediterranean food patterns are associated with a significant reduction in the risk of developing type 2 diabetes, and a number of other studies have demonstrated improved glycaemic control and insulin sensitivity.
- Common mechanisms linking obesity, metabolic syndrome and diabetes, especially insulin resistance, suggest that reducing symptoms in one of these disorders may reduce the risk of another.

10.1 Introduction

Obesity, metabolic syndrome and type 2 diabetes are major health problems both in developed countries and in developing parts of the world, and current treatment and prevention strategies have had only a limited impact. A number of epidemiological studies have shown an association between adherence to the MedDiet and a reduced incidence of these conditions. Because of the multifactorial nature of these disorders

Obesity ——→ Metabolic syndrome ——→ Type 2 diabetes

Figure 10.1   Relationship between metabolic disorders.

and their close inter-relatedness, it is not possible to precisely define how the MedDiet may afford protection, although reducing obesity is particularly important. Based on current evidence, it seems reasonable to conclude that the benefits of the MedDiet are most likely due to a favourable combination of several factors.

Obesity is a major risk factor for type 2 diabetes, and the close relationship between these two conditions is encapsulated in the hybrid word "diabesity". One of the major physiological changes that can occur in obese individuals is an increased resistance of some tissues in the body to the actions of insulin. Insulin resistance will progress to type 2 diabetes if the pancreas is unable to produce sufficient insulin to compensate for the body's reduced responsiveness. Insulin resistance can also lead to a spectrum of other conditions including hypertension and dyslipidaemia (high triglycerides and low high-density lipoproteins). When several of these metabolic conditions are present together, an individual may be clinically diagnosed as having "metabolic syndrome". Hence it is evident that obesity, metabolic syndrome and type 2 diabetes are closely-related conditions (Figure 10.1).

10.2   Obesity

10.2.1   Introduction

An estimated 300 million people around the world are obese (defined as having a BMI $\geq 30 \, kg/m^2$), and many more are overweight (BMI $\geq 25.0 \, kg/m^2$ or higher). The International Obesity Task Force's conservative estimate suggests that obesity levels will continue to rise in the early 21st century – with severe health consequences – unless urgent action is taken now [1].

It is unfortunate that adipose tissue is not able to store excess calories safely. Rather, being overweight or obese comes with an increased risk of a range of health problems. This is an important public health problem since obesity reduces life expectancy because of an increase in CVD and mortality, and an increased incidence and mortality of certain cancers. Some estimates of these risks are [2, 3]:

- a decrease in life expectancy (by 7 years at age 40 years)
- an increase in all-cause mortality of 30% and for CVD of 40% for each $5 \, kg/m^2$ increase in BMI above the nadir for risk
- the cause of 10% of all cancers amongst non-smokers (up to 40–50% of cancers of endometrium and adenocarcinomas of the oesophagus, 20–30% of kidney cancers and 20% of post-menopausal breast cancers are due to excess weight)
- a contributory factor in arthritis
- the main cause of metabolic syndrome

Obesity is now recognised as an epidemic all over Europe. But for a long time, Mediterranean countries escaped this problem. However, the prevalence of over-weightness and obesity among Mediterranean adults from Southern Europe (Greece, Italy, Spain) is now quite high, and figures for 2004 are shown in Figure 10.2 [4].

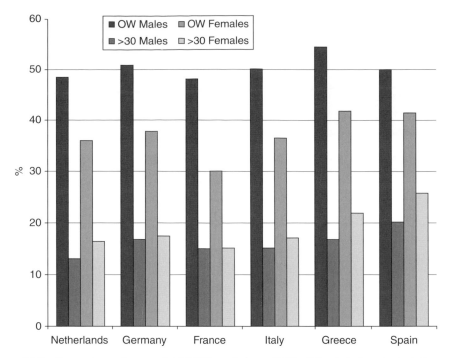

Figure 10.2 Percentage of overweight (OW) and obese (BMI >30) adults in selected European countries (adapted from [4]).

The WHO estimates that the prevalence of obesity in Greek adults (aged 30 y) is now 30%, whereas in Denmark it is 13%.

Childhood obesity is a particular problem in Mediterranean countries since childhood obesity is higher in these countries than in most other European countries, and it is still increasing. This is a consistent finding, despite the difficulty comparing studies due to the different cut-offs used to identify overweight and obese children. Whichever country is studied (Italy, Greece, Portugal or Eastern Mediterranean regions) or method used (such as those from the International Obesity Task Force or Communicable Diseases Center-USA cut-offs), it can be said from national studies that childhood obesity plus overweight prevalence is about 30% to 35%, of which 10% to 12% encompasses obesity (Figure 10.3) [5].

Multiple explanations have been proposed to explain obesity and overweight in Mediterranean countries, and some of these were disseminated in a press release by the FAO in 2008 [6]. In the 40 years to 2002, daily calorie intake in (15-nation) Europe increased by about 20%. But Greece, Italy, Spain, Portugal, Cyprus and Malta, who started out economically poorer than north European countries, increased their calorie intake by 30%. Higher calorie intake and lower calorie expenditure have resulted in Greece now being the EU member country with the highest average BMI and the highest prevalence of overweight and obesity. Today, three-quarters of the Greek population are overweight or obese. More than half of the Italian, Spanish and Portuguese populations are also overweight. At the same time there has also been, according to FAO, a "vast increase" in the overall calories and glycaemic load of the diets in the Near East-North Africa region. Spain was the country that registered the most dramatic increase, where fat made up just 25% of

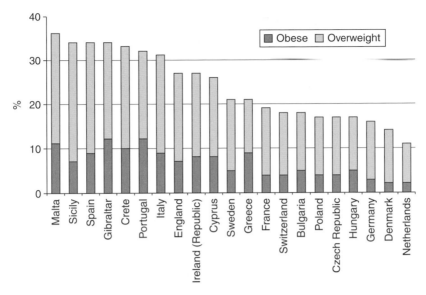

Figure 10.3 Percentage of school children aged 7–11 obese or overweight [5].

the diet 40 years ago, but now accounts for 40%. FAO attributes the change in eating habits not only to increased income but to factors such as the rise of supermarkets, changes in food distribution systems, working women having less time to cook, and families eating out more, often in fast-food restaurants. At the same time, calorie needs have declined, people exercise less and they have shifted to a much more sedentary lifestyle. In other words, they have lost the traditional Med-Diet and Mediterranean lifestyle.

10.2.2 Epidemiology

In a study of a French Mediterranean region, principal component analysis showed that loss of a MedDiet was associated with overweight in young adults whereas older adults (55 to 76 years of age) who maintained a better compliance with a MedDiet had a normal BMI [7]. In another study, there is an impressive difference in the prevalence of overweight and obesity (Figure 10.4) [8, 9] when Sardinia – where a traditional MedDiet is well maintained – is compared with Malta – where the traditional MedDiet and other correlated Mediterranean lifestyle factors have been lost [10, 11].

Several studies in Mediterranean countries have found that compliance with a traditional MedDiet is associated with lower overweight, obesity and central obesity [12–16]. However, in the analyses of the relationship of the M-MDS (see Chapter 8) with BMI and waist circumference in the EPIC-PANACEA cohorts (EPIC and Nutrition–Physical Activity, Nutrition, Alcohol, Cessation of Smoking, Eating Out of Home and Obesity) it was observed that there was no overall association with BMI and, in men only, there was a slight but significant positive correlation with normal BMI (18.5–25) [17]. However, there was a borderline significant overall negative correlation with waist circumference. The correlation was significant in all BMI categories (except <18.5), but larger in obese subjects, in Northern Europe, men and women, whatever level of physical activity. In Southern

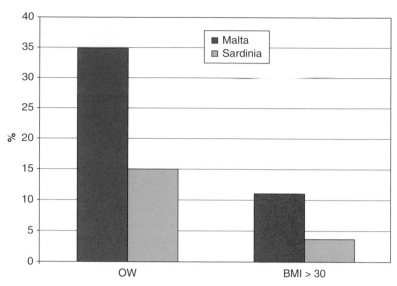

Figure 10.4 Percentage of overweight and obese children (7–11 years) from Malta and Sardinia [9].

Europe, the negative correlation was only observed in men and, when stratified on physical activity, only those with low activity. This extensive investigation is in line with previous observations that showed no association of BMI with MDS in a Greek population [14, 18].

A MedDiet intervention was tested in a weight loss trial [19]. In this 2-year trial, 322 moderately obese subjects (mean age 52 years; mean BMI 31; 86% males) were randomly assigned to one of three diets: low fat, restricted calorie; Mediterranean, restricted calorie; or low-carbohydrate, non-restricted calorie. The moderate fat, restricted calorie, MedDiet was rich in vegetables and low in red meat, with poultry and fish replacing beef and lamb. Energy intake was restricted to 1500 kcal per day for women and 1800 kcal per day for men, with a goal of no more than 35% of calories from fat; the main sources of added fat were 30–45 g of olive oil and a handful of nuts (5–7 nuts, <20 g) per day. The MedDiet group consumed the largest amounts of dietary fibre and had the highest ratio of monounsaturated to saturated fat ($p < 0.05$ for all comparisons among treatment groups). The mean weight loss was 2.9 kg for the low fat group, 4.4 kg for the MedDiet group, and 4.7 kg for the low carbohydrate group ($p < 0.001$ for the interaction between diet group and time); among the 272 participants who completed the intervention, the mean weight losses were 3.3 kg, 4.6 kg, and 5.5 kg, respectively. Among the 36 subjects with diabetes, changes in fasting plasma glucose and insulin levels were more favourable among those assigned to the MedDiet than among those assigned to the low fat diet ($p < 0.001$ for the interaction among diabetes and MedDiet and time with respect to fasting glucose levels).

In summary, the epidemiological evidence of an association between adherence to a Mediterranean-type diet and overweight/obesity is limited and somewhat conflicting and there are important methodological differences and limitations in previous studies that make it difficult to compare results [20]. An interesting point is that compliance with a diet representing the features of a MedDiet, as assessed by the M-MDS, is inversely and significantly associated with waist circumference, which characterises abdominal obesity, this type of obesity being related to two other metabolic disorders, namely metabolic syndrome and type 2 diabetes.

10.2.3   Mechanisms

An excess of energy consumption relative to energy expenditure is the primary cause of weight gain. With regard to energy consumption, the relatively low energy density (i.e. energy content per weight of food) of the MedDiet may be an important factor in reducing weight gain. The energy density of the MedDiet has been estimated at 5.23 kJ/g for men and 4.63 kJ/g for women, which is significantly lower than that reported for the US (7.98 kJ/g for men and 7.48 kJ/g for women) [21]. Although alcohol is a well-known source of calories, evidence linking red wine consumption and weight gain is inconclusive [21]. Apart from the food itself, the social environment in which a meal is consumed can also have a major influence on the level of consumption. Two other dietary components that have received attention in relation to weight gain that are worthy of further discussion are dietary fibre and fat.

Dietary fibre

Fibre induces a feeling of satiety, i.e. the satisfaction of appetite, and it has been suggested that the high intake of both soluble and insoluble fibre in the MedDiet is one reason for its association with reduced obesity. Several mechanisms have been proposed to explain the association between fibre intake and satiety [21]:

1. The requirement of fibre-rich foods for prolonged mastication. Mastication activates hypothalamic histamine neurons and these suppress the satiety centre in the hypothalamus. In addition, mastication increases saliva and gastric acid production which increase gastric distension contributing to the feeling of satiety.
2. Fibre-rich foods generally contain a large volume of water, and this will increase gastric distension.
3. Fibre increases the production of cholecystokinin. Cholecystokinin is a peptide produced in the small intestine that has been shown to induce a feeling of satiety.

Fats

Although fat consumption is generally associated with the risk of obesity, the overall effect of dietary fat on weight gain will depend on whether the fatty acids are deposited in adipose tissue or burnt by oxidation. Experimental studies *in vitro* and in animals have found that different types of fat have different predispositions to being stored or burnt. Properties of fatty acids that influence their metabolic fate include chain length, degree of unsaturation, and position and configuration of the double bonds [22]. Extrapolation of these experimental studies to epidemiological evidence is more controversial, and there is less consistent evidence linking consumption of particular types of fatty acids with weight gain or weight loss in humans. Some human studies have not controlled for the variable amounts of physical activity between individuals, although these will clearly affect overall weight gain or loss.

The MedDiet is characterised by a high fat intake (comprising about 35–38% of total energy), and has a particular characteristic fatty acid composition, namely:

- a relatively high consumption of MCFAs from goat and sheep milk
- a high consumption of MUFAs, especially oleic acid from olive oil
- a high consumption of long chain *n*-3 PUFAs (ALA, EPA and DHA)
- a relatively low consumption of *n*-6 PUFAs

Hence it is worth considering the possible fates of fats present in this diet.

Experimental studies, and some epidemiological studies, have shown that long chain saturated fatty acids (LCSFAs) (C14:0–C24:0) have a greater tendency to be stored than other types of fatty acids. Hence, the lower proportion of LCSFAs in the MedDiet relative to a "western" diet could be significant. By contrast, many fatty acids in the MedDiet have a greater tendency to be oxidised. For example, there is good evidence from both human and animal studies that MCFAs (C6:0–C12:0) are preferentially oxidised compared to LCSFAs [22]. MCFAs are transported directly to the liver via the portal system (rather than via the lymphatic system as is the case with LCSFAs). Once in the liver, MCFAs are preferentially oxidised in mitochondria, compared to LCSFAs, since they are not incorporated into esterified lipids and their transport to the mitochondrial matrix is not carnitine-dependent. In addition, there is some evidence that the net energy value of MCFA is only 5 kcal/g, much lower the usual 9 kcal/g of energy coming from oxidation of LCFAs see [22]. The high rate of oxidation of MCFAs, poor deposition in adipose tissue and lower level of energy per gram available for metabolism, may all contribute to favourable effects on final body weight reported in some studies when these types of fatty acids are consumed.

Several differences between SFAs and MUFAs in their metabolism have been identified that could explain the greater oxidation of MUFAs including differences in the way these FAs are packaged into lipoproteins, their rates of hydrolysis in triacylglycerol-rich lipoproteins by lipoprotein lipase and their rates of transport into oxidative tissues [23]. There is also evidence that olive oil consumption results in a diet-induced increase in thermogenesis [24]. Thermogenesis is heat production in response to diet or environmental temperature, and is one of three main ways that energy from fatty acid oxidation is utilised. (The other two are basic maintenance of cells and physical activity.) Thermogenesis stimulates the sympathetic nervous system (SNS) and the catecholamines that are produced stimulate lipolysis in fat cells (adipocytes). Adipocytes in the abdomen are known to be more responsive to stimulation of lipolysis by the SNS than fat cells on the hips, and this has been suggested as the mechanism that explains why administration of olive oil promoted postprandial fat oxidation in abdominally obese women [24].

There is some evidence from animal studies that dietary EPA, DHA and CLA have "anti-obesity" effects, although there is very little evidence of this from human studies [25].

In summary, the metabolic fates of different types of fatty acids present in the MedDiet are the result of complex processes. Experimental studies suggest that some of these fatty acids may contribute less to fat accumulation than the saturated fats that are more typical of a western diet.

10.3   Metabolic syndrome

10.3.1   Introduction

Metabolic syndrome is a condition that encompasses a cluster of symptoms associated with disorders of metabolism. It is described as a "syndrome" rather than as a disease since it is characterised by multiple symptoms. Various sets of criteria have been established in order to provide a means of making a clinical diagnosis of metabolic syndrome. One of the most widely-used sets of criteria was developed by the National Cholesterol Education Program Adult Treatment Panel III (ATP III) [26]. Their diagnosis is based on three or more of the following: abdominal obesity, elevated triglycerides, reduced HDL cholesterol, elevated blood pressure, and elevated fasting glucose (Figure 10.5). Although not required for the diagnosis, some hormonal changes are present in metabolic syndrome, especially a decrease of sex-hormone binding globulin [27].

Metabolic syndrome is associated with resistance to the actions of insulin in the body, and for this reason metabolic syndrome is also sometimes known as "insulin resistance syndrome" or "syndrome X". Insulin resistance increases the risk for a range of conditions, not only type 2 diabetes, but also CVD, essential hypertension, polycystic ovary syndrome, nonalcoholic fatty liver disease, sleep apnoea and certain forms of cancer [28]. Hence, metabolic syndrome frequently evolves towards type 2 diabetes, and/or cardiovascular complications, or cancers like breast cancer.

Currently, up to 30% of middle-aged people in more developed countries have several features of the metabolic syndrome. The prevalence is as high as 60% among individuals in the seventh decade of life. Only an estimated 30% of adults have no features at all [3].

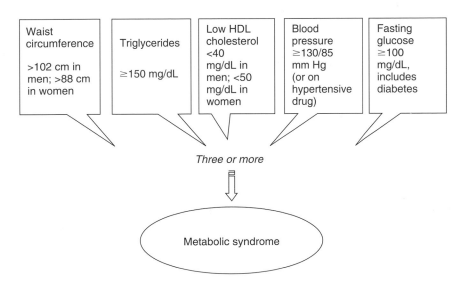

Figure 10.5   Diagnostic criteria for metabolic syndrome according to Adult Treatment Panel III (ATP III).

10.3.2 Epidemiology

"In the long run, the greatest benefit for those with metabolic syndrome will be derived from effective lifestyle intervention." [29]

Because of the multifarious nature of metabolic syndrome, choosing an appropriate endpoint is clearly an important issue for enabling a comparison between various interventions, and some commentators suggest that the primary endpoint for treatment of metabolic syndrome is to reduce the risk of CVD [30]. Other studies have focussed on other end-points such as a decrease in waist circumference and weight loss. Reviewing diets for treating metabolic syndrome with resolution of non-alcoholic fatty liver disease as an endpoint, it was concluded that diets are best tailored to the individual – although the MedDiet was recognised as a very promising approach [31]. Insulin resistance in an individual can be measured using HOMA. HOMA (homeostasis model assessment) is an empirical mathematical formula based on fasting plasma glucose and fasting plasma insulin levels.

Fibre

Fibre appears to be one of the most active nutrients for reducing different symptoms of metabolic syndrome. Total dietary fibre intake was clearly inversely associated with a reduction of several symptoms, namely elevated waist-to-hip ratio and blood pressure [32]. Evidence for an inverse association between total dietary fibre intake and hypertension was reported in a cohort study of young adults in the US [33]. This inverse association was found with non-soluble fibre, whereas only a trend was observed for soluble fibre. This association of fibre with blood pressure was independent of the observed inverse association of fibre with BMI. Two other epidemiologic studies in the US have provided evidence that body weight [33, 34] and waist-to-hip ratio [33] are inversely associated with total dietary fibre intake, whereas another study found no such relation [35]. Non-soluble fibre intake had the same inverse association with body weight and waist-to-hip ratio, whereas soluble fibre intake was associated with a lower risk of high waist-to-hip ratio only. Higher dietary fibre intakes from fruit, dried fruit, or nuts and seeds were associated with lower BMI and waist-to-hip ratio, whereas cereal fibre intake was associated with a low BMI only. This finding is in line with observations that whole grain intake is inversely associated with BMI, waist-to-hip ratio and metabolic syndrome [34, 36, 37]. In a Spanish study examining the association between the MedDiet and metabolic syndrome, high consumption of legumes was associated with a lower likelihood of having metabolic syndrome in a population of elderly men at high risk of CVD [38].

The mechanisms underlying the observed effects of dietary fibre on body fat stores have been discussed above, and might include reduced energy intake, increased fat excretion, and reduced chylomicron concentrations after high-fibre meals [39, 40]. In relation to insulin, a high-fibre meal may blunt postprandial increases in insulin, improve insulin sensitivity, and reduce insulinaemia [33]. McKeown et al. reported that whole-grain intake was also inversely associated with fasting glucose concentrations [36]. A few epidemiological studies [41] or clinical trials [42] have reported an association between higher fibre intakes and improved insulin sensitivity.

MUFAs

MUFAs have also been proposed to be an efficient way to improve metabolic syndrome. The KANWU study was pioneering work in this direction [43]. It included 162 healthy subjects chosen at random to receive a controlled, iso-energetic diet for 3 months containing either a high proportion of saturated fatty acids (SFA diet) or monounsaturated fatty acids (MUFA diet). Insulin sensitivity was significantly decreased by the SFA diet (−10%, p=0.03) but did not change on the MUFA diet (+2%, NS) (p=0.05 for difference between diets). Insulin secretion was not affected. The favourable effects of substituting a MUFA diet for an SFA diet on insulin sensitivity were only seen at a total fat intake below median (<37% fat). Here, insulin sensitivity was 12.5% lower and 8.8% higher on the SFA diet and MUFA diet respectively (p=0.03). Low density lipoprotein cholesterol (LDL) increased in the SFA diet (+4.1%, p < 0.01) but decreased in the MUFA diet (−5.2, p < 0.001), whereas lipoprotein (a) (Lp(a)) increased on a MUFA diet by 12% (p < 0.001). Thus decreasing SFA and increasing MUFA improves insulin sensitivity but has no effect on insulin secretion. A beneficial impact of the MUFAs on insulin sensitivity is not seen in individuals with a high fat intake (>37% of total energy).

Wine and alcohol

A meta-analysis of seven carefully selected studies (from 14 evaluated) showed that people who drink alcoholic beverages have a lower prevalence of metabolic syndrome compared with non-drinkers. The inverse relation of alcohol consumption and metabolic syndrome was significant in men who consumed <40 g/day (OR 0.84: CI 0.75–0.94) and non-significant for those consuming ≥40 g/day [44]. In women, the association was also significant for those who consumed <20 g/day. (OR 0.75: CI 0.64–0.89). However, the test of heterogeneity was significant in women. As discussed above, there is a close association between metabolic syndrome and CVD. A cross-sectional study was conducted with 808 high cardiovascular risk participants at the PREDIMED Centre[1]. Participants with the highest adherence to the MedDiet had 47 and 54% lower odds of having low HDL-cholesterol and elevated triglycerides [38]. Red wine along with olive oil and legumes were the components in the diet most closely associated with a reduced risk of metabolic syndrome. By contrast, a study in a cohort of elderly Italians (64–85 years of age) did not find any association between moderate alcohol intake (which was mostly wine taken with a meal) and the prevalence and incidence of metabolic syndrome [45].

Dietary pattern

Since fibre, MUFAs and wine are three major components of the MedDiet, it is reasonable to expect an inverse association between metabolic syndrome and adherence to a MedDiet, and several epidemiological studies have found such a relationship. Babio et al. conducted a cross-sectional study on 808 high

---

[1] The PREDIMED is a 5-year clinical trial that aims to assess the effects of the MedDiet on the primary prevention of CVD.

cardiovascular risk participants of the Reus PREDIMED Centre to evaluate the prevalence of the MS in association with metabolic syndrome, assessed by the MDS [38]. An inverse association between quartiles of adherence to the MedDiet (14-point score) and the prevalence of metabolic syndrome was observed (p for trend <0.001). The OR for metabolic syndrome in relation to MDS was decreased for the subjects with the highest MDS (OR 0.48: CI 0.29–0.78, trend 0.002). However, this was mainly due to the sub-group of men (OR 0.41: CI 0.20–0.87, trend 0.024), since there was no association in the group of women. When analysed by various symptoms of metabolic syndrome, the association was significant only for waist circumference and triglycerides blood levels, and only in men. The components of the MDS significantly associated with reduced metabolic syndrome risk were (a) olive oil used as the main culinary oil (OR 0.61: CI 0.38–0.97); (b) drinking ≥3 glasses of wine a week (OR 0.68: CI 0.48–0.95); and (c) having ≥3 serving of legumes (OR 0.62: CI 0.35–0.99). However, since these findings were only observed in men it needs confirmation, and since this study was cross-sectional it might be subjected to reverse causality (see Chapter 8), and requires analysis in a prospective study.

An MDS was also used in the Framingham Heart Study Offspring Cohort [46]. It was based on the recommended intake of 13 food groups in the Mediterranean diet pyramid, i.e. whole-grain cereals, fruit, vegetables, dairy, wine, fish, poultry, olives/legumes/nuts, potatoes, eggs, sweets, meat and olive oil. With the exception of olive oil, each food group was scored from 0 to 10 depending on the extent to which intake corresponded with the recommendation (e.g. consuming 60% of the recommended servings would result in a score of 6). Exceeding the recommendations resulted in a lower score proportional to the degree of over-consumption (e.g. exceeding the recommendation by 60% would result in a score of 4). A negative score due to this over-consumption penalty was defaulted to zero. Scorings for olive oil were: (1) exclusive use of olive oil – score 10; (2) the use of olive oil along with other vegetable oils – score 5; (3) no olive oil – score 0. The sum of the 13 component scores was standardised to a 0–100 scale and weighted proportionally by a continuous factor from 0 to 1, which reflected the proportion of energy intake attributed to the consumption of foods included in the Mediterranean diet pyramid. The total Mediterranean-style dietary pattern score (MSDPS) ranged from 0 to 100. This score was applied to 2730 participants of the Framingham Heart Study Offspring Cohort without type 2 diabetes and used to examine the association between MSDPS and symptoms for metabolic syndrome (mean follow-up time: 7 y), in 1918 participants free of the condition at baseline. All symptoms of the metabolic syndrome, except blood pressure but including insulin resistance, were significantly lower in subjects in the highest quintile of the MSDPS. In addition, participants in the highest quintile of the MSDPS had a lower incidence of metabolic syndrome than those in the lowest quintile (30.1% compared with 38.5%; p=0.01). Thus, the consumption of a diet consistent with the principles of the Mediterranean-style diet was shown to reduce metabolic syndrome risk factors and incidence in a US population.

A randomised single blind trial intended to assess the effect of a Mediterranean-style diet on endothelial function and vascular inflammatory markers in patients with the metabolic syndrome support these observational studies [47]. It was conducted among 180 patients (99 men and 81 women) with metabolic syndrome. Patients in the intervention group (n=90) were instructed to follow a

Mediterranean-style diet and were advised to consume at least 250 to 300 g of fruits, 125 to 150 g of vegetables, and 25 to 50 g of walnuts per day; in addition, they were also encouraged to consume 400 g of whole grains (legumes, rice, maize and wheat) daily and to increase their consumption of olive oil. Patients in the control group (n = 90) followed a prudent diet (carbohydrates 50–60%; proteins 15–20%; total fat <30%). All patients in both groups also received guidance on increasing their level of physical activity, mainly by walking for a minimum of 30 minutes per day but also by swimming or playing aerobic ball games. After two years, patients following the Mediterranean-style diet consumed more foods rich in monounsaturated fat, polyunsaturated fat, and fibre and had a lower ratio of n-6 to n-3 fatty acids. Total fruit, vegetable, and nut intake (274 g/d), whole grain intake (103 g/d), and olive oil consumption (8 g/d) were also significantly higher in the intervention group (p < 0.001). The level of physical activity increased in both groups by approximately 60%, with no difference between the two groups (p = 0.22). Mean [SD] body weight decreased more in patients in the intervention group (–4.0 [1.1] kg) than in those in the control group (–1.2 [0.6] kg) (p < 0.001). Compared with patients consuming the control diet, patients consuming the intervention diet had significantly reduced serum concentrations inflammatory cytokines as well as decreased insulin resistance (p < 0.001). Endothelial function score improved in the intervention group (mean [SD] change, +1.9 [0.6]; p < 0.001) but remained stable in the control group (+0.2 [0.2]; p = 0.33). At 2 years of follow-up, 40 patients in the intervention group still had features of the metabolic syndrome, compared with 78 patients in the control group (p < 0.001).

A comparative review found the MedDiet to be particularly effective in reducing metabolic syndrome compared to other dietary interventions and to various drug interventions [48] (see Figure 10.6). These interventions mostly used a decrease in waist circumference and weight loss as end-points.

In summary, these studies indicate that a Mediterranean-style diet might be effective in reducing the prevalence of the metabolic syndrome and its associated cardiovascular risk.

10.3.3 Mechanisms

Insulin signaling and insulin resistance

Although metabolic syndrome is a complex disorder, and hence there are many potential points of intervention, there is a general consensus that the major underpinning mechanism is likely to be insulin resistance. Thus, establishing the cause, or causes, of insulin resistance should contribute to understanding how constituents in the MedDiet may be acting to reduce metabolic syndrome.

Insulin resistance in the body is frequently due to defects in the insulin signalling pathway. This signalling pathway consists of a series of steps initiated by insulin binding to a cell surface receptor. The intracellular domain of the insulin receptor has an enzyme activity known as a protein tyrosine kinase. This enzyme phosphorylates tyrosine residues on insulin receptor substrate-1 (IRS-1). IRS-1 activates further "downstream" signaling molecules including protein kinase B (PKB) (also known as Akt). Akt/PKB enables the GLUT-4 transporter to translocate from the cytoplasm to the cell membrane thus allowing glucose uptake (Figure 10.7).

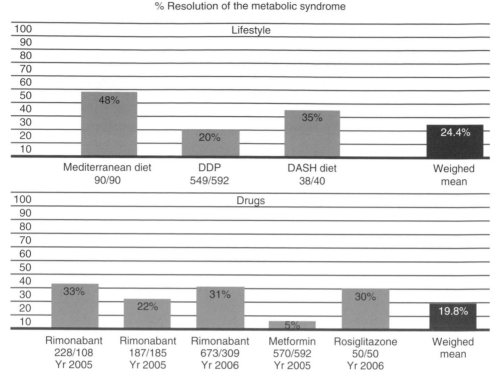

Figure 10.6   Effects of lifestyle changes or drugs on the % resolution of the metabolic syndrome (y axis) in placebo-controlled clinical trials. The numbers under the column heading indicate the size of interventional and placebo groups. The year is the year of publication of the study. DDP: Diabetes Prevention Program; DASH: Dietary Approach to Stop Hypertension [48].

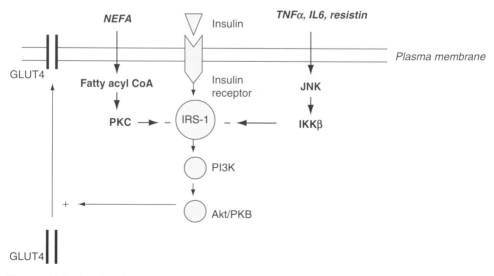

Figure 10.7   Insulin signalling and its inhibition. (IRS-1: insulin receptor substrate-1; NEFA: non-esterified fatty acids; PKC: protein kinase C; IKKβ: inhibitor of kappa B kinase β; PI3K: phosphatidylinositol-3-kinase; – inhibition; + activation.)

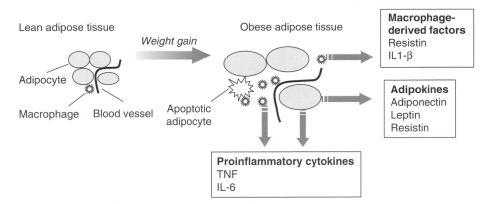

Figure 10.8   Adipokine and cytokine production by adipocytes and macrophages (redrawn from [51]). Reprinted with permission from Macmillan Publishers Ltd, copyright 2006 Nature.

Insulin resistance – the role of obesity

One of the main causes of defects in the insulin signalling pathway, and hence of insulin resistance, is obesity. Indeed, abdominal obesity has been estimated to account for more than three-quarters of all cases of metabolic syndrome [49].

Several mechanisms have been proposed to explain how abdominal obesity reduces insulin signalling and causes insulin resistance. Firstly, abdominal obesity is associated with the release of large amounts of non-esterified fatty acids (NEFAs) from adipose tissue. These accumulate in liver and muscle and are converted into metabolites which activate the enzyme protein kinase C. This enzyme phosphorylates IRS-1 on serine residues, rather than tyrosine residues, and this inhibits the activity of IRS-1 hence reducing the insulin signaling pathway (see Figure 10.7).

Another proposed mechanism linking obesity with insulin resistance arises from the increasing recognition that adipose tissue is not simply a passive store for fat, but rather acts as an important endocrine gland releasing various hormones into the circulation [50]. These hormones, known as adipocytokines or adipokines, can modulate insulin resistance. Adipokines include both conventional cytokines such as interleukins 1 and 6 (IL-1 and IL-6) and tumour necrosis factor α (TNFα), and factors more closely associated with adipose tissue such as leptin, adiponectin and resistin (Figure 10.8). Many of these factors are produced by the fat storage cells (adipocytes). It is now recognised that macrophages infiltrate adipose tissue, and these infiltrating macrophages also contribute to the pool of cytokines and adipokines (Figure 10.8). TNFα, IL-6 and resistin can activate an intracellular pathway that inactivates IRS-1, hence making the body less able to respond to insulin (Figure 10.7).

Reversing insulin resistance

Several mechanisms that link the MedDiet with a reduction in insulin resistance have been suggested. These include:

1. reducing adiposity
2. anti-inflammatory effects
3. restoring a normal insulin signalling pathway

1. Reducing adiposity

Weight loss has been shown to reduce insulin resistance [28] and this may therefore contribute to the improvements in clinical symptoms for metabolic syndrome in individuals on a MedDiet who lose weight. The relatively high proportion of calories from fat relative to carbohydrate in the MedDiet may also be significant. A high carbohydrate "prudent" diet (55–60% calories from carbohydrate, 25–30% from fat, 15% from protein) has been recommended in order to reduce intake of saturated fat. However, this proportion of calories from carbohydrate will lead to a significant increase in hyperinsulinaemia in individuals already showing some degree of insulin resistance and this could further exacerbate the condition. It has been suggested that saturated fat should be replaced by unsaturated fat rather than by carbohydrate, and this would more closely resemble the relatively high calorie intake from unsaturated fat present in the MedDiet. Increasing the proportion of calories from fat and protein rather than from carbohydrate was found to be an effective way of reducing obesity and of promoting a non-atherogenic lipid profile and to reduce fasting glucose levels [52].

2. Anti-inflammatory effects

The influx and activation of inflammatory cells into adipose tissue result in a number of adverse effects in the body. For example, pro-inflammatory cytokines inhibit the production of the adipokine adiponectin. Adiponectin normally has beneficial effects since it has insulin-like activity and sensitises the body to insulin. Hence, a reduction in adiponectin can increase the likelihood of insulin resistance. Increasing adiponectin may be a mechanism contributing to the beneficial effects of the MedDiet since a 2-year randomised controlled trial demonstrated that a MedDiet accompanied by increased physical activity significantly increased adiponectin concentrations in obese post-menopausal women, even after accounting for the decreased body weight associated with the intervention [47]. Many anti-inflammatory constituents have been identified in the MedDiet that could potentially suppress pro-inflammatory responses (see Chapter 9). For example, olive oil has anti-inflammatory effects by inhibiting the activation of the pro-inflammatory transcription factor NFκB [30].

3. Restoring a normal insulin signalling pathway

There is some experimental evidence that constituents in the MedDiet can restore a normal insulin signalling pathway, although clinical studies are often less consistent. Constituents in the MedDiet that have been implicated in modulating insulin signalling include:

(a) olive oil
(b) wine
(c) cinnamon
(d) green tea
(e) chromium

(a) **Olive oil**: Evidence from controlled intervention studies suggest that there are beneficial effects on insulin sensitivity when saturated fats and trans fats are replaced with MUFA or PUFA [53]. The evidence for a potential protective effect is stronger for *n*-6 PUFAs than for *n*-3 PUFAs, but more research is needed. Olive oil increases insulin sensitivity and one proposed mechanism is that oleic acid incorporated into cell membranes affects their fluidity causing favourable effects on the insulin receptor located there [30].

(b) **Wine**: Some intervention studies have found that moderate alcohol consumption increases production of adiponectin [54]. In another study, improvement of HOMA-score, i.e. insulin sensitivity, was observed after moderate alcohol consumption for 6 weeks [55]. Moderate alcohol consumption is associated with an increase in HDL cholesterol (low HDL cholesterol is one of the diagnostic criteria for metabolic syndrome). Some studies have suggested that red wine phenolics may exert additional benefits. Attention has focussed on resveratrol since feeding resveratrol to obese mice was found to increase their insulin sensitivity and overall longevity [56]. However, the relevance of this observation to humans consuming a MedDiet is uncertain since far higher levels of resveratrol were administered to the mice than would be consumed in red wine.

(c) **Cinnamon**: Cinnamon is a popular spice in some Mediterranean countries such as Greece. Cinnamon has insulin-sensitising properties [57] and polyphenols in cinnamon have been shown to increase the activity of the insulin signalling pathway which is required for cells to respond to insulin [30]. Clinical studies using cinnamon or cinnamon extracts have examined various parameters such as fasting blood glucose levels, glycated haemoglobin (HbA1c) and serum triglycerides, although results have been mixed [58].

(d) **Green tea**: Green tea, consumed in some countries in the southern Mediterranean basin, is another foodstuff known from experimental models to influence insulin signalling pathways [30].

(e) **Chromium**: Chromium has been shown to be required for insulin action. Indeed, the effects of chromium deficiency in the body are remarkably similar to those of metabolic syndrome, and include elevated fasting glucose, low serum HDL, elevated triglycerides, hypertension and visceral obesity [57]. Adequate intake of chromium will be important to prevent symptoms of metabolic syndrome associated with a deficiency. However, there is no consistent evidence that chromium deficiency is the dominant factor in most cases of metabolic syndrome, and chromium supplementation has not proven to be effective for treating metabolic syndrome in people who are not deficient in this mineral [58]. The chromium appears to be efficient only as picolinate and in subjects with high insulin-resistance [59]. The chromium content of the MedDiet has not been systematically studied, although pulses and some Mediterranean herbs such as mint are good sources [60].

10.4 Type 2 diabetes

10.4.1 Introduction

Diabetes mellitus is the major form of diabetes and refers to the sweet urine (hence *mellitus*) resulting from hyperglycaemia. There are more than 2.3 million people in the UK with diabetes, and it is estimated that by 2025 there will be 380 million people affected globally. There are two types of diabetes mellitus, types 1 (early onset diabetes) and 2. Type 2 diabetes is strongly associated with a Western lifestyle, especially obesity, lack of physical exercise, and consumption of a high fat, low fibre diet. Most of the evidence for benefits of a MedDiet are in relation to type 2 diabetes – a metabolic disorder, rather than type 1 – resulting from loss of cell function.

Type 2 diabetes occurs when two major abnormalities co-exist [61]:

- resistance of target tissues (skeletal muscle, adipose tissue and liver) to the actions of insulin
- a reduction in insulin secretion due to damage to the β cells in the pancreas

Insulin resistance results in a failure of muscle, adipose tissue and skeletal muscle to respond appropriately to glucose. Studies suggest that insulin resistance is an early phenomenon and occurs years before there is any evidence of glucose intolerance. The term "prediabetes" was adopted in 2002 for the state of impaired glucose tolerance in order to emphasise its serious nature. There may be a compensatory increase in insulin secretion during the early stages of the disease. A state of hyperinsulinaemia is also seen in metabolic syndrome. However, in the pathogenesis of diabetes, failure of the β cells to produce insulin eventually develops, and type 2 diabetes occurs when the pancreas is no longer able to produce sufficient amounts of insulin.

A large number of inherited gene defects have been identified that increase the risk of developing type 2 diabetes [62]. However, the stage or stages in the pathogenesis of diabetes where these defects act is not well defined. It is possible that some genetic factors act at later stages of the pathogenesis since not all people with obesity and insulin resistance will go on to develop diabetes.

10.4.2   Epidemiology

In view of the findings reported above on abdominal obesity and metabolic syndrome, and because components of a traditional Mediterranean dietary pattern were shown in short-term randomised experimental trials to improve insulin sensitivity and other vascular-metabolic risk factors [63–66], a strong relationship between adherence to a MedDiet and type 2 diabetes could be expected. However, only a few epidemiological studies are robust enough to support such a relationship. Rather, most studies relate to glycaemic control and evaluation of insulin and insulin-resistance. Insulin resistance can be assessed using homeostasis model assessment (HOMA) (see above) and by measuring glycated haemoglobin (HbA1c) which results from long- term exposure (several months) to high plasma glucose levels. A reduction in HbA1c is recognised by the US Food and Drug Administration as a clinically relevant marker of efficacy for diabetes treatment.

Adherence to a Mediterranean-type diet was assessed using the MDS in 901 out-patients with type 2 diabetes attending diabetes clinics located in Southern Italy in a cross-sectional analysis. Using multivariate analysis, mean HbA1c and 2 h post-meal glucose concentrations were significantly lower in diabetic patients with high adherence to a Mediterranean-type diet than those with low adherence: there was a difference in HbA1c of 0.9% (CI 0.5–1.2%, p <0.001) and 2 h glucose differed by 2.2 mmol/L (CI 0.8–2.9 mmol/l, p <0.001). The overall dietary pattern appeared to be most important since no strong associations were evident for individual components of the MedDiet score (there was a modest association with whole grains and the ratio of monounsaturated to saturated lipids) [67]. In the ATTICA study, 1514 men and 1528 women (18–89 years old) were enrolled. Both normo-glycaemic subjects and impaired fasting glycaemia or diabetic subjects in the upper tertile of the MDS had lower glycaemia, insulinaemia and HOMA scores. However, when multiple regression analysis (adjusted for age, sex, BMI, waist-to-hip ratio, physical activity, smoking status, and presence of hypertension and hypercholesterolemia) was performed, these associations were confirmed in normoglycaemic, but not in diabetic/impaired fasting glycaemia subjects suggesting a preventative role for the MedDiet [68]. In a study of 215 overweight newly-diagnosed patients with type 2 diabetes, putting them on a MedDiet delayed the need for anti-hyperglycaemic drugs [69].

As well as studying the potential benefits of the MedDiet in relation to glycaemic control, the overall beneficial effects of a diet rich in fruit and vegetable for diabetics was recently confirmed in a large multi-centre prospective cohort study, EPIC (European Prospective Investigation in Cancer and Nutrition) [70]. A cohort of 10,449 participants with self-reported diabetes within the EPIC study was followed for a mean of 9 y. Intakes of vegetables, legumes and fruit were assessed at baseline between 1992 and 2000 using validated country-specific questionnaires. A total of 1346 deaths occurred. An increment in intake of total vegetables, legumes, and fruit of 80 g/d was associated with a RR of death from all causes of 0.94 (CI 0.90–0.98). CVD mortality and mortality due to non-CVD/non-cancer causes were significantly inversely associated with intake of total vegetables, legumes and fruit (RR 0.88: CI 0.81–0.95 and RR 0.90: CI 0.82–0.99, respectively). Intake of vegetables, legumes and fruit was associated with reduced risks of all causes and CVD mortality in a diabetic population.

In the context of primary prevention, a few studies have shown that Mediterranean food patterns are associated with a significant reduction in the risk of developing type 2 diabetes. A study by Panagiotakos et al. [71] showed that a 10-unit increase in the diet score was associated with 21% lower odds of developing diabetes (p < 0.05), while individuals taking light physical activity were at 35% lower odds ratio of diabetes compared with sedentary individuals (p < 0.05). However, this was a cross-sectional study, and hence contributes only rather weak support for the relationship between adherence to a MedDiet and type 2 diabetes.

A prospective study of a cohort of 13,380 former Spanish university graduates (average age 38 years) without diabetes at baseline was followed up for a median of 4.4 years. Thirty-three cases of new onset type 2 diabetes were identified among 58,918 person years of follow-up. Incidence rate ratios adjusted for sex and age were 0.41 (CI 0.19–0.87) for those with moderate adherence (score 3–6) and 0.17 (CI 0.04–0.75) for those with the highest adherence (score 7–9) compared with those with low adherence (score <3). A 2-point increase in the score was associated with a 35% relative reduction in the risk of diabetes with a significant inverse linear trend (p = 0.04) in the multivariate analysis. The number of cases was very small, hence the large CI [72].

In an investigation of the role of dietary factors in the Mediterranean area, newly diagnosed individuals with type 2 diabetes, and individuals who had not known that they had diabetes, were found to have had a higher relative intake of total fat and SFA from animal fat sources compared with healthy controls [73].

Mozzafarian et al. [74] took advantage of the cohort of the GISSI intervention trial to study the development of diabetes and impaired fasting glucose in

8291 patients who had had a myocardial infarction within the previous three months, and who were free of diabetes at baseline (determined by medication use, a physician-reported diagnosis, or fasting glucose ≥ 7 mmol/L). Of the 7533 without impaired fasting glucose at baseline, 2514 (33%) developed new-onset impaired fasting glucose or diabetes rising to 3859 (62%) of 6229 with the lower cutoff for impaired fasting glucose of 5.6 mmol/L. The nutritonal data did not allow for the construction of an MDS, thus a substitute score was obtained according to consumption of cooked and raw vegetables, fruit, fish and olive oil. Independent lifestyle risk-factors included higher BMI, greater BMI gain during follow-up, current smoking, a lower MDS, and wine consumption of more than 1 L/day. Data for physical activity were unavailable, but inability to perform exercise testing was associated with higher incidence of diabetes and impaired fasting glucose. This study, although taking place in an unusual context (post-myocardial infarction), did show the beneficial effect of a diet presenting the main components of the MedDiet (except for grains, nuts or legumes.), and also other lifestyle factors associated with a Mediterranean dietary pattern.

A number of studies have shown that moderate alcohol consumption is associated with improved insulin sensitivity [75]. These studies may help explain the increasing number of studies that suggest that light to moderate alcohol consumption is associated with a lower risk of developing type 2 diabetes. A meta analysis of 15 prospective cohort studies found a J-shaped relationship between alcohol consumption and risk of type 2 diabetes [76]. For moderate consumption in three categories ranging from 6 to 48 g/day, the RR values for each of the three categories were very close to 0.70 (0.61–0.79). The risk of type 2 diabetes in heavy drinkers (≥ 48 g/day) was equal to that for non-consumers (RR 1.04; CI 0.84–1.29). However, controlling for food and energy consumption was only performed in two of the studies included in the meta analysis.

Long-term (>30 years) and moderate coffee consumption was also reported to be associated with a lower prevalence of type 2 diabetes in elderly people from the Mediterranean islands (the MEDIS study) [77].

10.4.3 Mechanisms

Glycaemic control

Rapid absorption of dietary glucose is associated with an increased risk of type 2 diabetes. Two mechanisms have been proposed to explain this: (a) excessive secretion of insulin eventually resulting in loss of this function by the pancreatic β-cells; (b) toxicity to the β-cells due to hyperglycaemia [78]. Irrespective of the underlying mechanism, the association between high dietary glucose and type 2 diabetes indicates that reducing glucose absorption will benefit diabetic patients.

One way to reduce glucose absorption is to replace carbohydrates with a high glycaemic index (GI) with ones with a lower GI in order to result in meals with a low glycaemic load. This has been found to benefit diabetic patients by improving glycaemic control in people treated with insulin, and also to reduce their hypogly-caemic episodes [78]. Although many carbohydrate-rich foods associated with the MedDiet have a relatively low GI, the GI values of honey and starchy foods such as potatoes and pasta are quite high (see Chapter 2). However, some preparation techniques used in Mediterranean cooking may modify the GI of these foods. For example, Italian potato dumplings (gnocchi), prepared by mashing potato with wheat flour, had a significantly lower GI value compared to plain mashed potato, possibly because access of α-amylase enzymes to the starch granules was reduced by protein from the cereal [79]. Various dietary factors including phytic acid and phenolics are inhibitors of α-amylase, although their role in reducing glucose absorption is unclear.

Fibre consumed as part of a meal can reduce the GI value of a carbohydrate-rich food. Various mechanisms have been suggested to explain this observation including:

- delaying gastric emptying (i.e. emptying of the stomach) – this is the major determinant of delivery of nutrients to the small intestine and may account for differences in the GI values between rice, bread and potatoes [80]
- slowing intestinal motility
- effects on hormones in the gut – these include hormones that increase the insulin response to food (so-called incretins), appetite-regulating hormones that stimulate food intake, such as ghrelin, and hormones that reduce food intake, such as cholecystokinin [81].

Glucose absorption across enterocytes mainly takes place in the proximal small intestine, via the sodium-glucose co-transporter (SGLT1) at the luminal membrane and via the glucose transporter GLUT2 at the basolateral membrane. Several dietary phenolics have been shown to interact with SGLT1 in experimental systems and hence lower glucose uptake, and it has been suggested that this could be a mechanism by which regular consumption of fruits and vegetables containing these phenolics could reduce the incidence of type 2 diabetes [82].

Although there is sound evidence that a MedDiet offers good glycaemic control, more research is required in order to establish whether or not it is better than current nutritional recommendations for type 2 diabetes.

Fats

The relatively high proportions of PUFAs and MUFAs in the MedDiet coupled with the low amounts of saturated fats and trans fatty acids has beneficial effects on insulin sensitivity and this is likely to reduce the risk of type 2 diabetes. Several mechanisms could be involved, including effects on membrane structure and function, PPARs and other receptor-mediated events [53].

Weight control

The term "diabesity" is used to highlight the close relationship between type 2 diabetes and obesity, and several mechanisms have been proposed to explain why obesity increases the risk of type 2 diabetes. One important effect of obesity is to increase insulin resistance, and this has been discussed above. Another consequence of obesity is that fat infiltrates into the pancreatic islet cells that produce insulin and this reduces their capacity to produce insulin. The preponderance of MUFAs and other fats in the MedDiet that have an increased tendency to be oxidised rather than stored, may contribute to the negative associations between the MedDiet and obesity observed in some epidemiological studies (see Section 10.2.2).

Coffee

Coffee consumption, which is high in some Mediterranean countries, is associated with a reduced risk of type 2 diabetes [77, 83]. Chlorogenic acid has a wide range of effects on glucose metabolism, and the high chlorogenic acid content of coffee may contribute to the association between coffee drinking and a reduced risk of type 2 diabetes [83]. Coffee is also a good source of magnesium, another substance that is associated with glucose homeostasis. There is less evidence for a role for caffeine since decaffeinated coffee is also associated with a reduced risk of type 2 diabetes.

Other nutrients

Chromium and cinnamon have been discussed above (see Section 10.3.3). Some studies have found that chromium improves glucose, insulin, HbA1c and cholesterol in diabetic patients, and cinnamon supplementation has also shown benefits, although results have been variable [57].

References

1. IOTF, *International Obesity Task Force* 2008 cited; Available from: http://www.iotf.org/
2. Teucher, B. et al. Obesity: focus on all-cause mortality and cancer. *Maturitas*, 65(2): 112–6.
3. Haslam, D.W., James, W.P. Obesity. *Lancet*, 2005. 366(9492): 1197–209.
4. Andreyeva, T. et al.Obesity and health in Europeans aged 50 years and older. *Public Health*, 2007. 121(7): 497–509.
5. IASO, International Association for the Study of Obesity. http://www.iaso.org/
6. FAO, FAO Newsroom. http://www.fao.org/index_fr.htm, 2008.
7. Scali, J. et al. Diet profiles in a population sample from Mediterranean southern France. *Public Health Nutr*, 2001. 4(2): 173–82.
8. Loviselli, A. et al. Prevalence and trend of overweight and obesity among Sardinian conscripts (Italy) of 1969 and 1998. *J Biosoc Sci*, 2010. 42(2): 201–11.
9. Velluzzi, F. et al. Prevalence of overweight and obesity in Sardinian adolescents. *Eat Weight Disord*, 2007. 12(2): e44–50.
10. Tessier, S., Gerber, M. Comparison between Sardinia and Malta: the Mediterranean diet revisited. *Appetite*, 2005. 45(2): 121–6.
11. Tessier, S., Gerber, M. Factors determining the nutrition transition in two Mediterranean islands: Sardinia and Malta. *Public Health Nutr*, 2005. 8(8): 1286–92.
12. Mendez, M.A. et al. Adherence to a Mediterranean diet is associated with reduced 3-year incidence of obesity. *J Nutr*, 2006. 136(11): 2934–8.
13. Panagiotakos, D.B. et al. Association between the prevalence of obesity and adherence to the Mediterranean diet: the ATTICA study. *Nutrition*, 2006. 22(5): 449–56.
14. Rossi, M. et al. Mediterranean diet in relation to body mass index and waist-to-hip ratio. *Public Health Nutr*, 2008. 11(2): 214–7.
15. Sanchez-Villegas, A. et al. Adherence to a Mediterranean dietary pattern and weight gain in a follow-up study: the SUN cohort. *Int J Obes (Lond)*, 2006. 30(2): 350–8.
16. Schroder, H. et al. Adherence to the traditional mediterranean diet is inversely associated with body mass index and obesity in a spanish population. *J Nutr*, 2004. 134(12): 3355–61.
17. Romaguera, D. et al. Adherence to the Mediterranean diet is associated with lower abdominal adiposity in European men and women. *J Nutr*, 2009. 139(9): 1728–37.
18. Trichopoulou, A. et al. Mediterranean diet in relation to body mass index and waist-to-hip ratio: the Greek European Prospective Investigation into Cancer and Nutrition Study. *Am J Clin Nutr*, 2005. 82(5): 935–40.
19. Shai, I. et al. Weight loss with a low-carbohydrate, Mediterranean, or low-fat diet. *N Engl J Med*, 2008. 359(3): 229–41.

20. Buckland, G. et al. Obesity and the Mediterranean diet: a systematic review of observational and intervention studies. *Obes Rev*, 2008. **9**(6): 582–93.
21. Schroder, H. Protective mechanisms of the Mediterranean diet in obesity and type 2 diabetes. *J Nutr Biochem,* 2007. **18**(3): 49–60.
22. Moussavi, N. et al. Could the quality of dietary fat, and not just its quantity, be related to risk of obesity? *Obesity (Silver Spring)*, 2008. **16**(1): 7–15.
23. Bergouignan, A. et al. Metabolic fate of saturated and monounsaturated dietary fats: the Mediterranean diet revisited from epidemiological evidence to cellular mechanisms. *Prog Lipid Res*, 2009. **48**(3–4): 128–47.
24. Soares, M.J. et al. The acute effects of olive oil v. cream on postprandial thermogenesis and substrate oxidation in postmenopausal women. *Br J Nutr*, 2004. **91**(2): 245–52.
25. Li, J.J. et al. Anti-obesity effects of conjugated linoleic acid, docosahexaenoic acid, and eicosapentaenoic acid. *Mol Nutr Food Res*, 2008. **52**(6): 631–45.
26. Grundy, S.M. et al. Clinical management of metabolic syndrome: report of the American Heart Association/National Heart, Lung, and Blood Institute/American Diabetes Association conference on scientific issues related to management. *Circulation*, 2004. **109**(4): 551–6.
27. Heald, A.H. et al. Low sex hormone binding globulin is a potential marker for the metabolic syndrome in different ethnic groups. *Exp Clin Endocrinol Diabetes*, 2005. **113**(9): 522–8.
28. Reaven, G.M. The insulin resistance syndrome: definition and dietary approaches to treatment. *Annu Rev Nutr*, 2005. **25**: 391–406.
29. Grundy, S.M. et al. Diagnosis and management of the metabolic syndrome: an American Heart Association/National Heart, Lung, and Blood Institute Scientific Statement. *Circulation*, 2005. **112**(17): 2735–52.
30. Minich, D.M., Bland, J.S. Dietary management of the metabolic syndrome beyond macronutrients. *Nutr Rev*, 2008. **66**(8): 429–44.
31. Zivkovic, A.M. et al. Comparative review of diets for the metabolic syndrome: implications for nonalcoholic fatty liver disease. *Am J Clin Nutr*, 2007. **86**(2): 285–300.
32. Lairon, D. Dietary fibres: effects on lipid metabolism and mechanisms of action. *Eur J Clin Nutr*, 1996. **50**(3): 125–33.
33. Ludwig, D.S. et al. Dietary fiber, weight gain, and cardiovascular disease risk factors in young adults. *Jama*, 1999. **282**(16): 1539–46.
34. Liu, S. et al. Relation between changes in intakes of dietary fiber and grain products and changes in weight and development of obesity among middle-aged women. *Am J Clin Nutr*, 2003. **78**(5): 920–7.
35. Wu, H. et al. Dietary fiber and progression of atherosclerosis: the Los Angeles Atherosclerosis Study. *Am J Clin Nutr*, 2003. **78**(6): 1085–91.
36. McKeown, N.M. et al. Whole-grain intake is favorably associated with metabolic risk factors for type 2 diabetes and cardiovascular disease in the Framingham Offspring Study. *Am J Clin Nutr*, 2002. **76**(2): 390–8.
37. Sahyoun, N.R. et al. Whole-grain intake is inversely associated with the metabolic syndrome and mortality in older adults. *Am J Clin Nutr*, 2006. **83**(1): 124–31.
38. Babio, N. et al. Adherence to the Mediterranean diet and risk of metabolic syndrome and its components. *Nutr Metab Cardiovasc Dis*, 2009. **19**(8): 563–70.
39. Cara, L. et al. Effects of oat bran, rice bran, wheat fiber, and wheat germ on postprandial lipemia in healthy adults. *Am J Clin Nutr*, 1992. **55**(1): 81–8.
40. Lia, A. et al. Postprandial lipemia in relation to sterol and fat excretion in ileostomy subjects given oat-bran and wheat test meals. *Am J Clin Nutr*, 1997. **66**(2): 357–65.
41. McKeown, N.M. Whole grain intake and insulin sensitivity: evidence from observational studies. *Nutr Rev*, 2004. **62**(7 Pt 1): 286–91.
42. Pereira, M.A. et al. Effect of whole grains on insulin sensitivity in overweight hyperinsulinemic adults. *Am J Clin Nutr*, 2002. **75**(5): 848–55.
43. Rivellese, A.A. et al. Type of dietary fat and insulin resistance. *Ann NY Acad Sci*, 2002. **967**: 329–35.
44. Alkerwi, A. et al. Alcohol consumption and the prevalence of metabolic syndrome: a meta-analysis of observational studies. *Atherosclerosis*, 2009. **204**(2): 624–35.
45. Buja, A. et al. Alcohol consumption and metabolic syndrome in the elderly: results from the Italian longitudinal study on aging. *Eur J Clin Nutr*, 2010. **64**(3): 297–307.

46. Rumawas, M.E. et al. Mediterranean-style dietary pattern, reduced risk of metabolic syndrome traits, and incidence in the Framingham Offspring Cohort. *Am J Clin Nutr*, 2009. **90**(6): 1608–14.
47. Esposito, K. et al. Effect of a mediterranean-style diet on endothelial dysfunction and markers of vascular inflammation in the metabolic syndrome: a randomized trial. *Jama*, 2004. **292**(12): 1440–6.
48. Esposito, K. et al. Mediterranean diet and the metabolic syndrome. *Mol Nutr Food Res*, 2007. **51**(10): 1268–74.
49. Mittal, S. *The metabolic syndrome in clinical practice*. 2008: Springer-Verlag, London.
50. Evans, R.M. et al. PPARs and the complex journey to obesity. *Nat Med*, 2004. **10**(4): 355–61.
51. Tilg, H., Moschen, A.R. Adipocytokines: mediators linking adipose tissue, inflammation and immunity. *Nat Rev Immunol*, 2006. **6**(10): 772–83.
52. Perez-Guisado, J. et al. Spanish Ketogenic Mediterranean Diet: a healthy cardiovascular diet for weight loss. *Nutr J*, 2008. 7: 30–6.
53. Risérus, U., Willett, W.C., Hu, F.B. Dietary fats and prevention of type 2 diabetes. *Prog Lipid Res*, 2009. 48(1): 44–51.
54. Hendriks, H.F. Moderate Alcohol Consumption and Insulin Sensitivity: Observations and Possible Mechanisms. *Ann Epidemiol*, 2007. **17**: pp. S40–S42.
55. Joosten, M.M. et al. Moderate alcohol consumption increases insulin sensitivity and ADIPOQ expression in postmenopausal women: a randomised, crossover trial. *Diabetologia*, 2008. **51**(8): 1375–81.
56. Baur, J.A. et al. Resveratrol improves health and survival of mice on a high-calorie diet. *Nature*, 2006. **444**(7117): 337–42.
57. Anderson, R.A. Chromium and polyphenols from cinnamon improve insulin sensitivity. *Proc Nutr Soc*, 2008. **67**(1): 48–53.
58. Potenza, M.V., Mechanick, J.I. The metabolic syndrome: definition, global impact, and pathophysiology. *Nutr Clin Pract*, 2009. **24**(5): 560–77.
59. Wang, Z.Q. et al. Phenotype of subjects with type 2 diabetes mellitus may determine clinical response to chromium supplementation. *Metabolism*, 2007. **56**(12): 1652–5.
60. Garcia, E. et al. Chromium levels in spices and aromatic herbs. *Sci Total Environ*, 2000. **247**(1): 51–6.
61. Virally, M. et al. Type 2 diabetes mellitus: epidemiology, pathophysiology, unmet needs and therapeutical perspectives. *Diabetes Metab*, 2007. **33**(4): 231–44.
62. Doria, A. et al. The emerging genetic architecture of type 2 diabetes. *Cell Metab*, 2008. **8**(3): 186–200.
63. Ryan, M. et al. Diabetes and the Mediterranean diet: a beneficial effect of oleic acid on insulin sensitivity, adipocyte glucose transport and endothelium-dependent vasoreactivity. *QJM*, 2000. **93**(2): 85–91.
64. Fuentes, F. et al. Mediterranean and low-fat diets improve endothelial function in hypercholesterolemic men. *Ann Intern Med*, 2001. **134**(12): 1115–9.
65. Perez-Jimenez, F. et al. A Mediterranean and a high-carbohydrate diet improve glucose metabolism in healthy young persons. *Diabetologia*, 2001. **44**(11): 2038–43.
66. Vincent-Baudry, S. et al. The Medi-RIVAGE study: reduction of cardiovascular disease risk factors after a 3-mo intervention with a Mediterranean-type diet or a low-fat diet. *Am J Clin Nutr*, 2005. **82**(5): 964–71.
67. Esposito, K. et al. Adherence to a Mediterranean diet and glycaemic control in Type 2 diabetes mellitus. *Diabet Med*, 2009. **26**(9): 900–7.
68. Panagiotakos, D.B. et al. The association between adherence to the Mediterranean diet and fasting indices of glucose homoeostasis: the ATTICA Study. *J Am Coll Nutr*, 2007. **26**(1): 32–8.
69. Esposito, K. et al. Effects of a Mediterranean-style diet on the need for antihyperglycemic drug therapy in patients with newly diagnosed type 2 diabetes: a randomized trial. *Ann Intern Med*, 2009. **151**(5): 306–14.
70. Heidemann, C. et al. Association of a diabetes risk score with risk of myocardial infarction, stroke, specific types of cancer, and mortality: a prospective study in the European Prospective Investigation into Cancer and Nutrition (EPIC)-Potsdam cohort. *Eur J Epidemiol*, 2009. **24**(6): 281–8.
71. Panagiotakos, D.B. et al. The epidemiology of Type 2 diabetes mellitus in Greek adults: the ATTICA study. *Diabet Med*, 2005. **22**(11): 1581–8.
72. Martinez-Gonzalez, M.A. et al. Adherence to Mediterranean diet and risk of developing diabetes: prospective cohort study. *BMJ*, 2008. **336**(7657): 1348–51.

73. Thanopoulou, A.C. et al. Dietary fat intake as risk factor for the development of diabetes: multinational, multicenter study of the Mediterranean Group for the Study of Diabetes (MGSD). *Diabetes Care*, 2003. **26**(2): 302–7.

74. Mozaffarian, D. et al. Incidence of new-onset diabetes and impaired fasting glucose in patients with recent myocardial infarction and the effect of clinical and lifestyle risk factors. *Lancet*, 2007. **370**(9588): 667–75.

75. Lippi, G. et al. Moderate red wine consumption and cardiovascular disease risk: beyond the "French paradox". *Semin Thromb Hemost*, 2010. **36**(1): 59–70.

76. Koppes, L.L. et al. Moderate alcohol consumption lowers the risk of type 2 diabetes: a meta-analysis of prospective observational studies. *Diabetes Care*, 2005. **28**(3): 719–25.

77. Panagiotakos, D.B. et al. Long-term, moderate coffee consumption is associated with lower prevalence of diabetes mellitus among elderly non-tea drinkers from the Mediterranean Islands (MEDIS Study). *Rev Diabet Stud*, 2007. **4**(2): 105–11.

78. Willett, W. et al. Glycemic index, glycemic load, and risk of type 2 diabetes. *Am J Clin Nutr*, 2002. **76**(1): 274S–80S.

79. Riccardi, G. et al. Glycemic index of local foods and diets: the Mediterranean experience. *Nutr Rev*, 2003. **61**(5 Pt 2): S56–60.

80. Rayner, C.K. et al. Relationships of upper gastrointestinal motor and sensory function with glycemic control. *Diabetes Care*, 2001. **24**(2): 371–81.

81. Anderson, J.W. Dietary fiber and associated phytochemicals in prevention and reversal of diabetes. In: *Nutraceuticals, glycemic health and type 2 diabetes*, V.K. Pasupuleti and J.W. Anderson, Editors. 2008, Wiley-Blackwell: Oxford. p. xvii.

82. Clifford, M., Brown, J.E. Dietary flavonoids and health - broadening the perspective. In: *Flavonoids: chemistry, biochemistry, and applications*, Ø.M. Andersen and K.R. Markham, Editors. 2006, CRC: Boca Raton, Fla.; London.

83. Pimentel, G.D. et al. Does long-term coffee intake reduce type 2 diabetes mellitus risk? *Diabetol Metab Syndr*, 2009. **1**(1): 6.

11 Cardiovascular Diseases

Summary

- The most prevalent form of CVD is coronary heart disease (CHD), and the main cause of CVD is atherosclerosis.
- An important interplay between the different FAs in the MedDiet contributes to its protective effects against CVD. Saturated fat is highly correlated with total cholesterol, whereas medium chain saturated fatty acids (<12 carbon atoms) – which are particularly rich in the MedDiet from goat and sheep milk products – are less atherogenic. PUFAs play a role in lowering total LDL-cholesterol, the more dangerous form of cholesterol. In contrast to PUFAs, oleic acid – the main FA in olive oil – does not lower more beneficial HDL-cholesterol.
- Long chain n-3 PUFAs have beneficial effects on myocardial rhythm and anti-inflammatory effects. Anti-inflammatory effects seem to be particularly important for eicosapentaenoic acid (EPA), whereas docosahexaenoic acid (DHA) appears to be more protective of the myocardium.
- Potassium has a specific role at the kidney and in sodium balance, and fibre decreases several risk factors for CVD. However, evidence for a role for many other micronutrients and phytochemicals found in fruits and vegetables is less consistent.
- Both the MUFA and phenolic components of olive oil contribute to a range of beneficial effects on risk factors for CVD seen in human intervention studies.
- In 2011 the European Food Safety Authority issued a general health claim on the polyphenol antioxidant and reduced LDL cholesterol effects of olive oil.
- There is good epidemiological evidence that tea drinking reduces the risk of CVD, although this evidence comes from non-Mediterranean countries. No clear pattern has emerged from studies on coffee consumption in various countries regarding risk of CHD or hypertension.
- Cardiovascular benefits of moderate consumption of red wine or other forms of alcohol relate mainly to reduced CHD and associated myocardial infarcts, and show a J-shaped curve with a reduced incidence at about 1–4 drinks per day (lower end for females). There is some evidence that daily moderate alcohol consumption is more cardioprotective than less regular consumption.
- Opinion remains divided whether or not wine confers additional cardio-protective benefits compared to a similar intake of alcohol from other types of drink. Part of the favourable effects of wine consumption could be related to the pattern of drinking wine daily with a meal.

- The most compelling mechanism to explain a protective effect of moderate alcohol/wine consumption is increased production of HDL-cholesterol. Moderate wine consumption also has a number of other beneficial effects including reducing LDL-cholesterol oxidation and anti-thrombotic effects, and these could be due to phenolics, especially in red wine.

- The complex interactions between nutrients in relation to CVD protection reinforce the need for a holistic/dietary pattern approach.

- Adherence to a Mediterranean dietary pattern, based on observational studies and using a MedDiet score (MDS), appears significantly protective for CVD in Mediterranean countries.

- When the MDS is modified for non-Mediterranean populations, it becomes similar to a "prudent" diet. This decreases CVD risk and mortality, but the decrease in risk is not as high as the one observed in Mediterranean countries with the MDS.

- Three major intervention studies with Mediterranean dietary patterns (Lyon study, Medi-RIVAGE and PREDIMED) resulted in a reduction in a range of risk factors for CVD.

11.1   Introduction

CVD is now the main cause of death in the Western world, and the World Health Organization predicts that CVD will also be the major killer globally within 15 years due to its rapidly increasing prevalence in developing countries and Eastern Europe and to the increase in obesity and diabetes in many parts of the world. Most forms of CVD result from atherosclerosis. The related term arteriosclerosis is used to describe the hardening (and loss of elasticity) of medium or large arteries due to any cause, and is the most frequent cause of coronary heart disease (CHD). Other clinically apparent signs of arteriosclerosis can include angina, a myocardial infarct, arterial thrombosis, embolism (blockage resulting from a clot migrating from one part of the body to another), stroke, or claudication (pain and/or cramping in the lower leg due to inadequate blood flow). The symptoms are generally progressive, except when the thrombosis occurs at a large artery when it is life-threatening.

The epidemiological study of atherosclerosis was facilitated by the recognition that hypercholesterolaemia is a major risk factor. Cholesterol is an easy-to-measure biological indicator, and levels are partly related to nutrition. Recommendations for the UK are not to exceed 5 mmol/L for total cholesterol (TC) (hypercholesterolaemia) (<4.0 mmol/L in individuals with established cardiovascular disease, diabetes, or at high risk of developing cardiovascular disease) and 3 mmol/L for LDL-cholesterol (<2.0 mmol/L in individuals with established cardiovascular disease, diabetes, or at high risk of developing cardiovascular disease). Other major measurable risk factors for arteriosclerosis are arterial hypertension (systolic ≥ 140 mmHg and diastolic ≥ 90 mmHg), and increased triglycerides (>2 mmol/L).

Other risk factors are obesity and a sedentary lifestyle, high intake of alcohol, high intake of salt, biological signs of inflammation (such as increased levels of C reactive protein), and an increase in plasma fibrinogen, A genetic predisposition is observed in people bearing the allele ε4 of APO-E. Several of these risk factors also occur in type 2 diabetes and metabolic syndrome, and these diseases are often complicated by CVD.

11.2   Nutrition and the biology of CVD

Atherosclerosis is a hardening of an artery specifically due to an atherosclerotic plaque (also known as an atheroma). Atherosclerosis is a progressive disorder associated with the accumulation of lipids in vessel walls and the subsequent thickening and hardening of the arterial intima (*sclerosis*). Atheromas protrude into and restrict blood flow in the lumen of arteries and weaken the underlying tissue. Atherosclerosis was long considered to be an age-related chronic degenerative disease but, more recently, attention has focussed on the inflammatory component of the disease, which is a response to damage of the intima. This damage can be caused by a range of factors including hypertension, oxidised lipoproteins, hyperglycaemia, tobacco and some bacterial infections.

Several of the risk factors for CVD such as tobacco use, sedentary lifestyle, excess alcohol and poor nutrition are modifiable. In relation to poor nutrition, salt intake should be reduced to prevent hypertension. Processed foods and bread are major contributors of salt intake.

11.2.1   Atherogenesis

Atheromatous plaques start with damage to the endothelium, followed by trapping of oxidised LDL-cholesterol in the intimal layer of the artery. These fatty streaks represent the initial lesion of atherosclerosis and occur at an early age. Around the fourth decade of life, fatty streaks convert into more complex lesions called fibrous plaques. These initially have a cap of connective tissue, but this can rupture resulting in the formation of a thrombus, which greatly increases the risk of the artery becoming occluded (blocked) which can precipitate a heart attack or stroke.

Reducing atheroma formation (atherogenesis) is a key aspect for protection by the MedDiet against CVD. Atherogenesis is thought to involve:

1. endothelial cell dysfunction
2. lipid deposition
3. inflammation

Endothelial cell dysfunction

Various factors can induce endothelial cell dysfunction including hypertension, LDL (see below discussion of lipoproteins), elevated homocysteine, diabetes or components in cigarette smoke. Although homocysteine can damage the vascular endothelium, and elevated levels are considered to be a risk factor for CVD, the importance of this in the aetiology of CVD needs clarification. Elevated homocysteine levels are associated, at least in part, with an inadequate intake of folates, and vitamins B6 and B12.

An important first line of defence against atheroma formation is maintaining a normal blood flow. The endothelial layer of blood vessels (see Anatomy of an artery below) helps maintain a normal blood flow by repelling blood cells and impairing clot formation. The anti-thrombotic effect is facilitated by endothelial cells producing the gas nitric oxide (NO) which inhibits platelet aggregation. NO also dilates blood vessels (vasodilation), and low levels of NO result in vasoconstriction, which increases blood pressure (hypertension) and the risk of atheroma formation. NO also reduces inflammation, an important pathological event in atherogenesis by decreasing leucocyte adhesion to blood vessels and inhibiting the production of inflammatory cytokines.

Anatomy of an artery

An artery consists of an inner layer known as the intima that consists of endothelial cells surrounded by a layer of vascular smooth muscle cells (VSMCs). Outside this is the media, which is surrounded by the adventitia consisting of loose connective tissue and nerves (Figure 11.1).

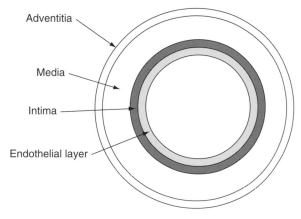

Adventitia

Media

Intima

Endothelial layer

Figure 11.1   Anatomy of an artery.

NO can react with superoxide to form the free radical peroxynitrite. Not only will this reduce the level of physiologically-active NO, but peroxynitrite can damage cells. Antioxidant phenolics in the MedDiet may play a role in protecting NO from oxidation [1]. Polyphenols in red wine also inhibit the production of endothelin-1, a vasoconstrictor that opposes the action of NO [2].

NO production is catalysed by the enzyme nitric oxide synthase (NOS). A constitutive form (eNOS) is produced by endothelial cells, and NOS can also be induced in VSMCs and macrophages (inducible NOS, iNOS). Since eNOS helps regulate many aspects of cardiovascular function, it has been suggested that modifying eNOS is a key mechanism for the cardio-protective effects of the MedDiet [1]. Although eNOS is produced constitutively, its expression – at least in cultured endothelial cells – can be increased by red wine polyphenols and *n*-3 fatty acids [1].

Platelet aggregation is also regulated by various eicosanoids. The *n*-3 fatty acids EPA and DHA are converted into the so-called series 3 eicosanoids which inhibit platelet aggregation. These eicosanoids are countered by the series 2 eicosanoids which are mostly pro-inflammatory, and promote platelet aggregation. Series 2 eicosanoids are derived from arachidonic acid (AA) which is found in red meat.

Lipoproteins and fat metabolism (from [3])

The basic composition of a lipoprotein is:

- a central lipid core consisting of cholesterol esters and TAGs
- an outer layer consisting of phospholipids, free cholesterol, apoproteins

The compositions of the various major forms of lipoproteins are shown in Table 11.1.

Table 11.1 Composition of plasma lipoproteins [3].

| | Composition (%) | | | | | |
	Cholesterol (free)	Cholesterol (esters)	TAG	PL	Protein	Major apolipoproteins
Chylomicrons	1	3	85	9	2	B_{48}, E, C-II
VLDL	7	13	50	20	10	B_{100}, E, C-II
IDL	12	22	26	22	8	B_{100}, E,
LDL	8	37	10	20	25	B_{100}
HDL	2	5	4	24	55	A-I, A-II

Apolipoproteins (apo), also known as apoproteins, are recognised by cell surface receptors and determine which cell type will take up the lipoprotein. Plasma lipoproteins transport fats in the circulation. These fats may have come from foods (exogenous fats) or have been synthesised by the body (endogenous fats).

Exogenous fats
Dietary fats (triglycerides, TAGs) and cholesterol are absorbed in the intestine. Dietary TAGs are digested to fatty acids, absorbed within the intestine and re-esterified to either glycerol to form triglycerides or to cholesterol to form cholesterol esters. TAGs and cholesterol esters are packaged with apoproteins to form chylomicrons. Chylomicrons are secreted into the lymphatics in the intestine and then carried to the thoracic duct and into the blood stream. TAGs in chylomicrons are hydrolysed in the blood stream to free fatty acids (FFAs) and delivered to muscle as fuel, or they can be re-esterified to glycerol and stored in adipose tissue. As they are hydrolysed, chylomicrons acquire cholesterol and apoE, and are now known as chylomicron remnants. These remnants are taken up by liver cells, a process requiring recognition between apoE and receptors on the surface of the liver cells.

Endogenous fats
Cholesterol and TAGs can also be synthesised by the liver, and are packaged into VLDLs for transport around the body. Hepatic TAGs are produced from fatty acids that originate either from adipose tissue or from carbohydrates (by lipogenesis). The key rate-limiting enzyme in cholesterol biosynthesis is HMGCoA reductase. TAGs in VLDLs are hydrolysed in the blood stream to FFAs. As they are hydrolysed, VLDLs acquire cholesterol and form IDLs. These cholesterol-rich IDLs can be further metabolised to LDLs or taken up by liver

cells by a recognition process that requires apoB on the IDLs and LDL receptors on the surface of liver cells.

LDL is the major form of cholesterol-carrying lipoprotein in the circulation and it carries cholesterol to peripheral tissues. LDL is taken up from the circulation by cells expressing LDL receptors. About 75% of LDL is cleared by liver cells and 25% is taken up by peripheral cells. Receptor-mediated LDL uptake is critical for regulating plasma cholesterol concentrations.

Cholesterol at peripheral tissues surplus to requirements is returned to the liver by HDL. (This process is referred to as reverse cholesterol transport.) HDL particles are synthesised in the liver and intestine and avidly take up cholesterol from the cell membranes of peripheral tissues. Most of the cholesterol in HDL is transferred to other lipoproteins and then taken up by the liver for excretion.

Lipid deposition

There is increasing recognition of the importance of oxidised LDL-cholesterol (LDL-C) in the pathogenesis of atherosclerosis, and elevated levels of circulating levels of oxidised LDL are predictors of CHD [4]. When plasma levels of LDL rise, the lipoproteins can infiltrate through the endothelium, and it is thought that oxidised LDL penetrates the arterial wall more readily than normal LDL. Oxidation of components of LDL particles (including FAs, cholesterol and apolipoprotein) is brought about by increased oxidative stress, including by macrophages which are a major source of reactive oxygen species (see Chapter 9). Macrophages also take up oxidised LDL, and this uptake is unregulated since the apolipoprotein on LDL (apoB100) is oxidised and interacts with scavenger receptors on macrophages that are not subject to normal negative feedback mechanisms. The macrophages become overloaded with lipids and change into foam cells (so-called because of their bubbly appearance). These are visible in the arterial walls as "fatty streaks". Dying foam cells release lipids that pool within the intima.

Oxidised LDL has a number of adverse effects on the propagation of atherogenesis including:

- induction of cell adhesion molecules on endothelial cells
- cytotoxic effects to endothelial cells
- mitogenic effecs to macrophages

The MedDiet may reduce the harmful effects of oxidised LDL by (1) influencing the relative proportions of LDL and HDL and (2) increasing the resistance of LDL to oxidation. Factors in the MedDiet that decrease LDL and/or increase HDL levels include the overall FA composition of the MedDiet (Section 11.3.1) and alcohol (Section 11.3.3). Various antioxidants present in the MedDiet that may reduce lipid oxidation are found in fruits and vegetables, virgin olive oil, wine and tea (see Sections 11.3.2 and 11.3.3).

Inflammation

Inflammation plays a fundamental role in atherogenesis [5]. Oxidised LDL is chemotactic for inflammatory cells such as monocytes and T-lymphocytes which infiltrate the atherosclerotic plaque. These inflammatory cells, together with VSMCs

Table 11.2 Inflammatory markers for CVD.

Marker	Role in CVD	Source
Interleukin-6 (Il.6)	Impairs endothelium-dependent dilation	immune cells, vascular cells (eg VSMCs)
C-reactive protein (CRP)	favours a proinflammatory and proatherosclerotic phenotype in endothelial cells	liver (+plaque?)
Fibrinogen	coagulation	liver
Soluble intercellular adhesion molecule-1 (sICAM-1)	increases adhesiveness of endothelial cells for inflammatory cells	endothelial cells and others
Soluble vascular cell adhesion molecule-1 (sVCAM-1)	increases adhesiveness of endothelial cells	endothelial and smooth muscle cells

and collagen, form a "cap" over the lipid pool which now constitutes a mature atherosclerotic plaque. The mature atherosclerotic plaque partially penetrates the artery wall and also reduces blood flow in the lumen of the artery. This can result in angina pectoris if the blockage is in the carotid artery supplying blood to the heart. In the legs, the patient experiences intermittent claudication. If the plaque remains stable, these symptoms can persist for many years. However, some plaques become unstable and rupture. This can trigger thrombosis (i.e. formation of a thrombus or blood clot) which can result in complete blockage of the artery and cause a heart attack, or a stroke if the artery is supplying the brain.

A plaque will rupture if the cap becomes sufficiently weakened. The main structural component of the cap is collagen, and this can be degraded by various enzymes including matrix metalloproteases (MMPs) produced by macrophages. Secretion of MMPs by macrophages is stimulated by cytokines produced by T lymphocytes. Hence, plaques that are rich in inflammatory cells and lipids are more prone to rupture than lipid-poor acellular plaques.

Several studies have suggested that a MedDiet is anti-inflammatory since consumption of a MedDiet has been found to lower levels of inflammatory markers, including some that are associated with CVD such as C-reactive protein and interleukin-6 [6, 7] (Table 11.2; see also Chapter 9). However, lowering inflammatory markers does not necessarily mean that this will protect against CVD, and indeed the association between lowering these markers and a reduction in CVD risk is inconclusive.

The MedDiet contains a favourable combination of foods that are associated with a lowering of inflammatory markers, and a low intake of foods that enhance inflammation (Table 11.3). For example, the MedDiet is associated with a low intake of industrially-produced trans fatty acids. Trans fatty acids have been found to raise serum levels of various inflammatory markers such as CRP, and markers of endothelial cell activation such as sICAM-1 and sVCAM-1. Elaidic acid, a trans fatty acid (TFA) originating from technological processes and found in some margarines, industrial confectionery and pastries, also increases cholesterol levels [8]. The MedDiet is relative low in foods with a high GI, and these are associated with a large postprandial rise in blood glucose and insulin that increase oxidative stress and promote lipid deposition. Some, but not all, studies have found that moderate red wine consumption reduces inflammatory markers associated CVD (see Section 11.3.3).

Table 11.3 Nutrients affecting inflammation.

Reduce inflammation	Enhance inflammation
low glycaemic index foods	high glycaemic index foods
cholesterol-lowering foods	trans fatty acids
n-3 fatty acids	
extra virgin olive oil	

11.2.2 Cardiac arrhythmias

Arrhythmias account for a large proportion of sudden cardiac death post a myocardial infarct. Numerous experimental studies have indicated that low concentrations of n-3 PUFAs, including ALA, reduce the severity of cardiac arrhythmias [9, 10]. It has been suggested that anti-arrhythmic effects of PUFAs are more important in relation to secondary cardiovascular protection than anti-thrombotic effects [11]. PUFAs are discussed in Section 11.3.1.

11.3 Epidemiological evidence and mechanisms

11.3.1 Fat and fatty acids

Elevated LDL-cholesterol (LDL-C) has long being recognised as a major risk factor for CHD, since high levels contribute to atherosclerosis, and oxidation of LDL-C may ultimately lead to plaque rupture. Saturated fat intake, found mainly in dairy products and meat, is highly correlated with total cholesterol, although not all saturated fatty acids (SFAs) are equally atherogenic (see Chapter 6). PUFAs play a role in lowering total LDL-C. Also, the beneficial role of a high level of HDL-C has been recognised as an important feature for predicting lower CVD risk. In this regard, olive oil has a beneficial effect since, in contrast to PUFAs, oleic acid does not lower HDL-C.

Later, it was observed that death following arrhythmias and fibrillation in the case of a myocardial infarct (MI), might be prevented by a high intake of fish. Fish is associated with a high intake of the n-3 fatty acids eicosapentaenoic acid (EPA) and docosahexaenoic acid (DHA). There is also now interest in n-3 fatty acids, and especially long chain n-3 PUFA (LC n-3 PUFA) for their regulatory properties in relation to myocardial rhythm and anti-inflammatory effects. Anti-inflammatory effects seem to be particularly important with respect to EPA, whereas DHA appears to be more protective of the myocardium [12].

This section considers the metabolic effects of fats on CVD, especially in terms of cholesterol levels, and in the context of total fat intake. The specific role of olive oil on other cardiovascular risk factors is discussed in Section 11.3.3.

Observational studies

Saturated fatty acids
Following on from the seminal work of the Seven Countries study [13, 14], data from a prospective study on 43,757 health professionals (aged 40 to 75 years, and diagnosed free of diagnosed CVD or diabetes) published in 1996 indicated that the

association between intake of saturated fat and risk of CHD was not as strong as had been suggested by international comparisons [15]. During the 6-year follow-up, 734 coronary events were documented, including 505 non-fatal myocardial infarctions and 229 deaths. After age and usual coronary risk factors were controlled for, men consuming 14.8% v 5.7% of energy as SFA showed a RR borderline significant for MI (1.22: CI 0.96–1.56) and significant for fatal CHD (2.21: CI 1.38–3.54). The risk associated with SFA intake decreased after adjustment for fibre intake. After adjustment for intake of fibre, the risks were 0.96 (CI 0.73–1.27) and 1.72 (CI 1.01–2.90) respectively for MI and fatal CHD. Thus, these data were compatible with the hypotheses that saturated fat intake affects the risk of CHD – as predicted by their effects on blood cholesterol concentration – but also suggested that concomitant intake of fibre in the diet attenuates this effect. Hence, this early study was already suggesting that a single nutrient alone could not explain CHD. Later studies drew attention to the importance of different foods, sources of nutrients and the distinction between various SFAs [16]. This had previously been suspected by Kromhout et al. in the Seven Countries study [8], due to differences between FAs in their hypercholesterolemic effect, namely that short-chain FAs (up to C10) are less, or not, hypercholesterolaemic.

Monounsaturated fatty acids (MUFAs)
There are no observational studies showing that MUFAs from sources other than olive oil were specifically involved in beneficial effects on CVD. On the contrary, it was shown in a pooled analysis, that substituting MUFAs for SFA did not show any protection [17]. In the Seven Countries studies, Keys et al. underline the importance of the ratio of MUFA:SFA for risk reduction of CVD and for reduction of overall mortality.

Polyunsaturated fatty acids (PUFAs)
Various studies have demonstrated the importance of dietary PUFAs. In the Western Electric Study, the percentage of CHD deaths was higher in those subjects with a lower intake of PUFAs [8]. The Atherosclerosis Risk in Communities (ARIC) study showed a significant inverse association between the carotid artery wall thickness of the high PUFA consumers (75th percentile) compared to that of the low consumers (25th percentile) for a difference of 3% of total energy between the two groups (mean consumption of the population sample 5% energy from PUFA) [18]. The Nurse's Health Study showed that for an increment of 5% of energy from PUFAs (81% linoleic acid) there was a 38% reduced risk of CVD (RR 0.62: CI 0.46–0.85, p=0.003) [19]. A subsequent review describing 11 prospective studies, found 9 showing a beneficial association between PUFA intake and CVD incidence and mortality [20]. Finally, a recent pooled analysis confirmed that replacing SFA with PUFAs had a beneficial effect on CHD mortality [17]. It is generally acknowledged that linoleic acid (LA) is the major constituent of the total PUFAs (about 80%) in these observational studies.

While food composition tables remain incomplete, it is difficult to address the specific role for most series of FAs using questionnaires. The roles of LC *n*-3 PUFAs are somewhat easier to confirm since LC *n*-3 PUFAs are essentially provided in the diet by fish. A meta-analysis of 13 cohorts, including 222,364 individuals with an average 11.8 years of follow-up, showed pooled multivariate RRs for CHD mortality of 0.89 (CI 0.79–1.01) for fish intake of 1–3 times per month, 0.85 (CI 0.76–0.96) for once per week, 0.77 (CI 0.66–0.89) for 2–4 times per week, and 0.62 (CI 0.46–0.82) for five or more times per week [21]. Each 20 g/d increase in fish intake was related to a 7% lower risk of CHD. A recent meta-analysis of nine prospective studies could even define an optimal amount of 400–500 mg/day of EPA+DHA provided by the diet for the protection of the general population against CHD [22]. In a Dutch population-based cohort study, EPA+DHA and fish intake were assessed at baseline among 21,342 participants aged 20–65 with no history of MI or stroke. Compared with the lowest quartile of EPA+DHA (40 mg/d), participants in the top quartile (234 mg/d) had a 49% lower risk of fatal CHD (CI 6–73%) and a 62% lower risk of fatal MI (CI 23–81%) [23]. There was an inverse dose-response relations for EPA+DHA intake and fatal CHD (p for trend=0.05) and fatal MI (p for trend=0.01). Results were similar for fish consumption (17.3 g/d versus 1.1 g/d). Non-fatal MI was not associated with EPA+DHA or fish intake.

In conclusion, EPA+DHA and fish may lower fatal CHD and MI risk in a dose-response manner. In future studies it will be possible to study the specific effects of these FAs through improvements in food composition tables and through the biochemical analysis of the FA composition of different tissues (plasma, erythrocytes, adipose tissue). Among the n-3 PUFAs, ALA with 18 carbon atoms and 2 double bonds is theoretically a precursor for EPA (20 C and 5 double bonds) and DHA (22 C and 6 double bonds). However, the conversion of ALA to EPA is rather low in humans (approx. 10%), and conversion of EPA to DHA is close to zero. Thus, although biochemically ALA is the only indispensable n-3 FA, EPA and DHA appear to be essential for CVD protection (and also for neurological development and health).

With regard to ALA, the results of observational studies analysing the effect of this FA in relation to CVD are inconsistent. Some studies have shown an increased risk, which may be related to the co-consumption of trans fatty acids (TFAs) in margarine [24–26], or insignificant results [15, 24, 27, 28], or a significant inverse relationship [29–32]. A beneficial effect was observed in two studies, but this was confounded by LC n-3 PUFA [33, 34]. One possible interpretation for this observation is that sufficient EPA can be synthesised from ALA when there is a high dietary intake of ALA and only a low intake of EPA+DHA.

TFAs were found to be a significant risk factor for CVD, with a risk comparable to that of SFAs [35].

Intervention studies

Intervention studies provide a more precise way than observational studies for determining the effects of different FAs. Most of these studies have selected LDL-C or LDL-C plus HDL-C as end-points. Later studies have used other markers such as apo-lipoprotein B, triglycerides, or markers of vascular tone and inflammation.

Most of the early intervention studies examined the effect of replacing a diet rich in SFA with either a diet rich in MUFAs – most often oleic acid of olive oil – or with a diet rich in n-6 PUFAs – most often sunflower oil containing a high percentage of LA. For a diet rich in MUFAs, LDL-C was not affected or slightly decreased, and HDL-C was maintained or increased, whereas in the n-6 PUFA rich diet, the LDL- C is generally significantly decreased and HDL-C maintained or slightly decreased. Thus, the principal role of LA appears to be to decrease plasma LDL-C.

These results have been confirmed in a recent meta-analysis of randomised controlled trials showing the beneficial effect of replacing SFA with PUFAs or *n*-6 PUFAs [36]. It has been shown that in situations of high intake of SFA and cholesterol, LA is more efficient than oleic acid for maintaining normal cholesterol levels, but that a high intake of LA is not necessary when the SFA intake is low [37]. This observation places FA consumption in the perspective of the overall dietary pattern, and demonstrates that consumption of specific FAs needs to be considered in the context of total fat intake. This is well illustrated by comparing the diet in the South-West region of France with the MedDiet: in SW France, fruit, vegetable and fish consumption is very close to that of the MedDiet, but the SFA and cholesterol intake is higher. However, sunflower oil (rich in LA) is also used, for example in salad dressings, and through the effect of LA on cholesterol, cholesterol plasma concentration and the incidence of CHD in SW France is very comparable to that of a Mediterranean country [38].

ALA has shown beneficial effects against cardiovascular parameters in several experimental animal models, although only two nutrition intervention studies using a modified diet enriched in ALA alluded to a possible beneficial effect of ALA [39, 40]. However, it is difficult to assign the beneficial effect specifically to ALA and, moreover, one of these studies has been judged invalid [41].

By contrast, intervention studies carried out with LC *n*-3 PUFA have provided more clear-cut evidence of beneficial effects. Two large studies, GISSI (Gruppo Italiano per lo Studio della Sopravvivenza nell'Infarto miocardico) and JELIS, support the beneficial effects of EPA and DHA given as fish oils [42, 43]. In the GISSI study, 11,323 randomised patients with CHD received 850 mg/d of EPA and DHA ethyl-ester or none. After 3.5 years follow-up, the total death rate and cardiovascular mortality were decreased by 14% and 17% respectively in the supplemented group compared to total death rate and cardiovascular mortality in the non-supplemented group. Survival curves for *n*-3 PUFA treatment diverged early after randomisation, and total mortality was significantly lower by 3 months of treatment (RR 0.5: CI 0.36–0.97) and the reduction in risk of sudden death was statistically significant even by 4 months after intervention (RR 0.47: CI 0.219–0.995) [44].

In the JELIS study, 18,645 Japanese patients presenting with hypercholesterolae-mia (>6.5 mmol/l) and being treated with statins, were randomised to two groups, one receiving EPA (1.8 g/day) and the other not receiving EPA. After 4.6 years of follow-up, there was a 19% decrease in coronary events, irrespective of the presence or absence of coronary antecedents in the patients. There was no effect on CHD death but this may be because the patients were treated with EPA only and, in addi-tion, there were only a low number of fatal events since the Japanese population is generally at low risk for CHD, and this resulted in a weak statistical power. Other trials have also been conducted with intermediary end-points related to cardiac rhythm (rate, atrial fibrillation) which are important for CHD [45], and also on triglycerides.

Intervention studies were conducted to determine the effect of TFAs, mainly technological TFAs, using the same design as for SFAs, i.e. by replacing TFAs in the diet with either SFAs, MUFAs or PUFAs. It was shown that TFAs had a higher negative impact on intermediary endpoints than SFAs, and this may be due to a unique cardio-metabolic effect via pathways linked to the metabolic syn-drome [46]. However, traditional MedDiets contain only very low amounts of natural TFAs, mainly found in milk products, and these do not appear to increase cardiovascular risk markers [47].

In summary, studying the relationship of CVD by nutrients has revealed a degree of complexity and the important interplay between the different FAs for the prevention of CVD, and this suggests the need for a new approach with regard to prevention of the general population. In relation to specific foods, these studies help explain how the unique fat profile of the traditional MedDiet, i.e. low-to-moderate animal foods from dairy products or meat (constituting the main sources of SFA intake), fish and – uniquely – olive oil, are likely to have contributed to the low rates of numerous chronic diseases observed in these populations [48]. Olive oil is discussed further in Section 13.3.3.

11.3.2 Plant food constituents

Several plant food constituents may be involved in the beneficial effects of plant foods against CVD, and also against metabolic disorders that increase CVD risk such as obesity and diabetes. Although the mechanisms are not fully understood, fibre, carotenoids and folic acid – all abundant in plant foods of the MedDiet – appear to play important roles in the prevention of these diseases.

Fibre

The beneficial effects of fibre have been revealed from analytical epidemiology. A study of 573 middle-aged adults reported a significant negative correlation between soluble dietary fibre intake with the total/HDL-C ratio [49]. In a pooled analysis of 10 prospective studies, cereal fibre was less protective for CHD than fruit fibre, and vegetable fibre was not at all protective [50]. Subsequently, Lairon and colleagues examined the relationship between the source or type of dietary fibre and CVD risk factors in a cohort of adult men and women, in the French SU.VI.Max (SUpplementation en VItamines et Mineraux AntioXydants) study [51]. In a cross-sectional study, quintiles of fibre intake were determined separately for 2532 men and 3429 women from dietary records, and several intermediary end-points were examined (BMI, waist-to-hip ratio, elevated blood pressure, Apo B, total cholesterol, triglycerides, fasting blood glucose, homocysteine). The authors observed a significant association of soluble fibre with homocysteine and waist/hip ratio, and a marginal association with blood pressure, Apo B and total cholesterol (Table 11.4). Soluble fibre, not being digested by intestinal enzymes, induces an increase in faecal bulk. It is reported to decrease post-prandial glucose and insulin peaks, as well as lowering serum cholesterol. Insoluble fibre was significantly associated with waist/hip ratio, blood pressure, BMI, Apo B and total cholesterol. Fibre from cereals was the only factor to be associated with lowering homocysteine concentrations. This association might be partly explained by the high vitamin content of plant foods, especially folate, which is a known down-regulator of homocysteine concentrations. However, the effect remained even after adjusting for folate intake.

An interesting observation is that nut and seed fibre intakes, even when low, could have beneficial effects on body weight, abdominal adiposity, apo B concentrations, and glycaemia, although further studies are needed to evaluate these possible specific effects. Several clinical trials support the effect of fibre-enriched diets for lowering

Table 11.4 Odds ratios (CI and trend) for the relative risk of abnormal markers of cardiovascular disease for soluble and insoluble fibre and dietary fibre intake from plant foods (data from [51]).

	Source of fibre							
	Soluble fibre	Insoluble fibre	Cereals	Vegetables	Legumes	Fruit	Dried fruit	Nuts
BMI		0.69 (0.53–0.90) 0.01	0.70 (0.55–0.90) 0.003		0.85 (0.71–1.02) 0.22		0.60 (0.50–0.73) 0.0001	0.60 (0.50–0.73) 0.0001
Waist/hip	0.80 (0.63–1.02) 0.03	0.55 (0.42–0.72) < 0.0001				0.71 (0.58–0.88) 0.0001	0.62 (0.51–0.76) 0.0001	0.72 (0.60–0.88) 0.001
Blood pressure	0.86 (0.68–1.10) 0.10	0.68 (0.52–0.89) 0.01	0.86 (0.67–1.10) 0.02	0.79 (0.64–0.97) 0.004		0.79 (0.64–0.97) 0.02	0.76 (0.62–0.92) 0.01	
ApoB	0.79 (0.59–1.05) 0.05	0.69 (0.49–0.95) 0.03		0.79 (0.62–1.01) 0.12			0.76 (0.60–0.97) 0.02	0.78 (0.62–0.99) 0.03
Total cholesterol	0.81 (0.65–1.01) 0.15	0.73 (0.57–0.93) 0.06					0.85 (0.71–1.02) T 0.22	
Tri-glycerides		0.65 (0.46–0.92) 0.01					0.72 (0.56–0.92) 0.01	

Glycaemia		0.34 (0.21–0.57) 0.0001	0.57 (0.37–0.90) 0.002
Homo-cysteine	0.52 (0.34–0.80) 0.005	0.52 (0.32–0.85) 0.01	0.73 (0.50–1.07) 0.02

OR were computed using the following cut-offs for high versus low intake of fibre (g/day):
Soluble dietary fibre: >5.2 versus <3.2 in men; >4.4 versus <2.7 in women
Insoluble dietary fibre: >22.1 versus <12.8 in men; >17.7 versus < 10.6 in women
Fibre from cereal: >10.6 versus <5.3 for men; >7.7 versus < 3.9 in women
Fibre from vegetables: >6.5 versus <3.0 in men; >6.0 versus <2.9 in women
Fibre from legumes: >2.13 versus 0.02 in men; >1.43 versus <0.01 in women
Fibre from fruit: >6.4 versus <1.9 in men, >5.5 versus <2.0 in women
Fibre from dried fruit: >0.38 versus <0.03 in men; >0.35 versus <0.04 in women
Fibre from nuts and seeds: >0.56 versus <0.05 in men; >0.48 versus 0.05 in women

cholesterol levels [52, 53]. Such an association was observed in a meta-analysis of clinical trials and in a study with whole grains [54].

In summary, it can be concluded that individuals with high intakes of dietary fibre appear to be at significantly lower risk of developing CHD, stroke, hypertension, diabetes, obesity and certain gastrointestinal diseases [55]. Increasing fibre intake lowers blood pressure and serum cholesterol levels, and increased intake of soluble fibre improves glycaemia and insulin sensitivity in non-diabetic and diabetic individuals. However, most studies have found that whole cereals appear to mitigate more strongly against cardiovascular risk than fibre.

Potassium

Potassium, abundant in fruit and vegetables, is another micronutrient for which there is good evidence for cardiovascular benefits. As early as the 1970s, it was observed in clinical studies that potassium plays a role in blood pressure, either by modifying renin secretion directly by acting on the juxtaglomerular cells or by a change in tubular reabsorption or secretion, or indirectly via an induced change in tubular sodium transport [56]. The role of potassium is now well substantiated from human studies, and has been recognised by the American Society of Hypertension as a major factor for the prevention and modification of elevated blood pressure [57].

Phytochemicals

Antioxidants in fruit and vegetables, including carotenoids and flavonoids, have long been recognised as being associated with lower CVD risk [58, 59]. These early pioneering studies on flavonoids were confirmed in 2007 in a prospective study of CVD in postmenopausal women [60], and were further extended to stroke in a recent meta-analysis of flavonol intake [61]. Comparing the highest range of intake (from 16 to 47 mg/day) with lowest category of intake (range 4 to 14 mg/day) for six independent estimates from six cohort studies produced an overall RR of 0.8 (CI 0.65–0.98). However, there was significant heterogeneity in some of the studies (i.e. the variation in study outcomes between the studies), which casts some doubt on their overall significance and suggests that other dietary factors might be confounding. This conclusion led to further studies being conducted. Whilst in the plasma, LDL is normally protected from oxidation by various antioxidants such as vitamin E and carotenoids[1] [62], and oxidised LDL-C is important in the pathogenesis of atherosclerosis. Hence, intervention studies were undertaken with various antioxidants such as vitamin E [42, 63], or multiple nutrients including β-carotene [64, 65]. The results of these studies do not support the conclusion that supplementation with antioxidants has a beneficial effect on cardiovascular risk. This suggests that a micronutrient that is not part of the food matrix may not have the same biological effect as when it is part of the whole food. Another possible explanation is that the global intake of several complementary phytochemicals is necessary for a preventative effect. There is some limited epidemiological evidence linking elevated plasma lycopene concentrations with a reduced risk for CVD, and this may be linked to a reduction in LDL-C levels, although this has not been studied specifically in the context of a MedDiet [66].

---

[1] However LDL that has diffused into the intima is much more susceptible to oxidation since the concentration of antioxidants here is far lower.

Quercetin and atherosclerotic plaques

A recent study offers an explanation as to how the flavonol quercetin can specifically target atherosclerotic plaques and so reduce CVD [67]. Quercetin 3-glucuronide (Q3GA), a major metabolite of quercetin found in the blood following a quercetin-rich meal, was shown to specifically accumulate in injured human aorta with atherosclerotic plaques (obtained during autopsy from patients with generalised arteriosclerosis) and not in normal aorta. This may be due to increased permeability of injured endothelial cell for Q3GA, whereas normal endothelial cells will not take up this metabolite. Once in the sub-intimal layer, the Q3GA may be cleaved by glucuronidases produced by inflammatory macrophages generating free quercetin. This may then be taken up by macrophages and decrease scavenger receptors (SR) for ox-LDL expressed on the surface of the macrophages. Hence, the macrophages will be less able to take up ox-LDL and so the formation of foam cells will be reduced. Also, it is possible that Q3GA may be directly taken up by the macrophages and converted to free quercetin inside the macrophages. Although this study needs confirmation, it provides a way of explaining how quercetin may help prevent CVD despite its extensive metabolism in the body.

Increased levels of homocysteine have been related to folate deficiency for a long time [68]. However, it is still unclear whether decreasing plasma levels of homocysteine through diet or drugs is paralleled by a reduction in cardiovascular risk. In a detailed review of epidemiological studies and large-scale trials with folic acid supplementation, Ciaccio and Bellia concluded that hyperhomocysteinemia might be related to mortality or to stroke but not to CHD, and that supplementation with folic acid did not consistently reduce the risk of vascular outcomes but did possibly reduce the risk of stroke [69]. The authors conclude, however, that dietary prevention might still be considered beneficial.

Conclusions

In summary, current evidence suggests that potassium has a specific role at the kidney and cellular level in sodium balance, and fibre decreases several risk factors for CVD. However, the evidence is less consistent for supporting a role for many of the other micronutrients and phytochemicals found in fruits and vegetables, and overall, the failure of antioxidant trials for CVD reinforces the need for a holistic approach to understand the relationship between disease and nutrition.

11.3.3   Whole foods

A number of studies have evaluated analysed whole foods, rather than the microconstituents and phytochemicals that they contain.

Plant foods

Consumption of fruit and vegetables has been shown to be inversely associated with a myocardial infraction (OR 0.70: CI 0.62–0.79) (in the so-called INTERHEART study) [70]. The proportion of MI in the study population that was attributable to lack of daily consumption was 13.7% (the so-called population attributable risk). The beneficial effect of a diet rich in fruit and vegetable was recently confirmed in the EPIC study (European Prospective Investigation in Cancer and Nutrition), a large multi-centre prospective cohort study [71]. A cohort of 10,449 participants with self-reported diabetes was followed for a mean of 9 y. Intakes of vegetables, legumes and fruit were assessed at baseline between 1992 and 2000 using validated country-specific questionnaires. A total of 1346 deaths occurred. An increase of 80 g/d in total intake of vegetables, legumes, and fruit was significantly inversely associated with CVD mortality (RR 0.88: CI 0.81–0.95). Legume consumption has been found to be specifically associated with low risk of CHD and CVD in the NHANES prospective study. Legume consumption (peas, several kind of beans and peanuts) four or more times per week compared with less than once a week reduced risk of CHD (RR 0.78: CI 0.68–0.90) and of CVD (RR 0.89: CI 0.80–0.98) [72]. Legumes, as well as being a good source of fibre, contain phytosterols and these may have beneficial effects by lowering cholesterol levels. Increasing chickpea consumption as part of a normal diet has been shown to be associated with a small decrease in total and LDL-cholesterol, although this was in a non-Mediterranean population [73].

Several large-scale prospective studies have associated the frequency of nut intake with a reduced risk of CVD [74]. An intervention study, the PREDIMED Study tested the efficacy of a traditional MedDiet on the primary prevention of CHD. Subjects were assigned to either a low-fat diet or one of two traditional MedDiets: one was supplemented with virgin olive oil and the other was supplemented with nuts. After the 3-month interventions, mean oxidised LDL levels decreased in both the traditional MedDiet+virgin olive oil (–10.6: Upper/Lower [–14.2 to –6.1]) and traditional MedDiet+nuts (–7.3: Upper/Lower [–11.2 to –3.3]) groups, without changes in the low fat diet group (–2.9: Upper/Lower [–7.3 to 1.5]) [75]. A meta-analysis of trials on walnut consumption and risk factors for CVD concluded that diets supplemented with walnuts resulted in a significantly greater decrease in total cholesterol and in LDL-cholesterol concentrations than control diets [76]. Walnuts also significantly improved markers for antioxidant capacity and reduced inflammation, and had no adverse effects on body weight. Walnuts have a particularly high content of ALA, and this fatty acid is associated with a reduced risk of CVD; this may be due to it either acting directly or after its partial conversion to EPA [77]. The high MUFA content of most nuts may also contribute to their cardioprotective effects [78].

Other plant foods studied in relation to CVD include onions and cereals. With regard to cereals, the prospective SUN study of 5880 Spanish men and women found that vegetable protein and fibre from cereal were inversely associated with the risk of hypertension [79].

Olive oil

Besides its important role in interacting with other FAs in the regulation of cholesterol levels (see above), olive oil consumption also reduces a number of other cardiovascular risk factors.

LDL-oxidation

There is some evidence that consuming extra virgin olive oil could increase the resistance of LDL to oxidative stress. Both the MUFA content and the antioxidant constituents in olive oil may contribute to this observation. Support for a role of the MUFA component of olive oil is suggested in reviews reporting studies that have shown that dietary MUFA formulations, as well as olive oil, increase the resistance of LDL to oxidation [80, 81]. There is also evidence that consumption of oleic acid results in it being incorporated into LDL particles. A randomised cross-over intervention study, the EUROLIVE study, conducted on 200 healthy male Europeans volunteers, found that consuming 25 mL olive oil for three weeks increased the oleic acid concentration in LDL (1.9%; p <0.001) accompanied by a reduction in the concentrations of linoleic acid (1.1%; p <0.002) and arachidonic acid (0.5%; p <0.001) [82]. The MUFA/PUFA and oleic/linoleic acid ratios in LDL increased after olive oil consumption. In addition, there was an inverse relationship between the oleic/linoleic acid ratio (i.e. MUFA/PUFA) and biomarkers of oxidative stress as assessed by isoprostane levels (one unit increase in the oleic/linoleic acid ratio was associated with a decrease of 4.2 µg/L in plasma isoprostanes). This suggests that oleic acid, with its single double bond, contributes to reduced oxidative stress, or that the decrease in PUFAs – which contain multiple double bonds and are more susceptible to oxidation – results in LDL particles with decreased susceptibility to oxidation.

The non-fat constituents in olive oil are also probably involved in the antioxidant effects of olive oil. Much of this work has focussed on the phenolic constituents. A comprehensive review of the effects of olive oils with different phenolic contents on markers of oxidative stress in human studies has provided convincing evidence that phenolics in olive oil are important for reducing oxidative stress. Statistically significant decreases in plasma levels of oxidised LDL after consuming high phenolic olive oil compared with low phenolic olive oil were seen in five out of six human intervention studies (the sixth study showed a reduction but was not statistically significant) [83]. For example, the EUROLIVE study, quoted above, found that consuming 25 mL olive oil with a medium or high phenolic content for three weeks decreased plasma oxidised LDL (−1.48: U/L [−3.6 to 0.6 U/L], and −3.21 U/L [−5.1 to −0.8 U/L], respectively),[2] as well as a number of other risk factors for CVD including the LDL/HDL ratio [84].

Candidate phenolics in virgin olive oil that may reduce oxidative stress include hydroxytyrosol and oleuropein. These are major constituents in olive oil (see Chapter 6), and inhibit LDL oxidation in *in vitro* studies [85]. Like many other phenolics, hydroxytyrosol and oleuropein are mainly present as conjugates in the body. Although it is generally thought that phenolics lose a lot of their potency as antioxidants when they are conjugated to chemical groups (see Chapter 9), a glucuronide conjugate of hydroxytyrosol was in fact found to be a more potent antioxidant than hydroxytyrosol itself [86].

As well as acting directly as antioxidants, olive oil phenolics may act by enhancing the body's own antioxidant defence mechanisms as two of the human studies discussed above reported an increase in levels of the enzyme glutathione peroxidase [83]. This suggests that phenolics in the olive oil can stimulate new gene expression (further evidence for this is also presented below).

Overall, these observations suggest that olive oil phenolics may be important contributors to the antioxidant effects of virgin olive oil observed in the human studies, although the mechanisms are not fully elucidated. It is important to note that these observations are mostly based on the effects of consuming *raw* virgin olive oil. Hydroxytyrosol and its derivatives in virgin olive oil are not very heat

---

[2] U: upper limit; L: lower limit.

stable, and levels were found to decrease by 40–50% following heating to 180C for 10 min [87]. Hence, consumption of virgin olive oil that has been used for frying may not have the same antioxidant benefits as raw virgin olive oil. This is also a potential confounding factor in observational epidemiological studies, since the state of the olive oil (used in cooking or raw, and also virgin versus non-virgin) is not usually determined.

Inflammation

Atherosclerosis is now considered to be an inflammatory disease (see Section 11.2.1). A number of intervention studies have shown that virgin olive oil reduces markers for inflammation, including thromboxane B2 (TBX2) and leukotriene B4 (LTB4) [88, 89]. These studies found that oils with a lower phenolic content were less effective, indicating that it is the polyphenols in virgin olive oil (VOO) that are important for the anti-inflammatory effects. One polyphenol that may be important is oleocanthal, which inhibits COX-1 and COX-2 and thus the generation of inflammatory cytokines [90] (see Section 9.4.4).

Many pro-inflammatory and pro-oxidatative processes are initiated via activation of the transcription factor NFκB (Section 9.4.4). Virgin olive oil has been shown to suppress NFκB activation. For example, meals rich in butter (i.e. high SFAs) or walnuts (high PUFAs) were found to transiently increase NFκB prior to a postprandial increase in markers for inflammation and oxidation, but this increase in NFκB was not observed following a meal rich in olive oil [91]. Hence, suppressing NFκB activation provides a common mechanism that may explain many of the diverse effects of virgin olive oil on markers for inflammation and oxidation.

Blood pressure

Intervention studies have found that olive oil reduces systolic blood pressure in healthy men [92] and in hypertensive patients with stable CHD (p=0.001) [93]. There is evidence that it is the oleic acid in olive oil – rather than the minor constituents – that is responsible for reductions in blood pressure since both oleic acid and virgin olive oil were found to cause similar reductions in blood pressure in experimental studies with rats [94]. Oleic acid may act by changing membrane structure, so affecting the activities of receptors in the membrane [94].

Anti-thrombotic effects

Formation of a thrombus (thrombogenesis) at an atherosclerotic plaque is a potentially life-threatening event. Thrombogenesis involves platelet activation (primary haemostasis) and coagulation (secondary haemostasis) and is countered by fibrinolysis (breakdown of a clot) which involves the generation of plasmin from plasminogen. Olive oil has been shown to help prevent a prothrombotic state. There were favourable effects on the procoagulant factors plasminogen activator inhibitor-1 (PAI-1) and factor VII (FVII) following consumption of a high phenol olive oil by hypercholesterolaemic individuals [95]. Consumption of high phenol olive oil has also been shown to decrease levels of thromboxane B2 (TXB2), which is the metabolic product of TXA2, an eicosanoid that increases platelet aggreggation [89]. A low phenol olive did not have this effect, thus suggesting that the phenolics in olive oil were responsible for these effects.

Gene expression

Consumption of VOO with a traditional MedDiet has been shown to modulate a number of proatherogenic genes. A 3-month intervention trial assessed the effects of a traditional MedDiet and virgin olive oil (VOO) on proatherogenic gene expression in peripheral blood mononuclear cells taken from healthy volunteers (n = 90) [96]. The MedDiet, especially together with a VOO rich in polyphenols, decreased the expression of a number of genes associated with oxidative stress and inflammation.

In conclusion, these studies demonstrate that both the MUFA and phenolic components of olive oil contribute to a range of beneficial effects on risk factors for CVD seen in human intervention studies.

Olives

There are no studies that have specifically examined the effects of consuming table olives on risk factors for CVD. This is surprising in view of the very high levels of potentially bioactive antioxidant phenolics, such as tyrosol and hydroxytyrosol, in olives relative to levels in virgin olive oil. For example, Greek olives were found to contain an average of 480 mg/kg of hydroxytyrosol (range 20–1140 mg/kg) in their flesh [97] which compares with about 15 mg/L in virgin olive oil. The traditional habit in some Mediterranean countries – typified by Greek men – of consuming a few olives before a meal would provide far more hydroxytyrosol than from a normal intake of olive oil, and without the danger of loss from degradation by cooking. Based on average figures, 31 g of olives – about 10 olives – would contain the same amount of hydroxytyrosol as 1 L of virgin olive oil. Moreover, phenolics in table olives have been shown to be readily bioavailable and to increase the total antioxidant capacity of the plasma of human subjects [98]. However, it should be noted that the salt content of table olives precludes high intake, especially in subjects at risk for high blood pressure.

Tea

Tea is perceived as a low calorie, healthy drink [99]. However, it is difficult to accurately evaluate tea in the context of a MedDiet since there are no epidemiological studies from the main tea-consuming nations of the Mediterranean basin. Rather, most studies on green tea originate from Asian countries (Japan or China), and studies on black tea are mostly from North European or North American populations. It has been suggested that there are parallels between tea and wine drinking, and this may contribute to why, despite having risk factors for CVD, certain Asian populations retain a low incidence of CVD [100].

There is good epidemiological evidence that tea drinking reduces the risk of CVD, and the American College of Cardiology Foundation Task Force now recommends moderate tea intake as possibly a useful part of a nutritional programme to reduce cardiovascular risk. However, in Morocco some of these benefits are compromised due to the custom of adding large amounts of sugar which has been identified as a possible cause of the increasing obesity in this country [101]. Both green and black tea have been shown to improve markers of cardiovascular function [102]. A review of the epidemiological data from between 1990–2004 linking black tea consumption to a reduced CHD risk concluded that this evidence was "robust", with one meta-analysis reporting an 11% decrease in the incidence rate of MI with an increase in black tea consumption of three cups per day [103]. One study found that the improved vascular effects of black tea consumption were completely prevented by the presence of milk [104], although others have concluded that milk is unlikely to reduce the bioactivity of tea flavonoids [103]. A review of randomised controlled trials (RCT) of green tea consumption conducted between 1966–2007 found that 17 out of 30 studies showed a statistically significant benefit, 11 showed no significant effect and 2 showed a harmful effect [105].

Mechanisms

A number of mechanisms may contribute to the protection against CVD observed in epidemiological studies. A meta-analysis suggested that chronic green tea consumption may significantly reduce LDL cholesterol concentrations, and it was estimated that this would require drinking 2–5 cups of green tea per day [106]. In experimental studies, EGCG has also been shown to prevent the oxidation of LDL, an important early step in atherosclerosis, as well as inhibiting other events associated with atherosclerosis including the proliferation and migration of smooth muscle cells [100].

Black tea has also been shown to reduce LDL oxidation *ex vivo* [103]. There is some evidence that black tea leads to acute rises in systolic and diastolic blood pressure independent of caffeine content, but that chronic intake of black tea has no overall effect on blood pressure [106]. Both green tea and black tea consumption have been shown in human studies to improve endothelial function as assessed by flow mediated vasodilatation (FMD) of the brachial artery [102, 107].

Coffee

No clear pattern has emerged from studies in various countries regarding risk of CHD or hypertension and coffee consumption [108]. In a case control study of a Greek population (who mainly consume boiled, unfiltered coffee) there was a J-shaped relationship between coffee consumption and risk of a myocardial infarct, with a reduced risk of 31% (OR 0.69: CI 0.50–0.86) relative to no risk at <300 ml coffee per day after controlling for various confounding factors [109].

The coffee diterpenes cafestol and kahweol have been shown to raise LDL cholesterol levels [108]. These diterpenes are extracted from ground coffee during brewing, and are present at relatively high levels in Turkish coffee (6–12 mg per cup) and at about 4 mg per cup in espresso (due to the smaller serving size). However, they are largely removed from coffee by filtration and during the production of instant coffee.

Wine and other forms of alcohol

The most consistent evidence for the cardiovascular benefits of moderate consumption of red wine and other forms of alcohol relates to reduced coronary heart disease (CHD) and associated myocardial infarcts. Studies on light-to-moderate alcohol consumption (any type) generally show reductions of about 30–35% in CHD [110, 111]. This follows a J-shaped curve, i.e. a reduced incidence at about 1–4 drinks per day (at the lower end for females) compared to no drinks, but a significantly increased risk at more than about four drinks per day. This trend is of most relevance for individuals >40 years of age since these are at most risk of CHD.

Only a few studies have specifically studied the role of wine in relation to cardiovascular protection within the context of a MedDiet. In a case control study conducted on a Spanish population, drinking wine during meals was associated with a reduced risk for CHD, but this reduced risk was similar to that of other alcoholic drinks (OR for low and high intake were 0.48 and 0.38 for wine; 0.42 and 0.55 for other drinks) [112]. A second study, the MEDIS study, evaluated whether alcohol consumption is associated with blood pressure [113]. MEDIS is a study conducted on elderly men and women from various MEDiterranean ISlands. Forty-four percent of men and 19% of women reported long-term consumption (at least 30 years) of alcohol, and this was mostly red or white wine or retsina, a uniquely Greek type of wine. There was a J-shaped association of alcohol intake with systolic ($p=0.001$), diastolic (p=0.02), mean (p=0.001) and pulse pressure (p=0.07) after adjusting for various confounding factors. This study suggests that long-term moderate alcohol consumption in the elderly can improve blood pressure levels and thus CVD prognosis. However, other studies have not found that moderate alcohol consumption is associated with decreased hypertension [114]. Indeed, consumption of wine at high levels – as for other forms of alcohol – is associated with an increased risk of hypertension [115].

There is some evidence that daily alcohol consumption is more cardioprotective than less frequent consumption [110]. In a case-control study nested in a large prospective studies on CHD risk in men (18,225 from the Health Professionals Follow-Up Study) and women (32,826 women from the Nurses Health Study), drinking frequency among both women and men tended to be associated with a lower risk of MI, with the lowest risks amongst those who drank 3–7 days per week (OR 0.70 CI: 0.57–0.85) for women and 0.86 CI 0.76–0.9 for men) [116]. The inverse association of frequent drinking with a lower risk of MI among women and men was no longer significant after further adjustment for levels of HDL cholesterol, haemoglobin A(1c), and fibrinogen, indicating that this association is apparently attributable to the relationship of alcohol with HDL cholesterol, fibrinogen, and haemoglobin A(1c). Because the effects of alcohol on HDL cholesterol, fibrinogen, and insulin sensitivity have been confirmed in randomised trials, these findings support the hypothesis that the inverse relation of alcohol use and MI is causal. In this study, where wine is the prevalent alcoholic beverage drunk by women, the effect is stronger in women than in men, suggesting that wine may have an additional effect over alcohol [116]. Not only may frequent consumption be more protective against CHD, but it also avoids the dangerous rise in blood pressure that can be caused by binge drinking. The consequences of this were starkly illustrated in a study that found that heart attacks in Northern Ireland peaked on Mondays and Tuesdays, due, it was concluded, to the effects of binge drinking on the previous Fridays and Saturdays [117].

Of particular note in the context of the MedDiet are studies showing that light-to-moderate alcohol is most cardioprotective when consumed before or during a meal [118]. It has been suggested that this may be related to improvements in postprandial glucose metabolism [110]. Drinking wine with a meal also raises the possibility for interactions between constituents in wine with other constituents in the MedDiet. A small study (15 people) that examined the short-term effects of consuming both red wine and olive oil found that there was a significant improvement in postprandial flow mediated dilatation (FMD) compared to either red wine or olive oil alone [119]. FMD is indicative of an improvement in endothelial function and is a technique that is based on ultrasound assessment of the diameter of the brachial artery.

Light-to-moderate alcohol consumption has also been found to reduce the risk of cardiovascular and all-cause mortality in patients already with a history of cardiovascular events. A meta-analysis of eight studies found a J-shaped relationship, with a significant maximal protection against cardiovascular mortality (of average 22%) at about 26 g alcohol per day [120]. However, there is no indication that controlling for food intake was performed in these studies.

Mechanisms

1. **Increased HDL:** The most compelling mechanism to explain a protective effect of moderate alcohol/wine consumption is increased production of HDL-cholesterol [121]. It has been suggested that this explains about 50% of the protective effect of moderate alcohol consumption (of any type) against coronary artery disease (CAD) [122]. Increased plasma cholesterol concentrations are a well-established risk factor for CVD, and HDL-cholesterol particles return cholesterol from peripheral tissues to the liver for disposal. The cholesteryl ester transfer protein is responsible for this efflux and is increased by alcohol [123]. Red wine was shown to have a slight additional beneficial effect over alcohol [124]. In addition, HDL-cholesterol has antioxidant properties due to its association with the enzyme paraoxonase which inhibits lipid peroxidation. It is not fully understood how alcohol increases HDL production although increasing the levels of apolipoproteins AI and AII (which form part of HDL particles) is one possibility [125].

2. **Reduced LDL-cholesterol oxidation:** Although a number of *in vitro* studies have demonstrated that wine phenolics have antioxidant activity, the relevance of this to humans is more controversial. Studies in humans have measured markers for oxidative stress in subjects given wine. One study found that after subjects drank wine, they had reduced urinary PGF2α, a marker for oxidative stress [126]. The effect was greater for red wine than white wine, perhaps due to the higher polyphenol content of red wine. Dealcoholised wine was found to retain antioxidant activity, suggesting that polyphenols in the wine, rather than the alcohol, may be responsible for the effect. Another study found that drinking red wine, but not white wine, increased the anti-oxidant capacity of blood and inhibited the oxidation of LDL-cholesterol [127]. It is also possible that several polyphenols in wine may interact synergistically to inhibit oxidative stress [126].

Despite these positive correlations, a number of other studies have found no reduction in oxidative stress after wine consumption [128]. Various differences in experimental design may contribute to the variability in results between studies, including dose and dosing (single dose or chronic administration) and type of wine, age and diet of the subjects, and the biomarker for oxidative stress that is measured. Based on their review of a number of studies, Covas et al. concluded that the oxidative status of the subjects was also important. These authors concluded that, although there is no overall evidence that sustained consumption of wine reduces oxidative stress in healthy individuals, there was better evidence that wine may afford protection under conditions of oxidative stress [128].

Oxidative stress may be induced by alcohol or by a meal. Postprandial oxidative stress can last for up to six hours after a meal and is recognised as a risk factor for atherosclerosis development. This emphasises the potential importance of context for drinking red wine, i.e. associated with a meal and the accompanying rise in postprandial oxidative stress.

Counterbalancing the anti-oxidant effects of wine are pro-oxidant effects. Ethanol can have pro-oxidant effects in the body due to metabolism by CYP2E1 which generates ROS, and also because of depletion of glutathione – a major protectant against oxidative stress in the body.

3. **Inhibition of vascular smooth muscle cells (VSMC):** The abnormal proliferation of VSMC in the arterial intima is thought to be a key step in the formation of the atherosclerotic plaque. Various phenolics in red wine have been shown in animal models to reduce the proliferation of VSMC [129].

4. **Vascular effects:** Correct regulation of vascular tone (i.e. the degree of constriction of blood vessels) is essential for a healthy vasculature. The endothelium helps regulate vascular tone by producing NO which relaxes the vasculature (i.e. NO is a vasodilator) and by producing endothelin-1, which is a vasoconstrictor. Both alcohol itself and phenolics in red wine increase levels of NO by increasing the activity of endothelial nitric oxide synthase (eNOS), the enzyme responsible for NO synthesis in endothelial cells [1, 130].

Some phenolics, and in particular proanthocyanidins, inhibit endothelin-1 and so reduce the vasoconstrictor activity in the endothelium [131]. It has been argued that inhibition of vasoconstriction by proanthocyanidins is an important mechanism for the cardioprotective benefits of red wine, and hence that wines rich in proanthocyanidins (such as those made from the Tannat grape) have particular health benefits [131]. However, current evidence suggests that the high molecular weight of proanthocyanidins precludes their absorption in their intact state.

5. **Anti-thrombotic effects:** Decreased platelet aggregation lowers plasma viscosity and is associated with a lower risk of CAD. Renaud and de Lorgeril in their discussion of the "French paradox" (see box below) concluded that consumption of red wine was possibly associated with reduced platelet aggregability rather than increased HDL [132]. Other studies have found that healthy volunteers who consume a daily glass of red wine have a significant reduction in plasma viscosity [133]. In one study, moderate wine consumption was shown to increase the production of nitric oxide (NO) which inhibits platelet aggregation [1]. Both *in vitro* incubation and oral supplementation with purple grape juice (PGJ) decreased platelet aggregation, increased platelet-derived NO release and decreased superoxide production. These findings may be a result of antioxidant-sparing and/or direct effects of select flavonoids found in PGJ providing evidence that the effects are due to phenolics and not alcohol [134].

6. **Anti-inflammatory effects:** Inflammation is now considered to be an important aspect of atherogenesis. Inflammatory markers (such as C-reactive protein and IL-6) have been found to decrease after moderate wine consumption, with superior effects shown for red wine [135]. However, not all studies have found that consumption of wine is associated with a decrease in inflammatory markers [136].

Inflammation and oxidative stress are closely inter-related processes, and some of the caveats discussed above that apply to studies of oxidative stress in humans may also apply to inflammation.

Wine versus other forms of alcohol
Opinion remains divided about whether or not wine confers additional cardio-protective benefits compared to a similar intake of alcohol from other types of drink. Part of the favourable effects of wine consumption could be related to the pattern of drinking wine daily with a meal, rather than the type of drink itself. It has been suggested that daily alcohol consumption may be most beneficial because favourable alcohol-induced changes to insulin sensitivity, HDL cholesterol, and inflammation are transient, reverting back to baseline within 24 hours [110]. Despite these reservations, several lines of evidence have been used to evaluate the contention that wine is more beneficial than other forms of alcohol.

Epidemiological evidence   The so-called "French paradox" (but see box below) has been linked to the high consumption of wine, particularly red wine. However, although some epidemiological studies have found red wine to be more beneficial than other types of alcohol, others have not [130, 137]. Intervention studies comparing wine with other types of alcohol could answer this question, but these are ethically difficult to undertake.

No French paradox?

The so-called "French paradox" is the reference to the reported low mortality rate from ischaemic heart disease among people in France despite the high amount of saturated fats in their diet. However, this concept disappears upon careful examination of the data: (i) a bias in death certificates was responsible for erroneous comparisons with other countries; (ii) France is a heterogeneous country in terms of food and drinking habits, and there is no French paradox when Northern France is compared with Belgium and Southern France with Spain; (iii) when controlling for food habits, the beneficial effect of wine drinking is confounded with healthy dietary habits [138].

Some studies have found an improvement in cardiovascular effects following acute consumption of red wine from which the alcohol has been removed. These alcohol-independent effects include decreased arterial stiffness and improved flow-mediated vasodilatation [139]. By contrast, a 4-week intervention study comparing red wine consumption with wine-equivalent red grape extract tablets suggested that the non-alcohol components in red wine were not responsible for the reduction in fibrinogen and increase in HDL cholesterol observed in the wine drinkers [140]. These studies suggest that only certain cardiovascular risk factors, such as some associated with vasodilatation, may be modifiable by the non-alcohol components in red wine.

Mechanisms   Whereas alcohol has a number of beneficial effects on the vasculature as discussed above, red wine phenolics influence a number of mechanisms that may confer additional cardiovascular benefits. These include decreasing the susceptibility of LDL to oxidation, reducing platelet aggregation and increasing fibrinolytic activity. Experimental studies have also shown that red wine phenolics increase the production of the vasodilatatory factor NO in cultures of endothelial cell and isolated arteries. A limitation of many *in vitro* experimental studies is their use of far higher concentrations of phenolics than are present in the blood after consumption of moderate levels of red wine. Hence their relevance to normal drinking patters is questionable. The phenolic resveratrol has attracted particular attention in these studies (see Chapter 7).

11.3.4   Dietary patterns

Analyses of the cardioprotective effects of foods, either by nutrients or by food sources, cannot give the full picture of the health effects of diet. This is due to complex interactions between constituents, a good example being the interplay between various FAs as discussed in Section 11.3.1. Hence, this prompted research towards another type of analysis, namely looking at the effects of dietary patterns.

Observational studies

One of the first reports on the association of dietary patterns with cardiovascular mortality was conducted in Denmark with a random sample of 3698 men and 3618 women aged 30–70 years [141]. A predefined healthy food index was used, which reflected daily intakes of fruits, vegetables and wholemeal bread, together with one based on principal component analysis that identified a "prudent" dietary pattern and a "Western" dietary pattern. The prudent pattern was positively associated with frequent intake of wholemeal bread, fruits and vegetables, whereas the Western pattern was characterised by frequent intake of meat products, potatoes, white bread, butter and lard. Among participants with complete information on all variables, 398 men and 231 women died during follow-up. The prudent pattern was inversely associated with cardiovascular mortality after controlling for confounding variables. Several subsequent analyses found that a prudent dietary pattern was associated with a lower risk of coronary heart disease (e.g. 0.70: CI 0.56–0.86, trend 0.0009), and a Western pattern with a higher risk of CHD (e.g. 1.64: CI 1.24–2.17, trend < 0.0001) [142–145].

With regard to the MedDiet and cardiovascular risk, observations with respect to a genuine Mediterranean dietary pattern are limited to Mediterranean countries, since observations are necessary over decades. Thus the *a priori* Mediterranean diet quality index was mainly used (see Chapter 8). Trichopoulou et al. were among the first to show the beneficial effect of the MedDiet score (MDS) on cardiovascular mortality. An inverse association between greater adherence to this diet and death due to CHD was evident in the Greek EPIC cohort (22,043 adults) (0.67 CI: 0.47–0.94]) [146]. The MDS was also applied to a Spanish population with the same results. This study evaluated the association between adherence to a MedDiet and the incidence of fatal and non-fatal cardiovascular events (100 cases) among 13,609, initially healthy, middle-aged adults (median age 38 y) from the Mediterranean area.

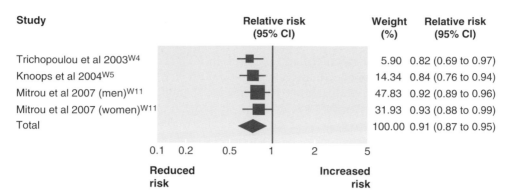

Figure 11.2 Risk of mortality from cardiovascular diseases associated with 2-point increase in adherence score for Mediterranean diet [151]. Squares represent effect size; extended lines show confidence intervals; diamond represents total effect size. With permission from BMJ Publishing Group Ltd.

In multivariate analyses, participants with the highest adherence to the MedDiet had a lower cardiovascular risk (HR 0.41: CI 0.18–0.95) compared to those with the lowest score. For each 2-point increment in the score, the adjusted HR were 0.80 (CI 0.62–1.02) for total CVD and 0.74 (CI 0.55–0.99) for CHD [147].

However, the MDS has to be modified (M-MDS) when applied to other European elderly cohorts of the EPIC study as described earlier (see Chapter 8) which leads to strong discrepancies in MDS values among countries [148]. This M-MDS does not appear to provide the same degree of risk reduction among the various countries with regard to survival after myocardial infarction among EPIC cohorts [149]. The mortality ratios associated with a 2-unit increment in M-MDS is 0.81 (CI 0.70–0.95) for the overall cohort and 0.44 (CI 0.22–0.87) for the Greek cohort. However, the aM-MDS, an MDS adapted to the US population (see Chapter 8) showed a risk reduction in the US NIH-AARP study of HR 0.78 (CI 0.69–0.87) [150]. A meta-analysis of the health effects associated with adherence to a MedDiet *a priori* defined by MDS (where MDS, M-MDS and modified M-MDS were mixed) was recently published [151]. Twelve studies that analysed prospectively the association between adherence to a MedDiet, mortality and incidence of diseases, with a total of 1,574,299 subjects followed for periods ranging from 3 to 18 years were included. The cumulative analysis among eight cohorts (514,816 subjects and 33,576 deaths) evaluating cardiovascular mortality in relation to adherence to a Mediterranean diet showed that an increase in the adherence score of two points was significantly associated with a reduced risk (pooled RR 0.91: CI 0.87–0.95) (Figure 11.2).

Considering these studies overall, adherence to a MedDiet appears significantly protective for CVD in Mediterranean countries. The slight change in the M-MDS (replacing MUFAs by unsaturated FA [UFA] in the ratio MUFAs/SFAs) does not modify the association observed in Mediterranean countries, but shows no association or a non-significant association of the M-MDS with CVD in non-Mediterranean countries. Three main explanations can be proposed to explain these observations. Firstly, difference in the actual FA exposure: in Mediterranean countries UFAs are mainly MUFAs from olive oil, whereas in other countries UFAs comprise PUFAs, from vegetable oils, and MUFAs from vegetable oils for a small part and from animal products for a large part. Secondly are the different cut-offs for score determination between the countries (lower for plant food and higher for animal food intake in non-Mediterranean countries). Thirdly, the unknown beneficial correlates of the *a priori* score that are present in Mediterranean countries and absent in non-Mediterranean countries (see Chapter 8). However, when the MDS is modified so as to adapt it to other populations, it becomes similar to a prudent diet, which was shown to decrease CVD risk and mortality, although the decrease in risk is not as high as the one observed in Mediterranean countries with the MDS.

Intervention studies

Only a few intervention studies in relation to CVD have been conducted using a holistic nutritional approach that covers intake of fruits, vegetables, grains, fatty acids and beverages. These have mostly used biomarkers in relation to primary prevention and survival as an end-point for secondary prevention.

In the Lyon study, a total of 605 patients (303 control subjects and 302 study patients) were studied over a mean period of 27 months [152]. The dietary pattern being tested was characterised by a low intake of total and saturated fats and an increased intake of marine or plant *n*-3 FAs and was not intended primarily to reduce blood cholesterol. The source of the plant *n*-3 FA, i.e. ALA, was a margarine (as a replacement for olive oil), which somewhat disqualifies this diet from the Mediterranean model. It also included a high intake of fresh fruits and vegetables, legumes and cereals, and contained large amounts of dietary fibre, antioxidants, minerals, vegetable proteins and B vitamins. Major primary end points (cardiovascular death and non-fatal acute myocardial infarction), secondary end points (including unstable angina, stroke, heart failure and embolisms) and minor end points (stable angina, need for myocardial revascularisation, postangioplasty restenosis and thrombophlebitis) were analysed separately and in combination. When major primary and secondary end points were combined, there were 59 events in the control subjects and 14 events in the study patients, showing a risk reduction of 76% (p<0.0001). When these end points were combined with the minor end points, there were 104 events in the control subjects and 68 events in the study patients, giving a risk reduction of 37% (p<0.005). The protective effect of this "MedDiet pattern" was maintained for up to four years after the first infarction, confirming previous intermediate analyses [39].[3]

In the Mediterranean Diet, Cardiovascular Risks and Gene Polymorphisms (Medi-RIVAGE) study, an actual Mediterranean-type diet was compared with the usually prescribed, low-fat/cholesterol diet in 212 volunteers (men and women) with moderate risk factors for CVD in a primary prevention context. The MedDiet was characterised essentially by the quality of fatty acids and their sources. Whole flour bread was recommended in the MedDiet group, together with olive oil as the more-or-less exclusive cooking oil (or canola oil as a second complementary choice), and oat bran-rich pasta. These two last foodstuffs plus tomato concentrate were provided to the MedDiet group. A special leaflet was provided with menus organised with weekly plans and by season so as to help the participants follow a MedDiet. Apart from these differences between the two groups, counselling and other recommendations were strictly identical in both groups, namely to increase fruit and vegetable intake, choose fish rather than meat, decrease calorie intake in those overweight or obese, and increase physical activity. The main factors measured were BMI, fasting lipids and lipoproteins, apolipoproteins,

---

[3] Another related study, the so-called Indo-Mediterranean study [40]. is not strictly relevant to the MedDiet pattern, and moreover has been judged invalid [153].

glucose, insulin and homocysteine [154]. After the 3-month dietary intervention, changes in risk factors were evaluated. Dietary questionnaires and plasma nutritional markers were used to test for compliance. Results could be analysed in 169 subjects. Fibre intake increased, with insoluble fibre being significantly higher in the MedDiet group, and fat quality improved, with the MedDiet-group showing a significantly higher intake of MUFAs, ALA and EPA. The other nutrients increased comparably in the two groups. BMI, total and triacylglycerol-rich lipoprotein cholesterol, triacylglycerols, apolipoproteins A-I and B, insulin and glucose levels and the HOMA score were significantly lower after three months in both groups, and the decrease was non-significantly higher in the MedDiet group. The reductions in total cholesterol, triacylglycerols, and insulin levels became significant after adjusting for BMI. The diet-by-time interaction was borderline significant for effect on LDL cholesterol ($p=0.09$). The data predicted a 9% reduction in CVD risk with the low fat diet and a 15% reduction with this particular MedDiet [155].

The PREDIMED multi-centre study, a three-group trial, has been conducted in Spain on 772 adults at high risk for CVD [156]. Participants were randomly assigned to a control group (n=257) or one of two MedDiet groups. Those allocated to the two Med-Diet groups received individual motivational interviews every three months. In addition, one MedDiet group (n=257) received free virgin olive oil (1 L/week), the other (n=258) received free mixed nuts (30 g/day). Participants in the control group received verbal instructions to reduce intake of all types of fat and a leaflet recommending the National Cholesterol Education Program. For total fat intake, these recommendations were opposite to those given to participants in the two MedDiet groups, who received instructions intended to increase the 14-item MDS, including increased consumption of vegetable fats and oils. There was no suggestion of any energy restriction. While the participants who were allocated to the low fat diet did not receive further intervention, those assigned to the two MedDiet groups had access to more intense intervention.

Compared with the low fat diet, the mean changes in the MedDiet + virgin olive oil group and the MedDiet + nuts group were: plasma glucose levels (mmol/L) −0.39 (CI −0.70 to −0.07) and −0.30 (CI −0.58 to −0.01), respectively; systolic blood pressure (mm Hg): −5.9 (CI −8.7 to −3.1) and −7.1 (CI −10.0 to −4.1), respectively; cholesterol/HDL–cholesterol ratio: −0.38 (CI −0.55 to −0.22) and −0.26 (CI −0.42 to −0.10), respectively. The MedDiet with olive oil reduced CRP levels by 0.54 mg/L (CI 1.04 to 0.03 mg/L) compared with the low fat diet. Using the same design, the effect of the three diets were also tested to assess their effects on *in vivo* lipoprotein oxidation in 372 subjects at high cardiovascular risk. After the 3-month interventions, mean oxidised LDL-cholesterol levels decreased in the MedDiet + virgin olive oil (−10.6 U/L [−14.2 to −6.1]) and MedDiet + nuts (−7.3 U/L [−11.2 to −3.3]) groups, without changes in the low fat diet group (v2.9 U/L [−7.3 to +1.5]). Change in oxidised LDL levels in the MedDiet + virgin olive oil group reached significance versus that of the low fat group (p: 02).

References

1. Leighton, F., Urquiaga, I. Endothelial nitric oxide synthase as a mediator of the positive health effects of Mediterranean diets and wine against metabolic syndrome. *World Rev Nutr Diet*, 2007. **97**: 33–51.
2. Corder, R. et al. Endothelin-1 synthesis reduced by red wine. *Nature*, 2001. **414**(6866): 863–4.

3. Wheatcroft, S. et al. The heart and blood vessels. In: *Clinical nutrition*, ed. M. Gibney, et al. 2005: Blackwell.

4. Steinberg, D. The LDL modification hypothesis of atherogenesis: an update. *J Lipid Res*, 2009. **50 Suppl**: S376–81.

5. Hansson, G.K. et al. Inflammation and atherosclerosis. *Annu Rev Pathol*, 2006. **1**: 297–329.

6. Salas-Salvado, J. et al. Components of the Mediterranean-type food pattern and serum inflammatory markers among patients at high risk for cardiovascular disease. *Eur J Clin Nutr*, 2008. **62**(5): 651–9.

7. de Lorgeril, M., Salen, P. Modified Cretan Mediterranean diet in the prevention of coronary heart disease and cancer: an update. *World Rev Nutr Diet*, 2007. **97**: 1–32.

8. Kromhout, D. et al. Dietary saturated and trans fatty acids and cholesterol and 25-year mortality from coronary heart disease: the Seven Countries Study. *Prev Med*, 1995. **24**(3): 308–15.

9. Benatti, P. et al. Polyunsaturated fatty acids: biochemical, nutritional and epigenetic properties. *J Am Coll Nutr*, 2004. **23**(4): 281–302.

10. Stark, A.H. et al. Update on alpha-linolenic acid. *Nutr Rev*, 2008. **66**(6): 326–32.

11. Patel, J.V. et al. Omega-3 polyunsaturated fatty acids: a necessity for a comprehensive secondary prevention strategy. *Vasc Health Risk Manag*, 2009. **5**: 801–10.

12. Rousseau-Ralliard, D. et al. Docosahexaenoic acid, but not eicosapentaenoic acid, lowers ambulatory blood pressure and shortens interval QT in spontaneously hypertensive rats in vivo. *Prostaglandins Leukot Essent Fatty Acids*, 2009. **80**(5–6): 269–77.

13. Keys, A. et al. The diet and 15-year death rate in the seven countries study. *Am J Epidemiol*, 1986. **124**(6): 903–15.

14. Kromhout, D. The 'Seven Countries Study': 40 years of research in coronary heart diseases in 7 countries. *Ned Tijdschr Geneeskd*, 1997. **141**(1): 7–9.

15. Ascherio, A. et al. Dietary fat and risk of coronary heart disease in men: cohort follow up study in the United States. *BMJ*, 1996. **313**(7049): 84–90.

16. Hu, F.B. et al. Dietary saturated fats and their food sources in relation to the risk of coronary heart disease in women. *Am J Clin Nutr*, 1999. **70**(6): 1001–8.

17. Jakobsen, M.U. et al. Major types of dietary fat and risk of coronary heart disease: a pooled analysis of 11 cohort studies. *Am J Clin Nutr*, 2009. **89**(5): 1425–32.

18. Tell, G.S. et al. Dietary fat intake and carotid artery wall thickness: the Atherosclerosis Risk in Communities (ARIC) Study. *Am J Epidemiol*, 1994. **139**(10): 979–89.

19. Hu, F.B. et al. Dietary fat intake and the risk of coronary heart disease in women. *N Engl J Med*, 1997. **337**(21): 1491–9.

20. Kris-Etherton, P.M. et al. Polyunsaturated fatty acids and cardiovascular health. *Nutr Rev*, 2004. **62**(11): 414–26.

21. He, K. et al. Accumulated evidence on fish consumption and coronary heart disease mortality: a meta-analysis of cohort studies. *Circulation*, 2004. **109**(22): 2705–11.

22. Harris, W.S. et al. Intakes of long-chain omega-3 fatty acid associated with reduced risk death from coronary heart disease in healthy adults. *Curr Atheroscler Rep*, 2008. **10**(6): 503–9.

23. de Goede, J. et al. Marine (n-3) fatty acids, fish consumption, and the 10-year risk of fatal and nonfatal coronary heart disease in a large population of Dutch adults with low fish intake. *J Nutr*, 2010. **140**(5): 1023–8.

24. Oomen, C.M. et al. alpha-Linolenic acid intake is not beneficially associated with 10-y risk of coronary artery disease incidence: the Zutphen Elderly Study. *Am J Clin Nutr*, 2001. **74**(4): 457–63.

25. Pedersen, J.I. et al. Adipose tissue fatty acids and risk of myocardial infarction–a case-control study. *Eur J Clin Nutr*, 2000. **54**(8): 618–25.

26. Pietinen, P. et al. Intake of fatty acids and risk of coronary heart disease in a cohort of Finnish men. The Alpha-Tocopherol, Beta-Carotene Cancer Prevention Study. *Am J Epidemiol*, 1997. **145**(10): 876–87.

27. Guallar, E. et al. Omega-3 fatty acids in adipose tissue and risk of myocardial infarction: the EURAMIC study. *Arterioscler Thromb Vasc Biol*, 1999. **19**(4): 1111–8.

28. Kark, J.D. et al. Adipose tissue n-6 fatty acids and acute myocardial infarction in a population consuming a diet high in polyunsaturated fatty acids. *Am J Clin Nutr*, 2003. **77**(4): 796–802.

29. Albert, C.M. et al. Dietary alpha-linolenic acid intake and risk of sudden cardiac death and coronary heart disease. *Circulation*, 2005. **112**(21): 3232–8.

30. Baylin, A. et al. Adipose tissue alpha-linolenic acid and nonfatal acute myocardial infarction in Costa Rica. *Circulation*, 2003. **107**(12): 1586–91.
31. Djousse, L. et al. Relation between dietary linolenic acid and coronary artery disease in the National Heart, Lung, and Blood Institute Family Heart Study. *Am J Clin Nutr*, 2001. **74**(5): 612–9.
32. Simon, J.A. et al. Serum fatty acids and the risk of stroke. *Stroke*, 1995. **26**(5): 778–82.
33. Lemaitre, R.N. et al. n-3 Polyunsaturated fatty acids, fatal ischemic heart disease, and nonfatal myocardial infarction in older adults: the Cardiovascular Health Study. *Am J Clin Nutr*, 2003. **77**(2): 319–25.
34. Mozaffarian, D. et al. Interplay between different polyunsaturated fatty acids and risk of coronary heart disease in men. *Circulation*, 2005. **111**(2): 157–64.
35. Willett, W.C. et al. Intake of trans fatty acids and risk of coronary heart disease among women. *Lancet*, 1993. **341**(8845): 581–5.
36. Mozaffarian, D. et al. Effects on coronary heart disease of increasing polyunsaturated fat in place of saturated fat: a systematic review and meta-analysis of randomized controlled trials. *PLoS Med*, 2010. **7**(3): e1000252.
37. Abbey, M. et al. Partial replacement of saturated fatty acids with almonds or walnuts lowers total plasma cholesterol and low-density-lipoprotein cholesterol. *Am J Clin Nutr*, 1994. **59**(5): 995–9.
38. Jost, J.P. et al. Comparison of dietary patterns between population samples in the three French MONICA nutritional surveys. *Rev Epidemiol Sante Publique*, 1990. **38**(5–6): 517–23.
39. de Lorgeril, M. et al. Mediterranean diet, traditional risk factors, and the rate of cardiovascular complications after myocardial infarction: final report of the Lyon Diet Heart Study. *Circulation*, 1999. **99**(6): 779–85.
40. Singh, R.B. et al. Effect of an Indo-Mediterranean diet on progression of coronary artery disease in high risk patients (Indo-Mediterranean Diet Heart Study): a randomised single-blind trial. *Lancet*, 2002. **360**(9344): 1455–61.
41. Horton, R. Expression of concern: Indo-Mediterranean Diet Heart Study. *Lancet*, 2005. **366**(9483): 354–6.
42. Anon. Dietary supplementation with n-3 polyunsaturated fatty acids and vitamin E after myocardial infarction: results of the GISSI-Prevenzione trial. Gruppo Italiano per lo Studio della Sopravvivenza nell'Infarto miocardico. *Lancet*, 1999. **354**(9177): 447–55.
43. Yokoyama, M. et al. Effects of eicosapentaenoic acid on major coronary events in hypercholesterolaemic patients (JELIS): a randomised open-label, blinded endpoint analysis. *Lancet*, 2007. **369**(9567): 1090–8.
44. Marchioli, R. et al. Early protection against sudden death by n-3 polyunsaturated fatty acids after myocardial infarction: time-course analysis of the results of the Gruppo Italiano per lo Studio della Sopravvivenza nell'Infarto Miocardico (GISSI)-Prevenzione. *Circulation*, 2002. **105**(16): 1897–903.
45. Calo, L. et al. N-3 Fatty acids for the prevention of atrial fibrillation after coronary artery bypass surgery: a randomized, controlled trial. *J Am Coll Cardiol*, 2005. **45**(10): 1723–8.
46. Mozaffarian, D. et al. Health effects of trans-fatty acids: experimental and observational evidence. *Eur J Clin Nutr*, 2009. **63 Suppl 2**: S5–21.
47. Malpuech-Brugere, C. et al. Differential impact of milk fatty acid profiles on cardiovascular risk biomarkers in healthy men and women. *Eur J Clin Nutr*, 2010. **64**(7): 752–9.
48. Kushi, L.H. et al. Health implications of Mediterranean diets in light of contemporary knowledge. 1. Plant foods and dairy products. *Am J Clin Nutr*, 1995. **61**(6 Suppl): 1407S–1415S.
49. Wu, H. et al. Dietary fiber and progression of atherosclerosis: the Los Angeles Atherosclerosis Study. *Am J Clin Nutr*, 2003. **78**(6): 1085–91.
50. Pereira, M.A. et al. Dietary fiber and risk of coronary heart disease: a pooled analysis of cohort studies. *Arch Intern Med*, 2004. **164**(4): 370–6.
51. Lairon, D. et al. Dietary fiber intake and risk factors for cardiovascular disease in French adults. *Am J Clin Nutr*, 2005. **82**(6): 1185–94.
52. Brown, L. et al. Cholesterol-lowering effects of dietary fiber: a meta-analysis. *Am J Clin Nutr*, 1999. **69**(1): 30–42.
53. Lairon, D. Dietary fibres: effects on lipid metabolism and mechanisms of action. *Eur J Clin Nutr*, 1996. **50**(3): 125–33.
54. McKeown, N.M. et al. Whole-grain intake is favorably associated with metabolic risk factors for type 2 diabetes and cardiovascular disease in the Framingham Offspring Study. *Am J Clin Nutr*, 2002. **76**(2): 390–8.

55. Anderson, J.W. et al. Health benefits of dietary fiber. *Nutr Rev*, 2009. **67**(4): 188–205.
56. Brunner, H.R. et al. The influence of potassium administration and of potassium deprivation on plasma renin in normal and hypertensive subjects. *J Clin Invest*, 1970. **49**(11): 2128–38.
57. Appel, L.J. ASH position paper: Dietary approaches to lower blood pressure. *J Am Soc Hypertens*, 2009. **3**(5): 321–31.
58. Bilton, R. et al. The White book on antioxidants in tomatoes and tomatoes products and their health benefits. A European Commission concerted action programme Fair CT 97–3233. 2001: CMITI Sarl, Avignon, France.
59. Hertog, M.G. et al. Dietary antioxidant flavonoids and risk of coronary heart disease: the Zutphen Elderly Study. *Lancet*, 1993. **342**(8878): 1007–11.
60. Mink, P.J. et al. Flavonoid intake and cardiovascular disease mortality: a prospective study in postmenopausal women. *Am J Clin Nutr*, 2007. **85**(3): 895–909.
61. Hollman, P.C. et al. Dietary flavonol intake may lower stroke risk in men and women. *J Nutr*, 2010. **140**(3): 600–4.
62. Willcox, B.J. et al. Antioxidants in cardiovascular health and disease: key lessons from epidemiologic studies. *Am J Cardiol*, 2008. **101**(10A): 75D–86D.
63. Stephens, N.G. et al. Randomised controlled trial of vitamin E in patients with coronary disease: Cambridge Heart Antioxidant Study (CHAOS). *Lancet*, 1996. **347**(9004): 781–6.
64. Tornwall, M.E. et al. Effect of alpha-tocopherol and beta-carotene supplementation on coronary heart disease during the 6-year post-trial follow-up in the ATBC study. *Eur Heart J*, 2004. **25**(13): 1171–8.
65. Czernichow, S. et al. Effect of supplementation with antioxidants upon long-term risk of hypertension in the SU.VI.MAX study: association with plasma antioxidant levels. *J Hypertens*, 2005. **23**(11): 2013–8.
66. Silaste, M.L. et al. Tomato juice decreases LDL cholesterol levels and increases LDL resistance to oxidation. *Br J Nutr*, 2007. **98**(6): 1251–8.
67. Kawai, Y. et al. Macrophage as a target of quercetin glucuronides in human atherosclerotic arteries: implication in the anti-atherosclerotic mechanism of dietary flavonoids. *J Biol Chem*, 2008. **283**(14): 9424–34.
68. Kang, S.S. et al. Homocysteinemia due to folate deficiency. *Metabolism*, 1987. **36**(5): 458–62.
69. Ciaccio, M., Bellia, C. Hyperhomocysteinemia and cardiovascular risk: effect of vitamin supplementation in risk reduction. *Curr Clin Pharmacol*, 2010. **5**(1): 30–6.
70. Yusuf, S. et al. Effect of potentially modifiable risk factors associated with myocardial infarction in 52 countries (the INTERHEART study): case-control study. *Lancet*, 2004. **364**(9438): 937–52.
71. Nothlings, U. et al. Intake of vegetables, legumes, and fruit, and risk for all-cause, cardiovascular, and cancer mortality in a European diabetic population. *J Nutr*, 2008. **138**(4): 775–81.
72. Bazzano, L.A. et al. Legume consumption and risk of coronary heart disease in US men and women: NHANES I Epidemiologic Follow-up Study. *Arch Intern Med*, 2001. **161**(21): 2573–8.
73. Pittaway, J.K. et al. Chickpeas may influence fatty acid and fiber intake in an ad libitum diet, leading to small improvements in serum lipid profile and glycemic control. *J Am Diet Assoc*, 2008. **108**(6): 1009–13.
74. Kris-Etherton, P.M. et al. The effects of nuts on coronary heart disease risk. *Nutr Rev*, 2001. **59**(4): 103–11.
75. Fito, M. et al. Effect of a traditional Mediterranean diet on lipoprotein oxidation: a randomized controlled trial. *Arch Intern Med*, 2007. **167**(11): 1195–203.
76. Banel, D.K., Hu, F.U. Effects of walnut consumption on blood lipids and other cardiovascular risk factors: a meta-analysis and systematic review. *Am J Clin Nutr*, 2009. **90**(1): 56–63.
77. Gebauer, S.K. et al. n-3 fatty acid dietary recommendations and food sources to achieve essentiality and cardiovascular benefits. *Am J Clin Nutr*, 2006. **83**(6 Suppl): 1526S–1535S.
78. Ros, E., Mataix, J. Fatty acid composition of nuts – implications for cardiovascular health. *Br J Nutr*, 2006. **96 Suppl 2**: S29–35.
79. Alonso, A. et al. Vegetable protein and fiber from cereal are inversely associated with the risk of hypertension in a Spanish cohort. *Arch Med Res*, 2006. **37**(6): 778–86.
80. Tsimikas, S., Reaven, P.D. The role of dietary fatty acids in lipoprotein oxidation and atherosclerosis. *Curr Opin Lipidol*, 1998. **9**(4): 301–7.

81. Perez-Jimenez, F. et al. Protective effect of dietary monounsaturated fat on arteriosclerosis: beyond cholesterol. *Atherosclerosis*, 2002. **163**(2): 385–98.
82. Cicero, A.F. et al. Changes in LDL fatty acid composition as a response to olive oil treatment are inversely related to lipid oxidative damage: the EUROLIVE study. *J Am Coll Nutr*, 2008. **27**(2): 314–20.
83. Racderstoiff, D. Antioxidant activity of olive polyphenols in humans: a review. *Int J Vitam Nutr Res*, 2009. **79**(3): 152–65.
84. Covas, M.I. et al. The effect of polyphenols in olive oil on heart disease risk factors: a randomized trial. *Ann Intern Med*, 2006. **145**(5): 333–41.
85. Boskou, D. Olive oil. *World Rev Nutr Diet*, 2007. **97**: 180–210.
86. Tuck, K.L. et al. Structural characterization of the metabolites of hydroxytyrosol, the principal phenolic component in olive oil, in rats. *J Agric Food Chem*, 2002. **50**(8): 2404–9.
87. Gomez-Alonso, S. et al. Changes in phenolic composition and antioxidant activity of virgin olive oil during frying. *J Agric Food Chem*, 2003. **51**(3): 667–72.
88. Visioli, F. et al. Virgin Olive Oil Study (VOLOS): vasoprotective potential of extra virgin olive oil in mildly dyslipidemic patients. *Eur J Nutr*, 2005. **44**(2): 121–7.
89. Bogani, P. et al. Postprandial anti-inflammatory and antioxidant effects of extra virgin olive oil. *Atherosclerosis*, 2007. **190**(1): 181–6.
90. Beauchamp, G.K. et al. Phytochemistry: ibuprofen-like activity in extra-virgin olive oil. *Nature*, 2005. **437**(7055): 45–6.
91. Bellido, C. et al. Butter and walnuts, but not olive oil, elicit postprandial activation of nuclear transcription factor kappaB in peripheral blood mononuclear cells from healthy men. *Am J Clin Nutr*, 2004. **80**(6): 1487–91.
92. Bondia-Pons, I. et al. Moderate consumption of olive oil by healthy European men reduces systolic blood pressure in non-Mediterranean participants. *J Nutr*, 2007. **137**(1): 84–7.
93. Fito, M. et al. Antioxidant effect of virgin olive oil in patients with stable coronary heart disease: a randomized, crossover, controlled, clinical trial. *Atherosclerosis*, 2005. **181**(1): 149–58.
94. Teres, S. et al. Oleic acid content is responsible for the reduction in blood pressure induced by olive oil. *Proc Natl Acad Sci USA*, 2008. **105**(37): 13811–6.
95. Ruano, J. et al. Intake of phenol-rich virgin olive oil improves the postprandial prothrombotic profile in hypercholesterolemic patients. *Am J Clin Nutr*, 2007. **86**(2): 341–6.
96. Konstantinidou, V. et al. In vivo nutrigenomic effects of virgin olive oil polyphenols within the frame of the Mediterranean diet: a randomized controlled trial. *Faseb J*, 2010. **24**(7): 2546–57.
97. Boskou, G. et al. Antioxidant capacity and phenolic profile of table olives from the Greek market. *Food Chemistry*, 2006. **94**: 558–564.
98. Kountouri, A.M. et al. Bioavailability of the phenolic compounds of the fruits (drupes) of Olea europaea (olives): impact on plasma antioxidant status in humans. *Phytomedicine*, 2007. **14**(10): 659–67.
99. Popkin, B.M. et al. A new proposed guidance system for beverage consumption in the United States. *Am J Clin Nutr*, 2006. **83**(3): 529–42.
100. Sumpio, B.E. et al. Green tea, the "Asian paradox," and cardiovascular disease. *J Am Coll Surg*, 2006. **202**(5): 813–25.
101. Benjelloun, S. Nutrition transition in Morocco. *Public Health Nutr*, 2002. **5**(1A): 135–40.
102. Bolling, B.W. et al. Tea and health: preventive and therapeutic usefulness in the elderly? *Curr Opin Clin Nutr Metab Care*, 2009. **12**(1): 42–8.
103. Gardner, E.J. et al. Black tea – helpful or harmful? A review of the evidence. *Eur J Clin Nutr*, 2007. **61**(1): 3–18.
104. Lorenz, M. et al. Addition of milk prevents vascular protective effects of tea. *Eur Heart J*, 2007. **28**(2): 219–23.
105. Kuriyama, S. The relation between green tea consumption and cardiovascular disease as evidenced by epidemiological studies. *J Nutr*, 2008. **138**(8): 1548S–1553S.
106. Hooper, L. et al. Flavonoids, flavonoid-rich foods, and cardiovascular risk: a meta-analysis of randomized controlled trials. *Am J Clin Nutr*, 2008. **88**(1): 38–50.
107. Jochmann, N. et al. The efficacy of black tea in ameliorating endothelial function is equivalent to that of green tea. *Br J Nutr*, 2008. **99**(4): 863–8.

108. Bonita, J.S. et al. Coffee and cardiovascular disease: in vitro, cellular, animal, and human studies. *Pharmacol Res*, 2007. **55**(3): 187–98.

109. Panagiotakos, D.B. et al. The J-shaped effect of coffee consumption on the risk of developing acute coronary syndromes: the CARDIO2000 case-control study. *J Nutr*, 2003. **133**(10): 3228–32.

110. O'Keefe, J.H. et al. Alcohol and cardiovascular health: the razor-sharp double-edged sword. *J Am Coll Cardiol*, 2007. **50**(11): 1009–14.

111. Gunzerath, L. et al. National Institute on Alcohol Abuse and Alcoholism report on moderate drinking. *Alcohol Clin Exp Res*, 2004. **28**(6): 829–47.

112. Fernandez-Jarne, E. et al. Type of alcoholic beverage and first acute myocardial infarction: a case-control study in a Mediterranean country. *Clin Cardiol*, 2003. **26**(7): 313–8.

113. Panagiotakos, D.B. et al. The J-shape association of alcohol consumption on blood pressure levels, in elderly people from Mediterranean Islands (MEDIS epidemiological study). *J Hum Hypertens*, 2007. **21**(7): 585–7.

114. Klatsky, A.L. Alcohol and cardiovascular diseases. *Expert Rev Cardiovasc Ther*, 2009. **7**(5): 499–506.

115. Zilkens, R.R. et al. Red wine and beer elevate blood pressure in normotensive men. *Hypertension*, 2005. **45**(5): 874–9.

116. Mukamal, K.J. et al. Drinking frequency, mediating biomarkers, and risk of myocardial infarction in women and men. *Circulation*, 2005. **112**(10): 1406–13.

117. Ferrieres, J. The French paradox: lessons for other countries. *Heart*, 2004. **90**(1): 107–11.

118. Rehm, J. et al. Alcohol and cardiovascular disease – more than one paradox to consider. Average volume of alcohol consumption, patterns of drinking and risk of coronary heart disease – a review. *J Cardiovasc Risk*, 2003. **10**(1): 15–20.

119. Karatzi, K. et al. Postprandial improvement of endothelial function by red wine and olive oil antioxidants: a synergistic effect of components of the Mediterranean diet. *J Am Coll Nutr*, 2008. **27**(4): 448–53.

120. Costanzo, S. et al. Alcohol consumption and mortality in patients with cardiovascular disease: a meta-analysis. *J Am Coll Cardiol*, 2010. **55**(13): 1339–47.

121. Suh, I. et al. Alcohol use and mortality from coronary heart disease: the role of high-density lipoprotein cholesterol. The Multiple Risk Factor Intervention Trial Research Group. *Ann Intern Med*, 1992. **116**(11): 881–7.

122. Klatsky, A.L. Alcohol, wine, and vascular diseases: an abundance of paradoxes. *Am J Physiol Heart Circ Physiol*, 2008. **294**(2): H582–3.

123. Fumeron, F. et al. Alcohol intake modulates the effect of a polymorphism of the cholesteryl ester transfer protein gene on plasma high density lipoprotein and the risk of myocardial infarction. *J Clin Invest*, 1995. **96**(3): 1664–71.

124. Senault, C. et al. Beneficial effects of a moderate consumption of red wine on cellular cholesterol efflux in young men. *Nutr Metab Cardiovasc Dis*, 2000. **10**(2): 63–9.

125. De Oliveira, E.S.E.R. et al. Alcohol consumption raises HDL cholesterol levels by increasing the transport rate of apolipoproteins A-I and A-II. *Circulation*, 2000. **102**(19): 2347–52.

126. Pignatelli, P. et al. Polyphenols synergistically inhibit oxidative stress in subjects given red and white wine. *Atherosclerosis*, 2006. **188**(1): 77–83.

127. Fuhrman, B. et al. Consumption of red wine with meals reduces the susceptibility of human plasma and low-density lipoprotein to lipid peroxidation. *Am J Clin Nutr*, 1995. **61**(3): 549–54.

128. Covas, M.I. et al. Wine and oxidative stress: up-to-date evidence of the effects of moderate wine consumption on oxidative damage in humans. *Atherosclerosis*, 2010. **208**(2): 297–304.

129. Cordova, A.C. et al. The cardiovascular protective effect of red wine. *J Am Coll Surg*, 2005. **200**(3): 428–39.

130. Lippi, G. et al. Moderate red wine consumption and cardiovascular disease risk: beyond the "French paradox". *Semin Thromb Hemost*, 2010. **36**(1): 59–70.

131. Corder, R. et al. Oenology: red wine procyanidins and vascular health. *Nature*, 2006. **444**(7119): 566.

132. Renaud, S., de Lorgeril, M. Wine, alcohol, platelets, and the French paradox for coronary heart disease. *Lancet*, 1992. **339**(8808): 1523–6.

133. Kloner, R.A., Rezkalla, S.H. To drink or not to drink? That is the question. *Circulation*, 2007. **116**(11): 1306–17.

134. Freedman, J.E. et al. Select flavonoids and whole juice from purple grapes inhibit platelet function and enhance nitric oxide release. *Circulation*, 2001. **103**(23): 2792–8.

135. Sacanella, E. et al. Down-regulation of adhesion molecules and other inflammatory biomarkers after moderate wine consumption in healthy women: a randomized trial. *Am J Clin Nutr*, 2007. **86**(5): 1463–9.

136. Walzem, R.L. Wine and health: state of proofs and research needs. *Inflammopharmacology*, 2008. **16**(6): 265–71.

137. Mukamal, K.J. et al. Roles of drinking pattern and type of alcohol consumed in coronary heart disease in men. *N Engl J Med*, 2003. **348**(2): 109–18.

138. Ruidavets, J.B. et al. Alcohol intake and diet in France, the prominent role of lifestyle. *Eur Heart J*, 2004. **25**(13): 1153–62.

139. Karatzi, K. et al. Effects of red wine on endothelial function: postprandial studies vs clinical trials. *Nutr Metab Cardiovasc Dis*, 2009. **19**(10): 744–50.

140. Hansen, A.S. et al. Effect of red wine and red grape extract on blood lipids, haemostatic factors, and other risk factors for cardiovascular disease. *Eur J Clin Nutr*, 2005. **59**(3): 449–55.

141. Osler, M. et al. Dietary patterns and mortality in Danish men and women: a prospective observational study. *Br J Nutr*, 2001. **85**(2): 219–25.

142. Fung, T.T. et al. Association between dietary patterns and plasma biomarkers of obesity and cardiovascular disease risk. *Am J Clin Nutr*, 2001. **73**(1): 61–7.

143. Fung, T.T. et al. Dietary patterns and the risk of coronary heart disease in women. *Arch Intern Med*, 2001. **161**(15): 1857–62.

144. Heidemann, C. et al. Dietary patterns and risk of mortality from cardiovascular disease, cancer, and all causes in a prospective cohort of women. *Circulation*, 2008. **118**(3): 230–7.

145. Hu, F.B., Willett, W.C. Optimal diets for prevention of coronary heart disease. *Jama*, 2002. **288**(20): 2569–78.

146. Trichopoulou, A. et al. Adherence to a Mediterranean diet and survival in a Greek population. *N Engl J Med*, 2003. **348**(26): 2599–608.

147. Martinez-Gonzalez, M.A. et al. Mediterranean diet and the incidence of cardiovascular disease: a Spanish cohort. *Nutr Metab Cardiovasc Dis*, 2010. **21**(4): 237–44.

148. Trichopoulou, A. et al. Modified Mediterranean diet and survival: EPIC-elderly prospective cohort study. *BMJ*, 2005. **330**(7498): 991.

149. Trichopoulou, A. et al. Modified Mediterranean diet and survival after myocardial infarction: the EPIC-Elderly study. *Eur J Epidemiol*, 2007. **22**(12): 871–81.

150. Mitrou, P.N. et al. Mediterranean dietary pattern and prediction of all-cause mortality in a US population: results from the NIH-AARP Diet and Health Study. *Arch Intern Med*, 2007. **167**(22): 2461–8.

151. Sofi, F. et al. Adherence to Mediterranean diet and health status: meta-analysis. *BMJ*, 2008. **337**: a1344.

152. de Lorgeril, M. et al. Mediterranean alpha-linolenic acid-rich diet in secondary prevention of coronary heart disease. *Lancet*, 1994. **343**(8911): 1454–9.

153. Bawaskar, H.S. Research fraud. *Lancet*, 2005. **366**(9491): 1076.

154. Vincent, S. et al. The Medi-RIVAGE study (Mediterranean Diet, Cardiovascular Risks and Gene Polymorphisms): rationale, recruitment, design, dietary intervention and baseline characteristics of participants. *Public Health Nutr*, 2004. **7**(4): 531–42.

155. Vincent-Baudry, S. et al. The Medi-RIVAGE study: reduction of cardiovascular disease risk factors after a 3-mo intervention with a Mediterranean-type diet or a low-fat diet. *Am J Clin Nutr*, 2005. **82**(5): 964–71.

156. Estruch, R. et al. Effects of a Mediterranean-style diet on cardiovascular risk factors: a randomized trial. *Ann Intern Med*, 2006. **145**(1): 1–11.

12 Cancers

Summary

- Cancers generally develop over many years and are multifactorial diseases caused by genetic and environmental factors.
- Cancer development (carcinogenesis) can be delineated into three stages: initiation (caused by a carcinogen triggering a genetic alteration) → promotion (clonal proliferation) → tumour progression (angiogenesis and spread to other tissues – metastasis). Nutrients can intervene at all of these steps.
- A large number of epidemiological studies have evaluated the cancer-preventative effects of food components (including fats, fibre, phytochemicals and nutrients) and foods (wine, fruits and vegetables, tea, coffee). However, various confounding factors have highlighted the difficulties associated with establishing a causal relationship between a particular nutrient or food and cancer.
- MedDiet scores (MDS) have been used to evaluate the global effect of dietary patterns on cancer mortality and incidence. Most of the time, the original MDS is associated with a higher risk reduction of cancer than when this score is modified for non-Mediterranean populations.
- A prudent diet pattern identified by principal component analysis in various non-Mediterranean populations has been shown to be associated with a reduced risk for cancer in some, but not all, studies, whereas the Western pattern was more consistently associated with an increased risk. However, when a prudent dietary pattern includes olive oil, and thus becomes comparable to a MedDiet, there is a stronger suggestion of a risk reduction for breast cancer.
- A number of biologically-plausible mechanisms can be proposed to explain how interactions between various constituents in the MedDiet pattern may reduce cancer risk.

12.1 Introduction

Dietary cancer prevention aims to prevent the initiation and development of pre-cancerous lesions before they develop into clinically overt cancer. Prevention may take several forms:

- Preventing healthy individuals from developing cancer (primary prevention).
- Preventing the further development of premalignant conditions. This targets individuals with premalignant conditions such as oral leukoplakia, prostatic

The Mediterranean Diet: Health and Science, First Edition. Richard Hoffman and Mariette Gerber.
© 2012 Richard Hoffman and Mariette Gerber. Published 2012 by Blackwell Publishing Ltd.

intraepithelial neoplasia and premalignant growths in the colon known as adenomatous polyps or adenomas.
- Preventing the recurrence of cancer in patients who have previously been treated for the disease.

This chapter discusses epidemiological evidence for the primary prevention of cancer by a MedDiet, and possible biological mechanisms for these effects. There is no convincing clinical evidence that dietary factors, including those in a MedDiet, can help treat someone who already has cancer [1]. Although experimental studies are useful for understanding mechanisms of action, extrapolating from observations in cell culture or animal models of cancer to explain human observations is fraught with difficulties, and for most dietary constituents a definitive understanding of how they work in humans has not been established. Nevertheless, experimental studies have elucidated a plethora of plausible biological mechanisms of action for phytochemicals (in fruits, vegetables, wine and virgin olive oil), fatty acids, vitamins, low glycaemic foods and fibre, which occur in the MedDiet. Of particular interest is how the unique combination of constituents in the MedDiet may interact to prevent cancer. However, understanding this is far from trivial since one estimate is that an average diet has 25,000 "bioactives" [2] and this gives rise to an enormous number of possible interactions.

12.2   Nutritional factors and the biology of cancer

12.2.1   Introduction

Cancer is not a unique disease: rather, different types of cancers exist that affect numerous organs and tissues in the body. Cancers are multifactorial, and it is generally acknowledged that cancers result from an interaction between genes and the environment. Since cancers generally evolve over several years or even decades, the probability of developing a cancer increases with age. Sporadic cancers are the most frequently occurring, and are strongly induced or influenced by the environment, either by environmental carcinogens (tobacco, chemicals, radiations, viruses) or by protective factors, mainly related to lifestyle. Genetic polymorphisms may play a role by enhancing susceptibility to these environmental factors through the modulation of detoxification mechanisms. Hereditary (familial) cancers represent 5–10% of all cases, and these are more likely to occur earlier in life. In these cancers, the person has inherited one or more genetic abnormalities (mutations). A meta-analysis of 10 studies showed that the risk of developing breast cancer in women carrying mutations on BRCA1 genes increases with age: 1.8% at 30 years of age, 12% at 40 y, 29% at 50 y, 44% at 60 and 54% at 70 y [3]. This demonstrates that age-related environmental factors increase the risk of cancer development, thus raising the possibility for prevention in familial cancers. Risk never reached 100%, demonstrating that both age and environmental factors interact with the genetic predisposition.

12.2.2   Carcinogenesis

Cancers result from the uncontrolled growth of cells due to changes in the their genetic information. About 5–10% of cancers are linked to the inheritance of a single genetic change which then gives rise to further changes, both genetic and non-genetic, later on in life (familial cancers). However, the majority of cancers are due to the cumulative effect of many genetic changes acquired during the lifetime of an individual (sporadic cancers). These genetic changes manifest in cellular changes that enable cells to develop into a malignant tumour, i.e. a cancer. Most of the growth of a cancer goes unnoticed, and by the time it is detected the cancer has already completed most of its life cycle. A typical small tumour weighing 1 g is the result of about 30 cell divisions from the time the first cell divides. After only another 10 divisions, the tumour would weigh 1 kg, a size that is incompatible with life. It is estimated that for many solid tumours, the period between the development of the first cancer cell and the onset of metastatic disease is 20 years or more.

Tumour development occurs in a series of stages, each characterised by different events. This process is known as carcinogenesis. The initiating event is caused by an exogenous agent, such as a chemical, damaging the DNA of a cell, or by an endogenous one such as an abnormal hormone metabolite. This essentially reprogrammes the cell so that it has a growth advantage over neighbouring cells. Further changes then occur to the growing cell mass, some of which are caused by environmental factors, such as certain chemicals, and some of which occur from signals from within the body, such as hormones. Eventually the tumour acquires the ability to invade underlying tissues and spread (metastasis).

The stages of cancer development are sometimes described schematically as initiation (triggered by an alteration in DNA), promotion and tumour growth (clonal expansion of cells), and progression (angiogenesis and spread to other tissues, i.e. metastasis), and these stages have been delineated in some animal models of cancer. However, using experimental models to study cancer in humans is limited because humans are exposed to multiple factors and represent a more complex organism than laboratory animals, and it is often difficult to discriminate these different stages. Nevertheless, discrete stages have been described in some cancers such as colorectal cancer, these stages being aberrant crypt → small adenoma → large adenoma → carcinoma [4]. The clinical diagnosis might be made early when there are clinically detectable intermediate steps (e.g. adenomas), but diagnosis is delayed when the early stages are silent. In breast cancer, clinical progression may occur as: dysplasia → atypical hyperpasia → cancer *in situ* → invading cancer/metastatic cancer, but these stages are not always observed in this sequence.

About 80–90% of all cancers originate from epithelial cells. These cancers are called carcinomas. Epithelial cells can change into a cancer precursor known as an intraepithelial neoplasia (IEN). IEN is observed histologically as moderate to severe dysplasia (Figure 12.1). Targeting IEN, either by preventing it from arising or by preventing its subsequent development, is extremely important for cancer prevention, and this was emphasised in the American Society of Clinical Oncology definition of cancer prevention as "a reduction in the risk of developing clinically evident cancer, whether first or second primary cancer, or of developing intraepithelial neoplasia (IEN)" [5].[1]

The 100 or so different human cancers have both common characteristics related to the basic mechanisms of carcinogenesis, and also specific characteristics related to the target tissue or organ, and/or to associated risk factors (e.g. for hormone-dependent

---

[1] Monitoring IEN is also very useful for chemoprevention trials. The standard end-point in chemoprevention trials is cancer incidence. However, using an intermediary endpoint such as IEN can greatly speed up the evaluation of a chemopreventative strategy and so greatly reduce costs.

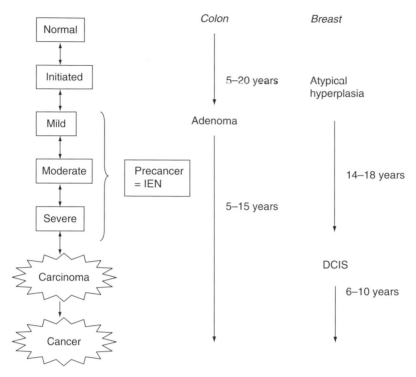

Figure 12.1 Targeting carcinogenesis with dietary prevention. Stages shown in boxes indicate where dietary intervention may be helpful. IEN: intraepithelial neoplasia; DCIS: ductal carcinoma *in situ*.

cancers). Hence, dietary constituents can help prevent a broad range of cancer types if they target one of the common features of cancer or precancerous cells. There is experimental evidence that the MedDiet can inhibit or delay all of the stages of carcinogenesis. However, early intervention is desirable since it is generally considered that the effectiveness in inhibiting carcinogenesis decreases as the tumour grows.

Some constituents may act on features specific to a particular cancer or cancer sub-type. Cancer sub-types could potentially have important implications for future dietary epidemiological studies. There is good evidence that components in the MedDiet have a great influence on oestrogen-receptor positive than oestrogen-receptor negative breast cancers. However, the majority of epidemiological studies measure the incidence of a particular cancer with no reference to sub-type. Hence, a dietary constituent that acts specifically on a target unique to a particular cancer sub-type may be missed if this sub-type only represents a small proportion of all of the sub-types for a particular cancer. There is some preliminary evidence that virgin olive oil shows selectivity for a minority sub-type of breast cancer (HER2 positive cells – see below).[2]

---

[2] This issue of selectivity for sub-types can be emphasised by considering the analogous situation that exists for new cancer therapeutics. Some of these do indeed have very specific targets. For example, a drug called Gleevec targets a specific change in a type of leukaemia called chronic myeloid leukaemia (CML), and Gleevec is ineffective against other forms of leukaemia. CML represents only 5% of all cases of leukaemia, and if Gleevec had been evaluated on patients with all types of leukaemia it may well have been concluded that it was an ineffective drug.

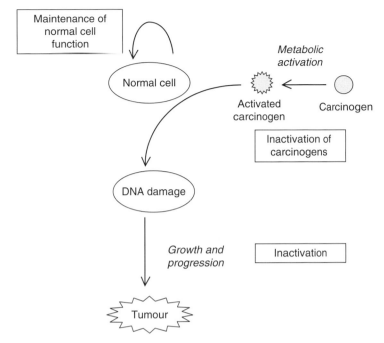

Figure 12.2 Events leading to a tumour that are potential targets for intervention by constituents of the MedDiet. The boxes represent possible sites for intervention.

Constituents in the MedDiet may prevent cancer by:

1. helping maintain the integrity of a normal cell
2. defending the cell against carcinogens
3. retarding the growth and progression of abnormal cells and tissues to more cancerous forms

These changes are possible targets for intervention by constituents in the MedDiet and are shown in Figure 12.2.

Maintaining normal cell function

Regulating genomic stability is key to maintaining the normal functioning of the 10^{13} cells that make up the human body. Although each cell contains the same genome (set of genes), the properties of an individual cell are due to the specific expression of a sub-set of genes within the genome of that cell. Gene expression, i.e. which genes are turned on and off, is regulated by transcription factors that bind to promotor regions on genes, and these genes are either switched on or off (see Section 9.6.2). Cell specific gene expression is responsible for the large variety of cell types in the body. The development of cells with specialised structure and function from unspecialised precursor cells is referred to as differentiation. Importantly, reduced differentiation of a cell often correlates with an increased proliferative capacity which in turn increases the likelihood of cancer development.

Some micronutrients affect transcription factors by either increasing or decreasing their ability to bind to promotor regions on genes. Transcription factors can be prevented from binding to promotor regions of genes by methylation (i.e. addition of a methyl group) of cytosine bases in the promotor region of the DNA[3]. This prevents the switching on of the gene: the gene is said to be "silenced". Silencing certain genes is an important mechanism for preserving the correct degree of differentiation of a cell. By contrast, insufficient methylation can result in the switching on of genes so that the cell becomes less differentiated, and this decrease in differentiation may increase the proliferative capacity of a cell, and so increase the risk of cancer. For example, hypomethylation of DNA is related to an increased risk of colon cancer. Some dietary constituents act as methyl donors. Folate is a particularly important methyl donor, and the MedDiet is an excellent source of folate, which is present in green leafy vegetables. Folate deficiency leads to hypomethylation of DNA and is associated with an increased risk of colon cancer.

Folate is also required for the synthesis of thymidine, one of the precursors for DNA synthesis. A lack of folate prevents thymidine being synthesised in sufficient amounts and this leads to genomic (DNA) instability and the resulting mutations can increase cancer risk.

Folic acid supplementation and cancer

Although folate is required for switching off certain genes which then helps preserve the correct degree of differentiation of a cell, genes normally involved in suppressing tumour growth may also be switched off. If folate results in these tumour suppressor genes being silenced, this will *increase* the risk of cancer. This double-edged effect may offer an explanation of why, despite the fact that sufficient folate is associated with a reduced risk of some cancers, folic acid supplementation has been found in some studies to *increase* cancer risk. For example, in a prospective study carried out on 25,400 women, folic acid supplementation (>400 µg) or supplementation plus the dietary contribution (>853 µg) significantly increased breast cancer risk [6]. Similarly, a randomised clinical trial with folic acid supplementation (1 mg/d) increased colorectal adenomas and prostate cancer [7].

Gene expression is also affected by changes to nuclear proteins called histones. DNA coils around histones, and the amount of acetylation (i.e. addition of an acetyl group) of histones controls how tightly DNA is able to coil around them. Increased acetylation of histones reduces the degree to which DNA can tightly coil, and this results in increased gene expression. By contrast, tight coiling of DNA reduces gene expression.

Acetylation of histones is increased by enzymes called histone acetyl transferases and deacetylation is increased by histone deacetylases. Experimental studies suggest that some dietary constituents inhibit histone deacetylases and so cause increased acetylation of histones and increased gene expression. This may be important for maintaining the correct degree of differentiation of a cell, although the precise role in cancer is not yet clear. Dietary constituents that inhibit histone deacetylases include butyrate (produced by probiotic bacteria in the colon) and some sulphur-containing phytochemicals such as diallyl sulphide found in garlic and sulforaphane in brassicas [8].

---

[3] Changing the functioning of a gene without affecting its nucleotide sequence is referred to as an epigenetic change.

Resveratrol has attracted a good deal of attention as an *activator* of a deacetylase called Sirt1. Sirt1 not only deacetylates certain histones but also deacetylates various transcription factors [9]. Sirt1 mediates responses associated with life extension, although it is uncertain whether sufficient resveratrol is consumed from a moderate intake of red wine to have these effects in humans.

Another important aspect of the normal homeostasis of cells is to prevent damage to DNA caused by normal cellular activities. Normal cellular function, especially that due to mitochondrial activity, continually generates free radicals, and these can oxidise bases in DNA. The best characterised product of this damage is 8-hydroxy-2′-deoxyguanosine (8-OHdG). 8-OHdG in DNA results in errors during normal replication and this may increase the risk of cancer. Ellagic acid (which is present in berries, pomegranates, red wine and nuts) is a potent inhibitor of 8-OHdG production and has been shown to induce DNA repair mechanisms in a mouse model [10]. A number of dietary substances in the MedDiet, such as lycopene and selenium, have been shown to decrease DNA damage and this may be due to the antioxidant activities of these substances.

In addition to increasing levels of 8-OHdG in DNA, oxidative stress can cause numerous other changes in cells that may predispose them to becoming cancerous. The relationship between oxidative stress and cancer is controversial, and it has been concluded that oxidative stress may be necessary, but is not in itself sufficient, for cancer development [11]. Besides oxidative damage to bases in DNA, oxidative stress is also associated with a number of other features of cancer progression such as suppressing apoptosis and promoting cell proliferation (see below).

Defending the cell against carcinogens

Carcinogens contribute in some way to the formation of cancer, and many are found in foods, such as heterocyclic aromatic amines (HAs) produced when meat is cooked at high temperatures. Many (but not all) carcinogens cause mutations in DNA. Some dietary carcinogens can act as initiating agents, whereas others cause changes at later stages in the process of carcinogenesis.

Enzymes, mostly in the liver, convert dietary carcinogens to forms that can be more readily excreted. However, during this process many dietary carcinogens are first activated from previously inactive forms, before they are subsequently converted into an excretable form. This activation of dietary carcinogens is catalysed by a group of enzymes known as phase 1 enzymes, particularly cytochrome P450 mixed function oxygenases (CYPs). There are multiple isoforms of CYPs. These enzymes generate electrophiles that can bind to and damage DNA.

Carcinogens that are activated by phase 1 enzymes are subsequently converted into excretable forms by phase 2 enzymes. Phase 2 enzymes conjugate the phase 1 metabolites to metabolites that can be excreted in bile or urine. Phase 2 enzymes include glutathione-*S*-transferases (GSTs), UDP-glucuronyltransferases, NAD(P) H:quinone oxidoreductase, and sulpho-transferases. Like phase 1 enzymes, phase 2 enzymes also exist in multiple isoforms.

Generally speaking, it is desirable to inhibit phase 1 metabolising enzymes (to prevent carcinogen activation) and to enhance phase 2 metabolising enzymes (to increase carcinogen excretion). The anti-cancer benefits of some nutrients in the MedDiet may operate through these mechanisms. There are a few reports of phytochemicals inhibiting CYPs. For example, naringenin and quercetin from citrus fruits inhibited the activity of CYP isoforms that activate a carcinogen in cigarette smoke, and this could

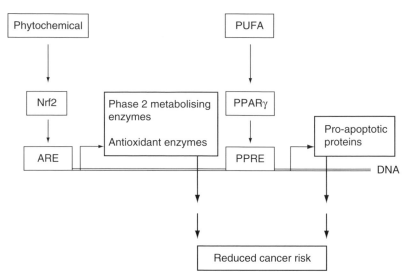

Figure 12.3 Induction of cancer prevention mechanisms by dietary constituents acting via the transcription factors Nrf2 and PPARγ. ARE: antioxidant response element; PPRE: peroxisome proliferator response element.

afford protection against cigarette-induced carcinogenesis [12]. There are, however, many more reports of phytochemicals inducing protective phase 2 enzymes.

Phytcohemicals induce the expression of phase 2 enzymes via the activation of transcription factors. Nrf2 is an example of one such transcription factor (see Chapter 9). Activated Nrf2 works by binding to the antioxidant response element (ARE) promoter region which is present in numerous genes encoding phase 2 metabolising enzymes and antioxidant enzymes (see left hand side of Figure 12.3). The resulting increased expression of these enzymes is associated with increased resistance to early stages of carcinogenesis, and has been dubbed a "cytoprotective effect" (see Chapter 9).

There is increasing evidence that polymorphisms in genes for phase 1 and phase 2 enzymes are important for the susceptibility of individuals to cancer. For example, a polymorphism resulting in a genetic deficiency in the GST isoform GSTM1 may result in a decreased ability to detoxify carcinogens and this has been associated with a moderately increased risk of cancers of the lung and bladder. Polymorphisms in phase 1 and phase 2 enzymes also interact with dietary factors in complex ways. Hence, polymorphisms may be important in determining the responses of individuals to anti-cancer constituents in the MedDiet and their susceptibility to cancer. Comparable epidemiological investigations of the MedDiet in relation to CVD have clearly revealed the importance of polymorphisms [13, 14].

Retarding the growth and progression of tumour cells

Even if the first defences of a cell have been breached, an initiated cell harbouring a single genetic mutation must still undergo many more changes before it can develop into a tumour. This next stage involves clonal expansion (proliferation of cells from a single precursor cell), and is also sometimes referred to as the "promotion" phase of tumour growth. Many factors can act to promote clonal expansion, most notably agents that stimulate cell proliferation and mechanisms involving inflammation. Many dietary substances have been identified that can inhibit these stages.

Tumour promoters
Although some carcinogens initiate cancer formation by causing mutations, other agents can only stimulate carcinogenesis once the initial mutagenic event has occurred. i.e. after the cell has been "initiated". These agents are non-genotoxic (do not cause mutations in DNA) and are known as tumour promoters. Alcohol acts as a tumour promoter in the mouth and throat by stripping away epithelial cells, and this triggers an increase in proliferation with the aim to replace the lost cells. Oestrogen and other steroid hormones also stimulate cell proliferation and are important tumour promoters. Bile acids and metabolites of bile acids may be important tumour promoters for colon carcinogenesis, and dietary fibre may, at least in part, reduce colon cancer by binding these tumour promoters.

Chronic inflammatory responses in the body to infection can act as tumor promotors and predispose to increased cancer risk. Good examples include *Helicobacter pylori* infection of the stomach and an increased risk of stomach cancer, and infection with papilloma virus and hepatitis virus with increased risks for cervical and liver cancers respectively. Other inflammatory conditions such as acid reflux in the oesophagus, chronic ulcerative colitis in the colon, asbestosis and prostatitis (inflamed prostate gland) also increase cancer risk.

Chronic inflammation is associated with an influx of macrophages and neutrophils. Activated macrophages produce tumour necrosis factor α (TNFα) which can induce COX-2 (see Figure 12.5 below). Induction of COX-2 in colon epithelial cells is thought to be important in colon cancer. COX-2 catalyses the formation of PGE$_2$ which promotes several stages of colon carcinogenesis including tumour growth and progression, and encourages metastatic spread [15]. The non-steroidal anti-inflammatory drug aspirin, an inhibitor of the activity of the COX-2 enzyme, is associated with a reduced risk of colon cancer. Several constituents in the MedDiet have also been found to inhibit the COX-2 enzyme in cell culture models of colon cancer, and these include oleocanthal, found in some virgin olive oils, and various quercetin conjugates [16]. Although there is epidemiological evidence that consumption of a MedDiet is associated with a lower incidence of colon cancer (see Section 12.3.2), it is difficult to disentangle COX-2 inhibition as a possible mechanism of action for this observation from other confounding factors (such as relatively low red meat consumption), and indeed many aspects of the Mediterranean dietary pattern may co-contribute.

Tumour progression
For the continually growing mass of tumour cells to become malignant, i.e. to become a cancer, it must acquire a number of key features. These features have been called the "hallmarks of cancer" and they are essential for solid cancers to develop (Figure 12.4) [17]. Correspondingly they are key targets for dietary intervention.

Cancer-related inflammation
Not only do some chronic inflammatory conditions such as various infections predispose to cancer (see above), but it is now clear that the growing tumour mass itself

Normal cell

↓ *Initiation*

- Free radicals
- Carcinogens (many require activation by phase 1 enzymes)

Initiated cell

↓ *Promotion*

- Chronic inflammation
- Growth factors

Clonally expanded

cell mass

Hallmarks of cancer:

1. Self sufficiency in growth signals
2. Insensitivity to inhibitory growth signals
3. Evasion of apoptosis
4. Immortality
5. Sustained angiogenesis
6. Invasion of tissues and metastasis
7. Chronic inflammation*

↓ *Progression*

Metastatic cancer

Figure 12.4   Events that drive carcinogenesis. *Originally six hallmarks of cancer were proposed [17], and chronic inflammation has recently been suggested as representing a seventh [18].

causes an influx of inflammatory cells. This inflammatory environment may be crucial to drive tumour growth [18]. TNFα produced by infiltrating macrophages activates the transcription factor NFκB. One of the genes induced by NFκB is that for COX-2. COX-2 catalyses the conversion of long chain PUFAs (LC PUFAs) into various eicosanoids. Some of these eicosanoids, such as PGE_2 can drive tumour growth by increasing cell proliferation, and metastasis by decreasing cell-cell contact (Figure 12.5).

Many dietary phytochemicals have been found to reduce COX-2 levels in cell culture by inhibiting the *transcription* of this enzyme, rather than by inhibiting the *activity* of the enzyme. These phytochemicals include luteolin, apigenin, resveratrol and green tea catechins [19]. The green tea catechins were also active in human tissue preparations of colon and colon carcinoma, adding further support that these effects may be relevant in humans.

The types of eicosanoids produced by COX-2 depend on the type of LC PUFA present in the cell membrane. LC *n*-6 PUFAs act as substrates for eicosanoids that have been shown to have adverse effects in animal models (e.g. PGE_2) whereas eicosanoids derived from LC *n*-3 PUFAs mostly have beneficial effects (see below). The relative proportions of these fatty acids in cell membranes is influenced by dietary intake, and the relatively high proportion of *n*-3 fatty acids relative to *n*-6 fatty acids in the MedDiet (compared to a Western-style diet) may be beneficial in relation to cancer.

Activated macrophage

↓

TNFα

↓

Tumour cell

↓

Activation of NFκB – **inhibited by dietary constituent**

↓

COX-2

↓

↓

PGE$_2$

↓

Increased cell proliferation, decreased cell-cell contact

↓

Cancer

Figure 12.5   Inflammation and tumour growth.

Wider implications of inhibiting NFκB activation   NFκB is a particularly versatile transcription factor and induces the transcription of many genes besides COX-2, including many genes that help drive tumour growth such as those associated with increased cell proliferation, decreased apoptosis and increased angiogenesis (see below). Hence, inhibiting the activation of NFκB could potentially have diverse beneficial effects that retard the growth of tumour cells (Figure 12.6).

A wide range of phytochemicals found in the MedDiet have been shown to inhibit NFκB activation in experimental systems (see Table 12.1), and many workers consider NFκB inhibition to be a likely target for the anti-cancer activities of some phytochemicals.

Selective activation of phenolics at tumour sites

Although most flavonoids circulate in the plasma as conjugates, there is some evidence that the conjugates can be cleaved back to the parent compound at specific sites such as tumours. Since the aglycones are generally considered to be more biologically active, this provides a means for selective production of the parent compound at a tumour site. For example, rats fed liver carcinogens had increased glucuronidase activity in their livers. When these rats were fed quercetin, they had increased production of quercetin aglycone relative to untreated animals which had been fed quercetin. This suggests that the increase in glucuronidase activity in the livers of the carcinogen-treated animals could convert quercetin glucuronides in the plasma back to the aglycone [20].

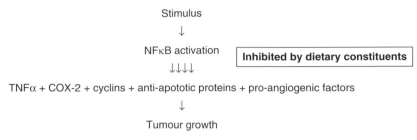

Figure 12.6   Diverse genes induced by NFκB.

Table 12.1   Some phytochemicals in the MedDiet that inhibit NFκB activation.

Phytochemical	Dietary source
Resveratrol	Grapes
Sulforaphane	Brassicas
Indole-3-carbinol	Brassicas
Caffeoylquinic acid	Quince
Anethole	Fennel
Ellagic acid	Pomegranate
Ursolic acid	Basil
Ursolic acid, oleanolic acid, triterpenoids	Prunes, plums
Catechins	Green tea
Lycopene	Tomato

Cell proliferation

The proliferation of normal cells is tightly regulated. A cell normally only divides when it is triggered by external growth signals. Undesirable replication is also prevented by growth inhibitory signals. A further check on the proliferation of normal cells is that they will only ever divide a limited number of times (about 60) before they undergo senescence and die, i.e. they have a finite replicative capacity.

Cancer cells can lose all of these checks. The consequences are increased cell proliferation and immortality. Cancer cells achieve this by (1) no longer requiring external growth signals for cell division, i.e. they become autonomous in growth signals, (2) becoming insensitive to inhibitory growth signals, and (3) acquiring the ability for unlimited replication. Many of these growth advantages are due to mutations in the normal genes, called proto-oncogenes, that produce growth regulatory proteins. These mutated proto-oncogenes genes are called oncogenes (literally cancer genes) and produce growth regulatory proteins in the cancer cells that are more active than the normal proto-oncogene products. In some cases, the sequence of the proto-oncogene may remain normal but multiple copies of the gene are expressed in the cancer cell, resulting in the production of increased amounts of the normal proto-oncogene product. In both cases, the result is increased cell proliferation. These proteins are important targets for the new generation of anti-cancer agents. In addition, there is now evidence that they are the target for constituents in the MedDiet. Inhibiting growth-promoting proteins in cancer cells not only stops them growing (called a cytostatic effect), but often results in the cells being triggered to undergo cell suicide, i.e. apoptosis.

A good example of an over-expressed growth promoting protein in cancer cells is a growth factor receptor called HER2. The HER2 receptor is over-expressed on the surface of breast cancer cells in about 20–30% of women with breast cancer (so-called HER2 positive breast cancer). Over-expression in HER2 occurs at an early stage in the carcinogenesis of breast cancer (before the tumour is clinically detectable), and targeting these HER2-expressing cells at this early stage may be an effective means of eradicating them before they have time to acquire other growth capabilities [21].[4]

Constituents in extra virgin olive oil have been found lower the incidence and number, compared to corn oil, of chemicelly induced mammary tumours in rats and decrease cell proliferation of HER2 positive breast cancer cells. Feeding rats extra virgin olive oil lowered the incidence and number of chemically-induced mammary tumours [22], and this effect may be due to the oleic acid inhibiting expression of HER2 [23]. Mixtures of phenolics from extra virgin olive oil containing either oleuropein and ligstroside or lignans (pinoresinol and acetoxypinoresinol) decreased cell proliferation of HER2 positive breast cancer cells in culture and induced them to undergo apoptosis; there was no effect on HER2 negative cells [24]. However, considerably higher concentrations of phenolics were needed than are likely to be achieved as part of a normal MedDiet. Nevertheless, some recent epidemiological studies have found that olive oil is an important component of dietary patterns and shows an inverse relationship with cancer (see Section 12.3.1), and one study found that a dietary pattern with a high consumption of raw vegetables and olive oil was more effective at preventing the development of HER2 positive breast cancer than of HER2 negative breast cancer (RR 0.25: CI 0.10–0.64, for the highest tertile, trend 0.001), whereas the effect was only borderline significant for HER-2-negative cancers (RR 0.71: CI 0.48–1.03, trend 0.07) [25]. Such an observation needs confirmation based on a larger number of cases and more work is needed to establish the precise role of olive oil in these observations. These observations do highlight the potential importance of dietary epidemiological studies considering tumour sub-types.[5]

Other dietary factors are important in decreasing cell proliferation, specifically in hormone-dependent cancers, because they interfere with steroid hormones which are important stimulators of cell proliferation ie they can act as mitogens in the human body. Oestrogen stimulates the proliferation of reproductive tissues in women during the monthly menstrual cycle. These tissues include epithelial cells lining the ducts of the breast and endometrial cells in the uterus. Oestrogen may also sustain the development of breast cancer once the process of carcinogenesis has been initiated. There is good evidence that a high lifetime exposure to oestrogen (for example, due to an early menarche or late menopause) increases the risk of breast cancer. Therefore, there is a good deal of interest in the role of dietary factors, such as lignans, that

---

[4] The potential importance of this early intervention can be illustrated by considering treating women with a drug that blocks this receptor, i.e. Herceptin. Although Herceptin is a promising approach for treating HER2 positive breast cancer, this therapy is not always curative, and one reason may be because the breast cancer cells have acquired other capabilities that enable them to proliferate.

[5] This is also very important for therapies that target specific oncogene products. Herceptin is ineffective in treating HER2 negative tumours, and if a trial with Herceptin had been evaluated against all sub-types of breast cancer it could well have concluded that Herceptin is not an effective therapy, hence missing the 20–30% of breast cancer cases where this is drug is having a major impact.

Table 12.2 Endocrine factors produced by adipose tissue that are associated with tumours in animal models.

Endocrine factor	Producing cells	Tumour association
Leptin	adipocytes	increased risk of breast, prostate, colon, endometrial tumour
Adiponectin	adipocytes	inversely correlated with breast, endometrial, and gastric tumours risk
Pro-inflammatory cytokines (TNFα, IL-6)	macrophages + adipocytes	increased risk of many types of tumours

modulate the effects of oestrogen (see Section 12.3.2.) Good sources of lignans in the MedDiet are whole grain products, virgin olive oil and sesame seeds.

The growth of the prostate is controlled by circulating testosterone. However, there is no clear relationship between levels of circulating testosterone and prostate cancer risk.

Obesity and cancer

Obesity is associated with increased risk of a number of types of cancer. Some epidemiological studies have shown an inverse association between the MedDiet and abdominal obesity (Chapter 10), suggesting that maintaining a correct BMI may be a contributory factor for the reduced cancer risk associated with consumption of a MedDiet.

Various mechanisms have been proposed to explain the link between obesity and increased cancer risk. Adipose tissue is now known to be a very metabolically active tissue, due to both the fat cells themselves (adipocytes) and to inflammatory cells that infiltrate the adipose tissue. Adipocytes are the main source of oestrogens in post-menopausal women, and obesity is associated with high levels of circulating oestrogens. The enzyme aromatase in adipocytes converts androgens into oestrogen (oestradiol). Oestradiol stimulates the proliferation of oestrogen-responsive tissues such as ovary, breast and endometrium. Increased circulating oestrogen is probably an important factor that contributes to the increased risk of oestrogen-responsive tumours. Various phytochemicals in red wine are reported to be inhibitors of aromatase activity [26]. However, any potential benefit from consuming red wine should be offset against the positive association between alcohol and breast cancer risk. Nevertheless, maintaining the body within the normal BMI range with a balanced diet – such as the MedDiet – and physical exercise is recommended both for primary prevention and for survival in breast cancer patients.

Various mechanisms have been proposed to explain the link between obesity and cancers in tissues that are not responsive to oestrogens. Adipocytes produce a range of endocrine factors and inflammatory cells produce cytokines, some of which can act in an endocrine manner (Table 12.2). Adipose tissue-derived cytokines contribute to a pro-inflammatory state in the overweight individual which is associated with cancer progression. In addition, leptin stimulates cell proliferation in various cancer cell types and levels are elevated in obese subjects [27].

Another important mechanism linking obesity with cancer is the association between obesity and increased resistance of the body to the actions of insulin. Various metabolic changes associated with obesity, such as increased levels of circulating triglycerides, are thought to increase insulin resistance in the body (see Chapter 10). Whatever the underlying cause, insulin resistance will trigger the body to produce more insulin (hyperinsulinaemia) to try and compensate for the failure of the body to respond to the insulin signal. Elevated circulating insulin can have direct effects of cancer growth since insulin can act as a growth factor for cancer cells. Insulin also acts indirectly by increasing production of the growth factor IGF-1 (insulin-like growth factor-1) and decreasing production of a protein called IGF-binding protein (IGFBP). IGFBP normally mops up up to 98% of the IGF-1 that would otherwise be free in the circulation. Unbound, active IGF-1 can act both to increase the proliferation of some cells and increase their survival. For example, increased circulating levels of IGF-1 are associated with an increased risk of men developing prostate cancer [28, 29].

There is increasing interest in the potential anti-cancer benefits of decreasing insulin resistance. It has been proposed that the MedDiet is particularly effective for achieving a reduction in insulin resistance [30] (see Chapter 10). Dietary constituents that have been found to decrease insulin resistance include cinnamon, chromium and the green tea catechin EGCG [31].

Apoptosis

Cells in the body that become damaged activate an internal programme that causes them to die. In effect, they commit suicide. This process is referred to as apoptosis, and is the main way by which damaged cells are eliminated from the body. Agents that damage cells include mutagens and free radicals. The intracellular pathways that cause apoptosis are frequently reduced in cancer cells, thus enabling cancer cells to undergo damage and yet survive. If this damage occurs in the DNA of the cell, the cancer cell will acquire new mutations. Some of these mutations may benefit the cancer cell, enabling it to flourish even more.

Studies using cancer cells grown in culture and animal models for cancer have demonstrated that many phytochemicals in the MedDiet promote apoptosis. Of course, eradicating cancer cells is only likely to benefit human health if it occurs without triggering apoptosis in normal cells. Importantly, it does appear that some phytochemicals can selectively induce apoptosis in cancer cells without affecting normal cells, at least in experimental systems. This may partly be due to cancer cells expressing higher levels of apoptosis-inhibitory proteins than normal cells and also because cancer cells are often – paradoxically – closer to undergoing apoptosis than normal cells[6]. Hence, although cancer cells are very successful, they are in a precarious situation, and a slight perturbation in apoptosis regulation could prove fatal. For example, Bcl-X_L is a protein that normally suppresses apoptosis, and this protein is over-expressed in some cancer cells, thus making them more resistant to apoptosis. EGCG (found in green tea) potently inhibits Bcl-X_L and inhibiting this protein in tumour cells can trigger apoptosis since these cells are, in other ways, already close to undergoing apoptosis. The triterpenoids maslinic acid and oleanolic acid found in

---

[6] This is at least in part thought to be due to cancer cells having a higher degree of oxidative stress than normal cells.

olives were reported to induce apoptosis in colon cancer cells at concentrations that are not non-specifically toxic [32]. The authors estimated that a moderate intake of olives and extra virgin olive oil (which also contains these triterpenoids) could be sufficient to achieve beneficial concentrations in the colon. However, at present no human investigations have been conducted.

Many other dietary phytochemicals have been found to induce apoptosis in cancer cells in culture or in animal models. These include EGCG in green tea, indole-3-carbinol and isothiocyanates in cruciferous vegetables, resveratrol in wine, luteolin in celery, lycopene in tomatoes, anthocyanins in pomegranates, delphinidin in purple fruits and vegetables and organo-sulphur compounds in garlic and onions [33].

Experimental studies, together with a limited amount of epidemiological evidence (see Section 12.3.1), suggest that *n*-3 LC PUFAs reduce cancer risk, and this may, at least in part, be mediated by inducing apoptosis. LC PUFAs and some metabolites of these PUFAs can activate peroxisome proliferator-activated receptors (PPARs) (Figure 12.3). PPARs are a family of transcription factors originally described in relation to lipid homeostasis (see Chapter 9), but PPARγ in particular has a broad range of effects in relation to cancer including inducing apoptosis [34]. For example, the LC PUFA docosahexaenoic acid induces cell death (apoptosis) in breast cancer cells through a PPARγ-dependent pathway.

PUFAs may also trigger apoptosis in response to oxidative stress, a risk factor for the conversion of normal cells into cancer cells. High oxidative stress results in the production of oxygenated metabolites of PUFAs (oxo-PUFAs) by cells. These oxo-PUFAs are potent ligands for PPARγ, and activated PPARγ triggers apoptosis. Hence PUFAs can act as sensors in the cell for oxidative stress and so prevent normal cells from embarking on the path to cancer.

Various phytochemicals, including carotenoids, also activate PPARγ, and although there have been favourable effects in cell culture models further work is needed to establish whether phytochemicals acting as PPARγ agonists are useful in humans as chemopreventative agents [35].

Angiogenesis

Cancer cells in the centre of a tumour mass larger than about $2\,mm^3$ need to have oxygen and nutrients supplied by new blood vessels because they have become too far away to be able to acquire oxygen and nutrients by diffusion from the existing vasculature. Vascularisation of a tumour mass can occur by stimulating the growth of new blood vessels from pre-existing vessels – a process termed angiogenesis – or by creating new blood vessels from infiltrating endothelial stem cells. Inhibiting angiogenesis is a very promising therapy for patients with cancer, and it is also now thought that inhibition of angiogenesis may contribute to the cancer-preventing actions of some phytochemicals.

Angiogenesis is regulated by both pro-angiogenic factors that stimulate angiogenesis and anti-angiogenic factors that inhibit angiogenesis. Both co-exist around tumours, and angiogenesis occurs when there is greater overall activity of pro-angiogenic factors compared to anti-angiogenic factors. This imbalance is termed the angiogenic switch. In theory, dietary factors could inhibit angiogenesis either by inhibiting pro-angiogenic factors or by stimulating the production of anti-angiogenic factors, although generally the former appears to be more common. Tumour cells and certain surrounding cells (so called stromal cells, the most important of which in the context of angiogenesis are macrophages) sense when there is insufficient oxygen (i.e. hypoxia) by producing hypoxia-inducible factor (HIF-1). HIF-1 then triggers the production of various pro-angiogenic factors, probably the most important of which is vascular endothelial growth factor (VEGF). VEGF then stimulates new blood vessel formation. Some phytochemicals that block HIF-1 and VEGF expression in tumour cells include catechins in green tea and apigenin, whereas other phytochemicals such as phenylethyl isothiocyanates and selenium inhibit the signalling pathway activated by VEGF [36]. However, the relevance of these actions for chemoprevention in humans is unclear.

Cancer stem cells and phytochemicals

Although cancer progression has been thought of as a linear process of continually changing cells (Figure 12.7a), there is now evidence that tumour growth is driven by a small population of self-renewing cells known as cancer stem cells (Figure 12.7b).

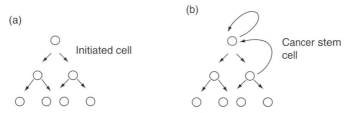

Figure 12.7 Traditional view (a) and stem cell hypothesis (b) for cancer growth.

   It is still too early to say if cancer stem cells represent an important target for phytochemicals although this is now attracting interest [37].

12.2.3   The issue of selectivity

Dietary constituents are only useful for preventing cancer if they inhibit cancer or precancerous cells at concentrations that do not detrimentally affect normal cell function. Differences in the types and amounts of proteins expressed in cancer cells versus normal cells may make this discrimination possible.

Oncogene addiction

One elegant hypothesis that may explain how some agents discriminate between normal and cancer cells is based on so-called "oncogene addiction" [38]. Oncogene addiction is the term used to describe differences between normal cells and cancer cells for their relative dependence on certain proteins in order to function. Cancer cells acquire various abnormal proteins – i.e. the products of oncogenes – as they develop. The scenario of oncogene addiction can be illustrated by considering the acquisition by a cancer cell of two abnormal proteins 1 and 2. The cancer cell exhibits oncogene addiction when acquiring abnormal protein 2 is only of benefit to it if it has previously acquired abnormal protein 1. In other words, the cancer cell is

Scenario 1 – *Cancer cell: no phytochemical*

Protein 1 – Over-active abnormal Ras benefits cancer cell

↓

Protein 2 – Over-active abnormal Myc benefits cancer cell as long as Ras is functioning

Scenario 2 – *Cancer cell: + phytochemical*

Protein 1 – Ras inhibited by phytochemical

↓

Protein 2 – Over-active abnormal Myc triggers apoptosis

Figure 12.8   Hypothetical scenario of how a phytochemical may inhibit a cancer cell with "onco-gene addiction" to functioning Ras. In scenario 1, alteration in a protein called Myc can stimulate cell proliferation as long as another protein called Ras is functioning. In scenario 2, Ras is inhibited by a phytochemical. Myc no longer stimulates cell proliferation but instead triggers apoptosis.

addicted to protein 1 for survival. Inhibiting protein 1 may now make protein 2 detrimental to the cell – such as by triggering cell death – rather than being beneficial (Figure. 12.8). Normal cells may not be affected to the same degree since neither protein is altered from normal.

It should be emphasised that, although evidence is accumulating that oncogene addiction may explain how some cancer therapeutics show selectivity for cancer cells versus normal cells [39], it is not known if a similar scenario may operate for dietary phytochemicals.

Oxidative stress

A second mechanism by which phytochemicals may discriminate between cancer and normal cells is by altering the redox status of cells. Although there is a good deal of evidence that phytochemicals can act as antioxidants (see Chapter 9 for discussion), there is also now evidence that the beneficial effects of some phytochemicals may be related to *prooxidant* activity. Somewhat confusingly, the same phytochemical may act as an antioxidant under certain circumstances (e.g. by scavenging ROS) and as a prooxidant under different circumstances (see [40]). For example, phenyl ethyl isothiocyanate (PEITC) (the active derivative from a glucosinolate present in some Brassicas) depletes glutathione – which normally helps maintain a reducing environment in the cell – hence creating a more prooxidant environment. Resveratrol can also act as a prooxidant under some circumstances [41], and indeed it has been suggested that prooxidant effects may be a general mechanism of action for many phytochemicals [42][7].

The outcome of these apparently contradictory effects may depend on the redox status of the cell. Normal cells with an intrinsic low level of oxidative stress can respond to increased prooxidant activity by inducing antioxidant enzymes: this is a

---

[7] In this regard, it is worth noting that all so-called antioxidants have the potential to act as prooxidants due to the inherent nature of redox (reduction-oxidation) reactions.

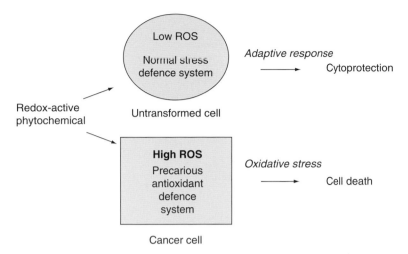

Figure 12.9 A model of how redox-active phytochemicals may trigger cell death in cancer cells.

homeostatic adaption that increases the resilience of cells (cytoprotection). However, it has been shown that cancer cells have a high intrinsic level of level of oxidative stress [43]. In order to survive, cancer cells have a correspondingly high reliance on antioxidant mechanisms. Depriving the cancer cell of these antioxidant defence mechanisms may expose it to a high level of oxidative stress, and it has been suggested that this may be sufficient to trigger the cancer cell to undergo apoptosis. For example, it is thought that some cancer cells have a high reliance on glutathione. Depleting glutathione with PEITC results in cancer cell death. Hence, cancer cells may be more easily pushed over the threshold of tolerance to oxidative stress and cell death than normal cells by dietary phytochemicals with pro-oxidant activity (Figure 12.9) [40].

12.2.4   Mediterranean dietary pattern and cancer prevention

"Food, Not Nutrients, Is the Fundamental Unit in Nutrition" [44]

There is good epidemiological evidence that adherence to an overall Mediterranean dietary pattern is protective against various cancers (Section 12.3.7), and some studies have found that there is a stronger positive correlation between adherence to an overall MedDiet and reduced cancer incidence than for any single component in the diet such as high fruit and vegetable intake [45].

Mechanistic findings from *in vitro* and animal models proposed to explain the relationship between phytochemicals and cancer are not always supported by human studies. For example, intake of a flavonoid-rich diet did not reduce oxidative DNA damage in healthy volunteers [46]. And single purified substances may be even worse, since there are dangers of *increased* cancer incidence (Section 12.3.2). Hence, workers have proposed that the health benefits of the MedDiet result from its unique combination of nutrients [47]. An hierarchy can be proposed, although this is probably not a linear progression (Figure 12.10).

Dietary constituents that are part of an overall dietary pattern may interact antagonistically, additively or synergistically in relation to the health benefits that they

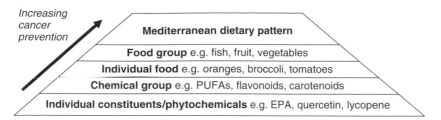

Figure. 12.10   A schematic representation of hierarchies in the prevention of cancer by nutrition.

confer. A good example of an antagonistic effect is the direct interaction between calcium and oxalic acid which reduces the bioavailability of calcium. Induction of metabolic enzymes by phytochemicals which increase the excretion of other phytochemicals may also be seen as an antagonist interaction, and may reduce the level of beneficial phytochemicals.

On the other hand, a number of synergistic interactions have been reported that could benefit cancer prevention. Synergism means "a greater than additive" effect, and dedicated computer programmes have been developed to distinguish between effects that are simply additive and those that are truly synergistic [48]. Synergism could, at least in theory, explain why mixtures of phytochemicals may have beneficial effects even though plasma levels of the individual phytochemicals obtained from dietary intake are too low on their own to produce an effect in experimental models. Similarly, it may not be necessary to consume the same amount of a phytochemical required in animal studies to achieve an effect if that phytochemical can interact synergistically with other constituents present in the diet.

It has been argued that some chronic diseases are due to "multiple parallel pathologic pathways" and therefore that combinations of agents are required in order to inhibit these and so effect a cure [49]. The complexities of cancer can be illustrated by a meta-analysis of microarray data from 22 different tumour types that found that no single common gene mutation is responsible for the onset of these tumours, but that shared functional modules exist between various cancer types [50]. However, these tumours also have unique characteristics. Hence a complex mixture of nutrients (aka a diet) may be required in order to target all of these changes and best prevent a wide range of cancers.

Many lines of evidence indicate that dietary factors target carcinogenesis in diverse ways, such as by changing redox status (either increasing or decreasing oxidative stress), modulating protein function and altering gene expression. Understanding the complex interactions between nutrients and these targets is still in its infancy. However, this understanding is expected to increase greatly over the next few years with the aid of "omics" research which can simultaneously measure large numbers of different variables such as genes (genomics), proteins (proteomics) and metabolic products (metabolomics).

Various relationships can be considered that exist between dietary factors and their cellular targets. Firstly, a single constituent may affect multiple targets (Figure 12.11). For example, quercetin has multiple cellular targets, including proteins that regulate apoptosis, growth, cell invasion and the expression of androgen receptors, and these may contribute towards the cancer-preventive effects of this phytochemical [51]. Microarray analysis provides an elegant way of determining multiple changes that can occur following consumption of a single phytochemical. One such study found

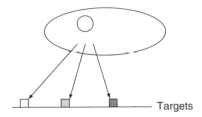

Figure 12.11   One nutrient, multiple targets.

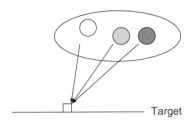

Figure 12.12   Multiple nutrients, one target.

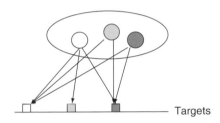

Figure 12.13   Multiple nutrients, multiple targets.

that oral administration of catechin to mice resulted in the modification of the expression of 450 genes [52].

A second scenario is where diverse nutrients act on a common target (Figure 12.12). This effect may be additive if various nutrients act on precisely the same target. Alternatively, a synergistic effect may be observed if the common target can be altered through various means. This latter scenario probably applies to phytochemicals that act through various means to create a particular redox status within a cell [53].

A third scenario is where diverse nutrients may have some common targets and some that are different (Figure 12.13). Clearly, this scenario is most likely to reflect the true situation in relation to diet, and it is the one most likely to result in synergistic effects. A good example of these complexities was shown in a study that compared the effects of feeding mice either a complex vegetable diet or individual vegetables present in the mixed vegetable diet on genes expressed in the colonic mucosa. The expressions of some genes were reduced following consumption of the complex vegetable diet compared to when individual vegetables were consumed, thus indicating that the complex diet can suppress genes as well as increase expression [54].

The situation may be further complicated by combinations of nutrients giving rise to *new* modes of action that are not seen by any of the individual components considered in isolation. One interesting perspective on this is as follows: "the application of drug combinations including phyto-pharmaceuticals does not necessarily mean the addition or multiplication of targets. It can lead to new modes of actions. Therefore, the demand to demonstrate the mode of action of each single component in a phyto pharmaceutical may not be obligatory any more" [49].

Experimental evidence for synergistic interactions

Constituents of many food groups have cancer-preventive effects, and it is likely that these effects can interact in favourable ways to reduce cancer [55]. However, at the moment, evidence for this is limited to experimental studies since human studies are not available. One constituent may favourably modify the metabolism of a second constituent, e.g. by increasing its absorption or by decreasing its metabolic inactivation. In relation to absorption, it is well known that the bioavailability of some nutrients is affected both by the food matrix and by the co-consumption of other foodstuffs. Olive oil probably has a significant effect on the cancer-preventive activity of vegetables by increasing the bioavailability of lipid soluble phytochemicals such as carotenoids (see Chapter 4). A study in rats found that the alcohol from red wine increases the absorption of the flavonoid quercetin [56]. In addition, red wine promoted the metabolism of quercetin to the flavonoids isorhamnetin and tamarixetin, and these flavonoids have potential protective effects against cancer. It is not known whether, for humans, drinking red wine with a meal may also increase the bioavailability of some phytochemicals present in vegetables.

There is some evidence from cell culture and animal models which suggests that synergistic interactions between phytochemicals may contribute towards cancer prevention, as shown in studies combining two or more pure phytochemicals and observing synergistic anti-carcinogenic effects [51]. However, not all such studies have found synergism, and in some cases it is not clear if this is because of a genuine lack of synergism or because the experimental design is inadequate. For example, a synergistic interaction was observed between epicatechin and EGCG in inducing apoptosis in gastric carcinoma cells *in vitro*, suggesting that drinking green tea may have superior benefits against gastric carcinoma than would be obtained from an equivalent amount of EGCG taken alone [57]. However, a study in rats found that for a realistic dietary intake of the two glucosinolate metabolites indole-3-carbinol and crambene there was not a synergistic effect in a short-term model for carcinogenicity [58]. This study highlights potential limitations of simply combining two phytochemicals. In the case of glucosinolate metabolites, this limitation may be because they require other nutrients, such as selenium, in order to be effective. For the glucosinolate metabolite sulforaphane, consuming an adequate amount of selenium is essential for the induction by sulforaphane of the selenium-containing cytoprotective enzymes thioredoxin reductase and glutathione peroxidase [59]. One cell culture study found that the synergistic induction of thioredoxin reductase by sulforaphane and selenium was due to sulforaphane enhancing the transcription of thioredoxin reductase and selenium enhancing the translation of the mRNA into protein [60].

Another approach used to study synergism is to see how a whole food compares with its putative active ingredients. Some of these studies have found a superior benefit of whole foods versus purified constituents. For example, when pomegranate juice was compared with some of its constituents, it was found that the juice had superior anti-proliferative, pro-apoptotic and antioxidant activities against various tumour cell lines compared to equivalent amounts of several of the major polyphenol constituents including punicalagin and ellagic acid [61]. However, a limitation of this and similar studies is that it is usually not possible to take into account all of the constituents that were originally present in the whole food.

This limitation can also be illustrated with red wine. Red wine consists of a complex mixture of phenolics and other constituents dissolved in alcohol. There are several reports suggesting that the antioxidant capacity of red wine is greater than the antioxidant activities due to the sum of individual phenolics present in the wine. In one study, reconstituting the main individual phenolics produced a slight synergistic effect since the combination had greater antioxidant activity than the sum of the individual constituents [62]. However, the combination still did not fully restore the expected antioxidant capacity present in the whole wine. This suggests that there were other unknown components present in the wine contributing to the antioxidant capacity, illustrating the problem with attempting to account for all the individual constituents in a whole food.

A good deal of scientific enquiry has been devoted to evaluating whether or not purified lycopene is as effective in reducing oxidative stress and carcinogenicity (especially in relation to prostate cancer) as eating tomato products that contain an equivalent amount of lycopene. Current epidemiological evidence suggests that tomato products are superior [63] (see Section 12.3.6). Synergistic interactions between lycopene and other constituents in tomato (vitamins C and E, phenolic acids, folates) may contribute towards this observation. For example, lycopene and other constituents act synergistically as antioxidants [64]. Also of relevance in relation to the MedDiet is the frequent consumption of tomatoes cooked in olive oil as this may enhance lycopene bioavailability.

A final example of possible synergy comes from studies investigating the induction of apoptosis in colon cancer cells by phenolics in virgin olive oil. Whereas the phenolic pinoresinol induced apoptosis in these cells, this effect was also achieved using substantially lower concentrations of a polyphenolic extract from the olive oil, leading the authors of the report to suggest that this may be due to a possible synergistic effect between the various polyphenols in the olive oil [65].

Supplements and cancer prevention

"The prospects for cancer prevention through micronutrient supplementation have never looked worse." [66]

Even though concentrations of phytochemicals that demonstrate anti-carcinogenic effects in cell culture models can be achieved in humans given supplements [67], achieving relevant plasma concentrations may not in itself be sufficient to produce a cancer-preventive (chemopreventive) effect in humans since a number of results from clinical trials and observational studies from supplementation with micronutrients, including vitamins (C, D, and E), selenium, calcium and folate, report no benefit - and in a few cases, possible harm (see Table 12.3). This highlights the importance of diet, rather than supplements, for cancer prevention.

Table 12.3 Results of studies using micronutrient supplements (2008–2009) (adapted from [68]). With permission from Oxford University Press.

Supplement	Cancer	Outcome	Study type
Multivitamin	all cancers in women	no effect	observational
Selenium	prostate	no effect	intervention
Vitamin C	all cancers in men	no effect	intervention
Vitamin E	prostate, all cancers in men	no effect	intervention
Calcium + vitamin D	breast in women	no effect	observational
Folate	prostate	more incidence	intervention
Selenium + vitamin E + β-carotene	gastric prostate	fewer deaths increased risk	intervention
Vitamin D	prostate	no effect	case-control
Folate + vitamin B$_6$ + vitamin B$_{12}$	breast in women, all cancers in women	no effect increased risk	intervention

It is worth noting that prevention strategies that use supplements may only be appropriate for a population deficient in a particular nutrient and not exposed to environmental carcinogens (e.g. tobacco, asbestos). Although folate supplements may help prevent colorectal cancer in individuals with low folate levels, they have been found to increase the risk of recurrence of premalignant adenomas in patients with resected adenomas [7].

12.3 Epidemiological evidence and mechanisms

This section reviews current epidemiological evidence for cancer prevention by individual constituents in the MedDiet, whole foods and the Mediterranean dietary pattern.

12.3.1 Fats

The implications of fat intake for cancer development have long been a matter of debate. Fat is the highest contributor to energy intake by weight, since 1 g of fat provides 9 kcal, whereas 1 g of protein or carbohydrate provides only 4 kcal. Thus, fat intake is highly correlated with energy intake, especially in the Western diet, and energy intake can be a confounding factor when studying the relationship between fat and disease. Obesity is a risk factor for several cancers (see Section 12.2.2) and, apart from genetic factors, energy imbalance is the major factor in the development of obesity. Specific statistical techniques have clearly shown that if total fat intake has an impact on the risk or some cancers, it is in proportion to its contribution to calorie intake and/or to an energy-dense food pattern. This is especially true for colorectal cancer [69], and there is limited, but suggestive, evidence that it is also the case for female cancers in which body fatness is an important risk factor [70]. In intervention studies showing a risk reduction of breast cancer incidence [71] or relapse [72], the low fat diet was also a low-energy diet and participants lost some weight. Hence, it is difficult to disentangle the specific effect of fat from that of decrease in body fatness.

The situation of calorie intake as a confounding factor similar to total fat arises when studying the role of SFAs, although the results of two large cohort studies on breast cancer suggest a possible relationship between high saturated fat intake and a modest increase in breast cancer risk [70].

For MUFA, results are heterogeneous. For most North American and North European countries, the relationship between MUFA and breast cancer is similar to that observed with total fat and/or SFA. This was also the case in two recent case control studies in France [73] and the US [74], and in one cohort study [75]. It should be noted that the major contributors to MUFA intake in these countries were meat and hard fatty cheese. By contrast, in Mediterranean countries, where olive oil is the major contributor to MUFA intake, MUFA intake was associated with a reduced risk of breast cancer [76, 77]. The food analysis showed that olive oil was responsible for the risk reduction effect. Two more recent case-control studies support the observations of these earlier studies [78, 79].

Mechanisms

The beneficial effect of olive oil might be attributed to one or more of the following:

- the presence in olive oil of oleuropein, a phenolic compound capable of phase 1 and 2 enzymes modulation [80] (see Chapter 9)
- the presence of oleocanthal and its potential anti-inflammatory effect [81]
- promoting the proteasomal degradation of HER2 protein (see Section 12.2.2) [25]
- an effect of substituting plant fat for animal fat: Rasmussen et al. showed that a test meal with butter is followed by a higher peak of insulinaemia than a test meal with olive oil [82]
- the context of the Mediterranean dietary pattern might either participate in or confound the effect.

In spite of several experimental *in vivo* and *in vitro* studies showing a deleterious effect of *n*-6 PUFA, there is no data for such an effect in humans [70]. In relation to *n*-3 LC-PUFA, many *in vivo* and *in vitro* studies show a beneficial effect. Some studies suggest that there exists a delicate balance between *n*-6 PUFA and *n*-3 LC-PUFA, especially with regard to breast cancer risk [83]. However, data in humans are scarce and heterogeneous, even though the level of evidence for a risk reduction of colon cancer related to high intake of fish is probable [70]. In addition, it should be noted that fish is also a main contributor in vitamin D intake, and is quoted in the WCRF/AICR report of 2007 as being inversely associated with colorectal cancer (the only vitamin associated inversely with cancer risk) [84].

The WCRF/AICR panel concluded that any effect of *trans* fatty acids on cancer risk is not known. However, there are some studies showing an increased risk for prostate cancer [70], and this is supported by evidence of pro-inflammatory effects of TFAs [85]. It should be remembered that a traditional MedDiet contains only natural TFAs.

12.3.2 Plant food constituents

Fibre

Fibre has long been suspected of reducing the risk of colon cancer in ecological and case-control studies. However, subsequent analytical epidemiological studies have not yielded consistent results. In the EPIC study, a large prospective study with 1065 colorectal cancer cases in a study population of 520,000 individuals throughout Europe, the risk of colorectal cancer was reduced by 40% in the highest versus the lowest quintile of fibre intake (RR 0.58: CI 0.41–0.85) [86]. By contrast, in the National Institutes of Health–AARP Diet and Health Study, which evaluated 2974 colorectal cancer case patients in a cohort of 490,000 men and women older than 50 years, total dietary fibre was not associated with risk of colorectal cancer (RR for the highest versus the lowest quintile of fibre intake 0.99: CI 0.85–1.15) [87]. A pooled analysis of 13 prospective cohorts that used study- and sex-specific quintiles of dietary fibre intake to investigate colorectal cancer risk found no overall association in a multivariable analysis (RR for highest versus lowest quintile of intake 0.94: CI 0.86–1.03) but observed an increased risk of colorectal cancer among those who consumed less than 10 g of fibre per day compared with those who consumed 10–15 g of fibre per day (RR 1.18: CI 1.05–1.31) [88]. A study of 37,562 individuals who were screened for colorectal adenoma in the Prostate, Lung, Colorectal, and Ovarian Cancer Screening Trial observed an inverse association between fibre intake and colorectal cancer risk (RR for highest versus lowest quintile of intake 0.73: CI 0.62–0.86) [88]. Recently, Dahm et al. examined the association between dietary fibre intake and colorectal cancer risk [89]. They conducted a prospective case-control study nested within seven UK cohort studies, which included 579 case patients who developed incident colorectal cancer and 1996 matched control subjects. They used standardised dietary data obtained from 4- to 7-day food diaries that were completed by all participants to calculate the OR for colorectal, colon and rectal cancers with the use of conditional logistic regression models that adjusted for relevant covariates. They also calculated OR for colorectal cancer by using dietary data obtained from food-frequency questionnaires that were completed by most participants. Intakes of absolute fibre and of fibre intake density, ascertained by food diaries, were statistically significantly inversely associated with the risks of colorectal and colon cancers in both age-adjusted models and multivariable models that adjusted for age, anthropomorphic and socioeconomic factors, and dietary intakes of folate, alcohol and energy. The multi-variable adjusted odds ratio of colorectal cancer for the highest quintile (24.1 g/d) versus the lowest quintile (8.9 g/d) of fibre intake density was 0.66 (CI 0.45–0.96). However, no statistically significant association was observed when the same analysis was conducted using dietary data obtained by food-frequency questionnaire (multivariable OR 0.88: CI 0.57–1.36). Such a demonstration of the nullifying effect of measurement error has been noted previously in a study of breast cancer and saturated fatty acid intake [90]. In conclusion, fibre appears to be significantly associated with a reduced risk with colorectal cancer, as has been observed for CVD (see Chapter 11).

For other cancers, the 2007 WCRF report was inconclusive, although several pieces of evidence suggest a relationship with breast cancer [91]. The recent report by the National Institutes of Health-AARP Diet and Health Study conducted on 185,598 women (mean age 62 y) showed an association with a reduced risk for breast cancer (RR 0.87: CI 0.77–0.98, p for trend 0.02 for an intake of 26 g/d versus 11 g/d) with a stronger association for oestrogen receptor negative (ER-) cancers (RR 0.56: CI 0.35–0.90, p for trend=0.008). Soluble fibre appeared to be responsible for this effect [92].

Mechanisms

By increasing stool bulk, dietary fibre may reduce colorectal cancer due to the dilution of potential carcinogens. Dietary fibre may also bind potential carcinogens including bile acids, and also prevent the formation of metabolites of bile acids that can act as tumour promoters. It should be noted that the mechanisms for colon cancer prevention by fibre are not fully understood. Other mechanisms, such as the production of short-chain fatty acids (particularly butyrate), from colon bacteria acting on fibre, which can induce apoptosis and cell cycle arrest in colon cells, may also be important [93].

For breast cancer, although the epidemiological evidence is limited, the biological mechanisms supporting a beneficial effect of fibre intake are very plausible, and these include a reduction and/or reversion of insulin resistance and obesity (see Chapter 10), and possible effects on the colon microflora by enhancing the prevalence of bacteria without glucuronidase activity, thus decreasing the recirculation of oestrogens in the blood and so facilitating faecal excretion [91].

Micronutrients and phytochemicals

Few plant micronutrients or phytochemicals are specifically recognised as being significantly associated with a reduction in cancer risk. The WCRF/AICR in its 2007 report does not specifically recognise any micronutrients or phytochemicals specifically associated with cancers, but only foods containing micronutrients (see below). For example, there is good evidence that foods containing vitamin C reduce the risk of oesophageal cancer and some evidence for protection against other cancers. The WCRF also concluded that there is "limited evidence" that foods rich in quercetin protect against lung cancer in humans [84].

Carotenoids

Carotenoids were among the first phytochemicals to be thoroughly studied. However, their relative ubiquity among plant foods has led to erroneous interpretation because of confounding by other factors in the plant foods. A relationship between β-carotene consumption and reduced cancer risk, especially of lung cancer, was observed in several studies [94], and hence β-carotene appeared to be the first "magic bullet" against cancer [95]. As a consequence, intervention studies were undertaken with β-carotene combined with other nutrients. Two studies of note were the ATBC study with heavy smokers, and the CARET study with smokers and subjects exposed to asbestos; both used high doses of β-carotene (20 mg/day) in order to increase the chances of showing a protective effect. But these studies produced unexpected and somewhat paradoxical results. The incidence of lung cancer was higher in the groups treated with β-carotene than in the placebo groups: 18% higher in the ATBC study [96] and 28% higher in the CARET study [97]. At the same time, another intervention study of a Health Professionals group, which included less than 10% smokers, did not show any effect, neither beneficial nor deleterious [98].

There are several possible explanations for the absence of a beneficial effect:

(i)   β-carotene is a marker for numerous fruits and vegetables that contain other micro-constituents, which might be responsible for beneficial effects
(ii) β-carotene in plasma is very sensitive to oxidation by tobacco compounds, which makes it a good marker of exposure to tobacco carcinogens without necessarily being protective against these carcinogens [99].

Furthermore, the deleterious effect might be explained by the ability of β-carotene to become a pro-oxidant in the presence of other chemicals [100, 101] (see Section 12.2.3). This can result in the induction of intracellular signal pathways (via the transcription factor NFκB) that promote the growth of transformed cells (see Figure 12.6). In both the ATBC and CARET studies, test subjects had been exposed to carcinogens (tobacco and asbestos), and were very likely to harbour already-transformed lung cells. This possibility is supported by observations from the French EPIC cohort of women, the so-called E3N cohort [102]. In this cohort, β-carotene intake was inversely associated with risk of tobacco-related cancers among non-smokers (HR 0.44: CI 0.18–1.07) with a statistically significant dose-dependent relationship, whereas high β-carotene intake was directly associated with risk among smokers (HR 2.14: CI 1.16–3.97), where the high intake corresponded to both dietary intake and use of supplements (β-carotene ≥3 times a week).

In order to try and circumvent these difficulties, the dose of micronutrients was reduced to be comparable to dietary intake (i.e. 6 mg β-carotene/day, although vitamin E was double the RDA at 30 mg/day), and multiple compounds were given (vitamin E, selenium, zinc). This seemed justified since in vitamin- and antioxidant-deficient populations, supplementation has been shown to be protective against those cancers associated with protection by antioxidants [103, 104]. However, even in the context of multiple compounds given at normal dietary doses, studies have found an increase in skin cancers in women [105, 106] and prostate cancers in men who had high levels of PSA [107]. These observations are in line with the association of high levels of vitamin E and poor relapse-free survival in breast cancer [108] and to the findings of the SELECT study showing an increase in prostate cancer in the group treated by vitamin E [109]. A possible mechanism would be an anti-apoptotic effect of vitamin E as has been demonstrated in animal models [110].

Phenolic compounds
Among phenolic compounds found in the MedDiet, some human studies have found flavonols and lignans to be associated with a reduced risk of some cancers. Flavonols were suggested to be protective against various cancers [111], but this effect disappeared in studies with improved methodology, such as after having adjusted for fibre intake [112]. By contrast, lignans appeared to be associated with a risk reduction for breast cancer, independent of fibre. In the French E3N EPIC cohort, 1469 cases of breast cancer were diagnosed. Compared with women in the lowest quartile of total plant lignan intake, those in the highest quartile (>1395 μg/day) had a reduced risk of breast cancer (RR 0.83: CI 0.71–0.95, p for trend=0.02), as did those in the highest quartile of lariciresinol intake (RR 0.82: CI 0.71–0.95, p for trend=0.01) [113]. The inverse associations between enterolignan intake and postmenopausal breast cancer risk were limited to ER+ and progesterone receptor positive (PR+) tumours

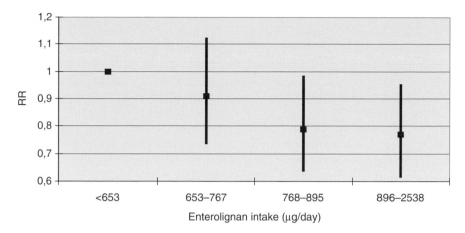

Figure 12.14 RR of postmenopausal ER+/PR+ breast cancer and enterolignan intake (μg/day). Drawn from [113].

(RR for highest quartile of total enterolignan intake [896–2538 μg/day] versus lowest quartile [<653 μg/day] was 0.77; CI 0.62– 0.95, p for trend=0.01) (Figure 12.14). Although needing confirmation, this observation suggests that lignans might act as phytoestrogens by modulating hormone metabolism (see below).

Buck et al. included 21 studies (11 prospective cohort studies and 10 case-control studies) in a meta-analysis [114]. Lignan exposure was not associated with an overall breast cancer risk (risk estimate, RE: 0.92: CI 0.81–1.02, p for heterogeneity 0.004). However, in postmenopausal women, high lignan intake was associated with a significantly reduced risk of breast cancer (13 studies: RE 0.86: CI 0.78–0.94, p for heterogeneity 0.32). Breast cancer risk was also inversely associated with estimated enterolignan exposure (ie enterolactone and enterodiol in the gut, produced from dietary lignans) (4 studies: RE 0.84: CI 0.71–0.97) but not with blood or urine enterolactone concentrations. The associations were not significantly different between ER status subgroups (6 studies). Because of this last finding, a residual confounding by fibre is unlikely.

Mechanisms

Lignans may act as oestrogen antagonists and so block the effects of oestrogens. However, the evidence for this as a mechanism *in vivo* is not conclusive. Another possible mechanism is that lignans increase the maturation (increased tissue differentiation) in pre-pubertal breast tissue, making it more resistant to cancerous change in later life [115]. If this is the case, it highlights the importance of a healthy diet from an early age. Lignans also favour the metabolism of oestrogen to 2-hydroxyoestrone rather than to 16- hydroxyoestrone, the former having less oestrogenic activity than the latter [116, 117].

Minerals

Investigations on the potential role of minerals have mostly focussed on selenium and calcium. Selenium was found to be inversely associated with prostate cancer in some studies, but intervention studies are not conclusive [109, 118]. Calcium has been shown in intervention trials to inhibit progression from small adenoma to large adenoma, which is a key step in the carcinogenesis of colorectal cancer [119, 120]. By contrast, calcium has been shown in some studies to *increase* the probability of prostate cancer. But when this effect is observed, it cannot be distinguished from the effects of milk or dairy products – the main dietary sources of calcium [121]. Even though contradictory studies exist [122, 123], a follow-up of participants in an earlier trial with calcium supplements did not observe any increase of prostate cancer incidence thus supporting the hypothesis for a possible association between milk consumption and increased levels of circulating insulin-like growth factor-1 (IGF-1) (see below) [124].

The MedDiet has a moderate intake of dairy products (mainly from goat and sheep milk products). On the other hand, it also includes constituents that are known to reduce calcium absorption, including oxalic acid and phytate [125]. The MedDiet has a relatively high intake of oxalic acid due to the high consumption of greens, some of which – such as spinach and wild greens – are particularly rich sources. Cheeses are often eaten combined with greens in Mediterranean dishes (such as in traditional "green" pies) and this could possibly help reduce the overall absorption of excess calcium. It should also be noted that sufficient calcium is an important part of osteoporosis prevention [126].

Mechanisms
The protein constituents of milt, especially essential amino acids, make it a potent stimulator of IGF-1 synthesis [127, 128]. Selenium may reduce prostate cell proliferation and induce apoptosis [129], however this *in vitro* data is not supported by the SELECT interrention study [130].

12.3.3 Tea

Results from the many studies on the effects of tea on cancer risk are inconclusive. A Cochrane review in 2009 on green tea included 27 case-control studies, 23 cohort studies and one randomised control trial (RCT) [131]. The RCT found that a preparation of green tea catechins reduced the risk of progression of high grade prostate intra-epithelial neoplasia to prostate cancer (p<0.01) [132]. However, attempts to draw conclusions based on reviewing data from cohort and case control studies of tea consumption have been inconclusive [131, 133].

These studies are subject to a number of potential confounding factors that may explain some of the variability seen between epidemiological studies. Some human studies indicate that protective effects are only seen where there is pre-existing oxidative stress [134]. The antioxidant status of consumers may also be confounding since green tea was shown in one study to be more effective in individuals with a lower antioxidant status. This suggests that green tea phenolics may be acting via antioxidant action in individuals in whom protection against oxidative stress is otherwise inadequate [134]. Analysing data on smoking in relation to tea drinking, Ju and co-authors pointed out that green tea was protective against oesophageal cancer in women, who mostly did not smoke (OR 0.5: CI 0.3–0.83) whereas in men, who mostly did smoke, there was no protective effect [134]. In addition to smoking, a number of other confounding factors may be important when interpreting epidemiological studies on tea. These include the type of tea (black or green), its quality, preparation method, the amount consumed, and whether or not it is consumed with milk. Milk proteins bind polyphenols and this might be expected to reduce the bioavailability and subsequent plasma antioxidant activity of (black) tea polyphenols. However, studies in humans have not reached a consensus on this [135]. Other factors in the diet may also interact mechanistically with tea constituents [134]. Genetic polymorphisms between consumers may be important since these can influence the rate of metabolism of catechins, putative protective factors.

Mechanisms

Many studies in animal models have found that tea and tea products inhibit tumour development [134]. These effects are mostly attributed to EGCG, the major polyphenol in green tea. The actions of EGCG may be related to its ability to directly bind to a number of proteins associated with tumour formation. The anti-tumour effects of EGCG may also be mediated via inhibiting the activity of various enzymes, including protein kinases involved in cell signalling, matrix metalloproteases (enzymes involved in cancer cell invasion) and enzymes involved in regulating the cell cycle. A human trial and an *in vitro* study indicated a 20% reduction in levels of DNA damage by green tea [136]. It is likely that the anti-tumour effect of EGCG operates through several of these mechanisms. Although it is not clear which mechanisms are most important, it is likely that they include those which are affected by the lowest concentration of EGCG. Since many of the protein targets for EGCG are also present in normal cells, it is of great interest to elucidate how EGCG, and other phytochemicals with multiple targets, can selectively kill tumour cells whilst not affecting normal cells. Interestingly, a receptor for EGCG (the metastasis-associated 67 kDa laminin receptor) has been identified on cancer cells, suggesting a means for selective uptake of EGCG by cancer cells versus normal cells [137, 138].

12.3.4 Coffee

Early studies suggested an inverse relationship between coffee consumption and risk of colorectal cancer [139]. However, a more recent meta-analysis of 12 prospective cohort studies found that coffee intake was not significantly associated with colorectal, colon or rectal cancer risk in men and women [140]. There are a number of potential confounding factors in some of these studies such as smoking and alcohol, as well as differences between countries in terms of the type of coffee consumed, and brewing method.

12.3.5 Wine and alcohol

A number of epidemiological studies have established a positive association between alcohol and some types of cancer, especially cancers of the upper aero-digestive tract, but also of the colon and breast. This section will discuss some of these studies, especially those relating to moderate levels of wine consumption, since these are the ones most relevant in the context of the MedDiet.

Only a few epidemiological studies have examined the risk of cancer from alcohol and wine consumption in Mediterranean populations. In the Greek cohort of the prospective EPIC study there was a decreased risk of cancer with an overall higher adherence to a MedDiet [45]. Specific analysis of the alcohol component in the diet found that it was neutral for cancer risk (HR 1.0: CI 0.96–1.04) when alcohol intake was moderate (defined as men consuming 10 g to less than 50 g per day and women consuming 5 g to less than 25 g per day) [45]. Although there was no analysis either by cancer sites nor by types of alcohol consumed, an earlier analysis of this cohort found that wine constituted 67% of total alcohol consumption in the women and 57% in the men [141]. Several case-control studies were conducted on a population of women in Mediterranean countries with regard to breast cancer and observed a moderate risk increase for all alcoholic beverages, including wine [142, 143]. A study in Southern France examined the effect of drinking pattern on breast cancer risk. Women who consumed one glass of wine per day (10 to 12 g ethanol) at least five times a week had a lower risk (OR 0.51: CI 0.30–0.91) of breast cancer when compared with non-drinkers, whereas risk increased when frequent consumption rose above two glasses/day (OR 1.72: CI 0.87–3.42 [144]. This study suggests that there is a minimum intake of wine ("threshold effect") before breast cancer risk increases.

A study examining breast density as a surrogate marker for breast cancer risk in American women found that removing consumption of one glass of red wine from the analysis had no effect on the data, suggesting that red wine consumption was neutral in this study [145]. However, the protective effect of a MedDiet was slightly improved by removing all alcohol from the analysis, suggesting that in this cohort of women alcohol is associated with an increased risk of breast cancer even in those consuming a MedDiet, albeit in a non-Mediterranean country.

In contrast to the limited studies in Mediterranean populations, a large number of epidemiological studies conducted in non-Mediterranean countries have found positive associations between alcohol consumption (all types) and cancer incidence. Studies that have looked at the relationship between cancer risk and the total intake of all forms of alcohol over a period of time have shown that with increasing alcohol intake, including wine, there is an increased risk of cancers of the mouth, pharynx and larynx, oesophagus, colon, rectum and breast (and probably liver) [146, 147]. The WCRF concluded that for all of these cancers, with the possible exception of colorectal cancer, there was no threshold of alcohol consumption below which there was no risk of cancer [84]. The recent Europe-wide EPIC study also found that lifetime alcohol consumption was significantly positively associated to colorectal cancer risk (HR 1.08: CI 1.04–1.12 for 15 g/day increase) [148]. A large prospective study of over one million middle-aged women in the United Kingdom (the "Million Women Study") found that low-to-moderate (1 to 2 glasses a day) consumption of any type of alcohol – including wine – was associated with a statistically significantly increased risk of some cancers. However, there was no adjustment for diet. The highest risk was observed for upper aero-digestive tract cancers (as is the case for men) (1.56: CI 1.26–1.94 for oesophageal adeno-carcinoma) and breast cancer (1.13: CI 1.10–1.16), but there was no effect for colon cancer (as opposed to men) [149]. The trend was significant in every case, indicating the absence of threshold. The Million Women Study is one of the few that specifically examined the role of wine: the finding was that breast cancer risk was similar in women who drank white wine, red wine or a mixture of both [149], as described earlier for Mediterranean countries [142, 143]. A large American prospective study (San Francisco Bay Area) found an increased risk of breast cancer with a possible threshold somewhere below one and two drinks daily (relative risks (CI) for breast cancer versus lifelong abstainers were: 1.08 (0.95–1.22) at <1 drink per day, 1.21 (1.05–1.40, p=0.01) at 1–2 drinks daily and 1.38 (1.13–1.68, p=0.002) at >3 drinks daily) A[150]. In this study, the effect of alcoholic beverages was mainly observed in patients with ER+ tumours

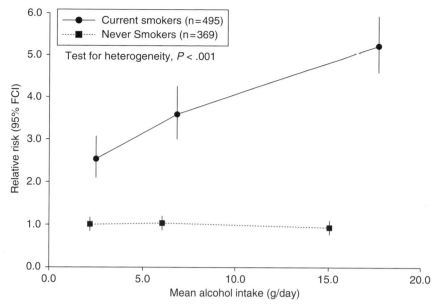

Figure 12.15   Relative risk (floated confidence interval, FCI) of cancers of the aerodigestive tract by moderate alcohol intake and smoking [149]. With permission from Oxford University Press.

(HR 1.4: CI 1.1–1.7), and this is consistent with possible mechanisms for the carcinogenic effects of alcohol in relation to breast cancer discussed below. The EPIC study on breast cancer found that all types of alcoholic beverages increased cancer risk [151]. For prostate cancer, an American prospective study found no effect on risk of prostate cancer with moderate red wine consumption [152].

The role of possible confounding factors has been examined in some of these studies. Smoking is a very important additional or multiplying factor, particularly in relation to cancers of the aerodigestive tract (i.e. cancers of the oral cavity, pharynx, larynx and oesophagus). Although there was a strong positive association between alcohol consumption and risk of aerodigestive cancers in the Million Women study, this association was only observed in smokers and there was no increased risk of aerodigestive cancers for non-smokers with increased alcohol consumption up to 15 g/day (equivalent to about 1.5 drinks per day) (Figure 12.15).

However the large prospective San Francisco Bay Area study quoted above did not show that breast cancer risk increased statistically significantly with tobacco smoking compared with never drinkers) [150].

Mechanisms

Evidence suggests that it is not ethanol *per se* that is carcinogenic, but rather the ethanol metabolite acetaldehyde produced by the enzyme alcohol dehydrogenase [153] (see Chapter 7). Acetaldehyde is subsequently detoxified by conversion to acetate by the enzyme acetaldehyde dehydrogenase (ALDH). The importance of ALDH for detoxifying acetaldehyde is highlighted by studies showing that individuals with forms of ALDH with reduced activity are at increased risk of oesophageal cancer [153]. If acetaldehyde is produced in high amounts due to high alcohol consumption, the acetaldehyde may saturate the detoxifying capacity of ALDH, and so acetaldehyde will accumulate, not only due to high levels of production but also due to a detoxifying system that has become saturated [154]. Alcoholic drinks are also a direct source of acetaldehyde. Levels vary widely depending on the type of drink, with fortified wines containing especially high levels. It is possible that preformed acetaldehyde could be an important carcinogen for oral cancer, and this mechanism is thought to contribute to the carcinogenicity of the apple brandy calvados (a speciality of Northern France) [155].

As well as acting as a source of acetaldehyde, there is evidence that ethanol modulates oestrogen metabolism, and since enhanced oestrogen is an important risk factor for breast cancer this may contribute to the particularly strong positive associations found in some studies between alcohol consumption and breast cancer risk. Alcohol has been shown to increase the levels of circulating oestrogens in women, and oestrogen also increases the expression of oestrogen receptors on breast cancer cells grown in culture [156]. Interestingly, the MedDiet has been shown to decrease the levels of circulating oestrogens (by 40%) in healthy post-menopausal women [157], but it is not known whether this may counterbalance any increase in oestrogen levels due to alcohol consumption. However, it is worth bearing in mind that the prevalence of breast cancer is lower in Mediterranean countries compared to Northern Europe (see below).

Some, but not all, epidemiological studies have found that dietary folates reduce the increased risk of cancer due to alcohol consumption at various sites, including breast [151, 158–160], colon [161] and ovary [162]. Folates are destroyed by acetaldehyde, and adequate dietary folates may be required to compensate for this loss. Folates are required to prevent the activation of genes associated with carcinogenesis, although it is not known if this is directly relevant to breast and other cancers. Adherence to a MedDiet has been found to strongly correlate with the degree of consumption of folates [163]. This raises the theoretical possibility that by providing an adequate supply of folates, a MedDiet may offset some of the increased risk of breast and other cancers associated with alcohol consumption [164].

Smoking is widely recognised as an additional or multiplying factor in epidemiological studies of cancer and alcohol consumption (see above). Beside its own role as a carcinogen, it has been suggested that alcohol may increase the risk of aerodigestive cancers by acting as a "solvent", thus facilitating the penetration of carcinogens from cigarette smoke into epithelial cells of the aerodigestive tract [84]. Hence, drinking and smoking at the same time are a particularly dangerous combination in relation to cancers of the aerodigestive tract. This suggests that the same amount of alcohol may have different degrees of carcinogenicity depending on whether or not an individual is also smoking at the same time.

Red wine consumption increases the plasma levels of uric acid – a metabolic product of alcohol metabolism (see Chapter 7) [165]. Uric acid is an important antioxidant in the plasma and the increased antioxidant capacity in the plasma could conceivably be beneficial against cancer associated with oxidative stress. However, the significance of changes in uric acid in relation to red wine consumption are unclear.

Wine, and especially red wine, is distinguished from other alcoholic beverages by its high content of phenolics. Several of these, such as resveratrol, have been shown to inhibit carcinogenesis in experimental models for cancer by acting as antioxidants and through modulating various signaling mechanisms. However, it is not known to what extent, if any, these phenolics may "offset" the pro-carcinogenic action of ethanol (see Chapter 7 for further discussions).

12.3.6   Plant foods

Besides examining specific nutrients in plant foods discussed earlier, studies have attempted to establish the overall impact of consuming fruits and/or vegetables. In the 1997 WCRF report, the overall category "Fruit and Vegetables" was concluded to be either "convincingly" or "probably" or "possibly" protective for most cancers. However, in the 2007 edition, no fruits or vegetables were found to be protective with a convincing level of evidence, and there were differences between fruits and vegetables [84]. For example, fruit was stated as probably reducing the risk of lung cancer, whereas there was no evidence for a protective effect of vegetables. More precise protective effects of cereals, fruits and vegetables were described. For example, garlic and foods containing fibre were said to probably decrease the risk of colorectal cancer, and foods containing carotenoids to probably decrease the risk of cancers of the mouth, pharynx, larynx and lung.

Since the WCRF/AICR 2007 report, the EPIC study of a cohort of 10,449 diabetic patients below 70-years-old found there was no risk reduction in cancer mortality for an increment of 80 g/day of fruit, vegetables and legumes [166]. The report from the EPIC study on the relationship between total fruit and vegetable consumption and overall cancer risk on the entire cohort of approximately half a million men and women showed negative results [167]. However, other reports from the EPIC study have shown beneficial effects of fruit and vegetables on some specific types of cancer, including lung cancer [168] and colorectal cancer [169]. Hence these data emphasise the need to consider cancers not as a single entity, but rather to consider cancers at each site separately.

A number of other studies have examined the effects of specific vegetables. There is some limited evidence that a diet which includes regular consumption of onions is associated with a reduced risk of cancer at several sites. A study conducted in Italy found that moderate consumption of onions reduced the risk of colorectal, laryngeal and ovarian cancers [170]. The WCRF concluded that it is "probable" that garlic consumption protects against both stomach and colorectal cancer risk [84]. The bacterium *Helicobacter pylori* is a known causal factor in stomach cancer and the anti-bacterial properties of garlic may contribute to this protection [171]. More recently, the Korean FDA, claiming to use the methodology of the US Food and Drug Administration (FDA), stated that "There was no credible evidence to support a relation between garlic intake and a reduced risk of gastric, breast, lung, or endometrial cancer"[172]. Very limited evidence supported a relationship between garlic consumption and reduced risk of colon, prostate, oesophageal, larynx, oral, ovary or renal cell cancers. However, the review includes various garlic supplements together with dietary intake, and this introduces strong heterogeneity into the analysis.

The WCRF/AICR concluded that there is a "probable" decreased risk of colorectal cancer from consuming foods rich in fibre, which may include cereals (see Section 12.3.2). However, the report concluded that the overall evidence for an association between cereal consumption itself and reduced cancer risk is "unimpressive". Most associations with disease and mortality are weak when cereals are scored for in relation to adherence to a MedDiet. For example, high cereal consumption was only weakly associated with reduced mortality in the Greek EPIC cohort [173]. There are, however, problems associated with studying cereals. Firstly, cereals are heterogeneous in nature and composition. Different forms of cereal have different health effects and this may depend on both the degree of refining of the grain and the product itself. For example, processed cereals have a higher GI than whole grains, and glycaemic control is important for preventing many disorders (see Chapter 10). Secondly, the method of preparation and consumption of cereals varies widely. For example, on the one hand cereals might accompany a vegetable dish, whereas they are also a component of pastries and may be consumed together with trans FAs which may influence cancer in the opposite way. Assessing cereals in a questionnaire is especially sensitive to these types of confounding factors.

For nut consumption and possible reduced risk of cancers of the colon, rectum and prostate, the results are not conclusive, although mechanistic observations in experimental models provide biological plausibility [174].

A large body of research has investigated the possible link between tomato and/or lycopene intake and protection against prostate cancer. However, two large reviews of the data have drawn conflicting conclusions. The 2007 WCRF/AICR report concluded: "There is a substantial amount of consistent evidence, in particular on tomato products, from both cohort and case-control studies. There is evidence for plausible mechanisms. Foods containing lycopene probably protect against prostate cancer" [84]. In 2004, the US FDA received requests from manufacturers of tomato products to allow them to put health claims on their products. In response to these requests, the FDA undertook an evidence-based review to examine the evidence that tomato consumption can reduce the incidence of various cancers [175]. The conclusions in their 2007 report are more equivocal than the WCRF/AICR, and they state that "very limited and preliminary scientific research suggests that eating one-half to one cup of tomatoes and/or tomato sauce a week may reduce the risk of prostate cancer. The FDA concluded that there is little scientific evidence supporting this claim". The FDA also concluded that there was very limited evidence for associations between tomato consumption and reduced risk of lung, ovarian, gastric and pancreatic cancers. However, their stringent conditions for including studies might explain this statement. For example, with regard to lung cancer, they eliminate studies where subjects were exposed to strong environmental carcinogens (coal fumes, tobacco). For gastric cancer, no prospective studies were retained, and no consistency among the findings observed in sub-groups in case-control studies. In relation to lycopene, the FDA concluded that "there was no credible evidence supporting a relationship between lycopene consumption, either as a food ingredient, a component of food, or as a dietary supplement, and any of the cancers evaluated in the studies" [175]. The main argument, which is also contained in the statement of the WCRF on "lycopene-rich food", is that it was not possible to accurately determine whether any of the associations between lycopene and cancer risk were due to: (1) lycopene alone; (2) interactions between lycopene and other nutrients; (3) other nutrients acting alone or together; or (4) decreased consumption of other nutrients or substances contained in foods that may have been displaced from the diet by an increased intake of lycopene-rich foods.

Evidence for an association between tomato consumption and a reduced risk of prostate cancer is stronger for data obtained from some Mediterranean populations. A case control study in Greece that included 320 prostate cancer case patients and 246 control subjects reported that intake of cooked tomatoes was inversely associated with prostate cancer risk (OR for the highest tertile of intake versus the lowest tertile of intake = 1.91: CI 1.20–3.04). However, they found no association between intake of raw tomatoes and prostate cancer risk [176]. This may be linked to the greater bioavailability of lycopene in processed tomatoes compared with raw tomatoes.

An EPIC study found only weak correlations between lycopene plasma levels and dietary intake of specific tomato products [177], and this might explain the difficulty in assessing an association between cancer and lycopene intake based on plasma levels. This study found a better correlation between lycopene plasma levels and tomatoes by summing the intake of *cooked and processed* tomato intake rather than for total tomato consumption (Pearson correlation coefficients 0.37 and 0.33 respectively). Total tomato consumption includes raw tomatoes which, when assessed separately, had a poor correlation with plasma lycopene levels (Pearson correlation coefficient 0.16). Indeed, the highest plasma lycopene levels were for the population from Southern Italy whose total tomato consumption was relatively low but who had a high consumption of cooked tomato products. One study found that more lycopene is absorbed by the body via tomato sauce or pizza compared with eating raw tomatoes [178].

The wide variety of antioxidants in tomatoes raises the possibility that they can interact synergistically as antioxidants [64]. For example, the antioxidant properties of lycopene have been found to be enhanced by vitamin E in experimental systems. But whether or not it is the antioxidant properties of tomato phytochemicals that are responsible for preventing prostate cancer is not clear since lycopene may have other beneficial effects such as improving the immune system, lowering inflammation, and suppressing the stimulation of prostate cancer cells caused by IGF-1.

Another important consideration when assessing the health benefits of tomato consumption is the wide variation between tomatoes in their phytochemical content (see Chapter 5). Factors that affect the bioavailability of phytochemicals are another important consideration (see Chapter 4). Fat both increases the release of carotenoids such as lycopene from plant cells and increases absorption. An illustration of this is from a study that found that eating diced tomatoes cooked in olive oil greatly increased the absorption of lycopene compared to when diced tomatoes were cooked without olive oil [179]. However, fats that are not absorbed by the body, or are absorbed by the body to only a limited extent (such as those found in some new types of slimming foods), may carry carotenoids through the gut, and this can result in substantially reduced plasma carotenoid concentrations, hence decreasing their potential benefit. [180].

In summary, variations in the levels of phytochemicals between types of tomatoes, method of preparation, and fat in the diet are all factors that may contribute to the conflicting epidemiological studies linking tomatoes and health. Also, it is known that there are inter-individual variations in the rate of absorption of some phytochemicals in tomatoes, including lycopene.

Intervention studies
Only a few intervention studies have been undertaken with diets rich in plant food. A study examining the effect of a diet low in fat and high in fibre and fruit and vegetables failed to demonstrate an effect on the recurrence of colorectal adenomas, a precancerous state of colon cancer [181]. One explanation is that fibre may prevent the progression of an adenoma to colon cancer but not affect the occurrence of adenomas. By contrast, a later study did find that fibre could reduce the risk of

adenoma recurrence [182]. In another study on breast cancer survival a randomised controlled trial (the Women's Healthy Eating and Living Study) compared a putative cancer prevention diet with a diet of five servings of vegetables and fruit daily and intensive counselling and a comparison group who received a notebook containing dietary guidelines from the USDA and the NCI. The intervention diet failed to show any benefit on survival [183]. However, a summary measure of cumulative plasma carotenoid levels during follow-up was undertaken in both groups to assess the compliance to the diet and it was observed that a higher biological exposure to carotenoids, when assessed over the time-frame of the study, was associated with a greater likelihood of breast cancer-free survival regardless of study group assignment (plasma total carotenoids lowest tertile [<1.656 μmol/L] versus medium/high [>1.656 μmol/L] HR 0.67: CI 0.54–0.83) (after adjustment for tumour characteristics, cholesterol concentration and BMI) [184].

Conclusions

These studies illustrate the difficulties associated with establishing a relationship between a nutrient or food and cancer. For example, the stage of the "natural history" of the cancer might play a role (whether the tumour is at initiation, promotion, progression, or it has already metastasised). Indeed, a nutrient that is beneficial at one stage of carcinogenesis might be detrimental at another. Another consideration is that a food chosen to be assessed for cancer prevention might not be the correct one: the food may have been selected since it is associated with a marker for decreased cancer risk, but that decreased risk might in fact have been due to another food. Another issue when considering cancers at different sites is the biological mechanism at work. In the report on lung cancer, the protective effect is greater in smokers, indicating the possible interaction of plant foods and their constituents with carcinogens in tobacco [168]. Finally, a nutrient shown to be protective might be relevant in a certain population because it is part of a globally beneficial diet, whereas the same nutrient as part of a different diet might not show any protective effect.

These considerations highlight the importance of an integrative approach combining nutrition with other lifestyle factors in order to comprehend all the factors involved in a disease such as cancer that is associated with multifactorial risks.

12.3.7   Dietary patterns

As for CVD, MedDiet scores (*a priori* approaches) and principal component analyses (*a posteriori* approaches) (see Chapter 8) have been used to evaluate the global effect of dietary patterns on cancer mortality and incidence.

A priori approaches

Adherence to an MD-QI was analysed in the Greek cohort of the EPIC study (22,043 adults). An inverse association with greater adherence to the MedDiet was evident for death due to cancer (0.76: CI 0.59–0.98) [185]. This was also the case for cancer incidence from a later analysis of the Greek EPIC cohort (10,582 men, 15,041 women: medically confirmed cancer in 421 men and 430 women) [45]. A higher degree of adherence to the MedDiet was associated with lower overall cancer incidence. A 2-point increase in the MDS corresponded to a 12% reduction in

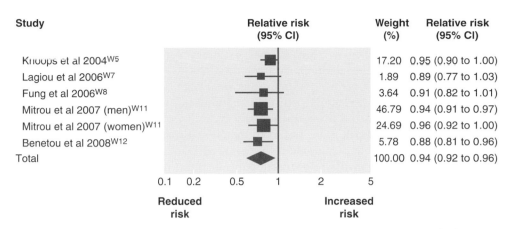

Study	Relative risk (95% CI)	Weight (%)	Relative risk (95% CI)
Knoops et al 2004[W5]		17.20	0.95 (0.90 to 1.00)
Lagiou et al 2006[W7]		1.89	0.89 (0.77 to 1.03)
Fung et al 2006[W8]		3.64	0.91 (0.82 to 1.01)
Mitrou et al 2007 (men)[W11]		46.79	0.94 (0.91 to 0.97)
Mitrou et al 2007 (women)[W11]		24.69	0.96 (0.92 to 1.00)
Benetou et al 2008[W12]		5.78	0.88 (0.81 to 0.96)
Total		100.00	0.94 (0.92 to 0.96)

Figure 12.16   Risk of occurrence of or mortality from cancer associated with two point increase in adherence score for Mediterranean diet. [190]. Squares represent effect size: extended lines show confidence intervals: diamond represents total effect size. With permission from BMJ Publishing Group Ltd.

cancer incidence (adjusted HR 0.88: CI 0.80–0.95). The association was exposure-dependent and stronger among women (HR 0.84: CI 0.74–0.95 for a 2-point increase and HR 0.76: CI 0.63–0.93 for the highest tertile compared to the lowest tertile of adherence to the MD-QI).

Recently, the MDS was used to estimate the effect of adherence to a traditional Med-Diet on breast cancer incidence in the Greek EPIC cohort which followed 14,807 women over 9 years and observed 240 cases [186]. Among the post-menopausal women, those with the highest conformity to a traditional MedDiet were at lower risk for breast cancer (HR for a score 6–9 0.59: CI 0.34–1.03; HR=0.78 for every 2 points increase in the MDS; CI 0.62–0.98, p for interaction by menopausal status=0.05). None of the individual foods was significantly associated with breast cancer. Thus, in spite of some limitations in the study (modest size, absence of ER and/or PR determination, menopausal status imprecise) it reinforces the interest of working with dietary patterns.

An adaption of the MDS, the M-MDS [187], was applied to the Nurses' Health Study (3580 cases of breast cancer: 2367 ER+ and 575 ER-). There was no association between the modified M-MDS and total or ER+ breast cancer [188]. However, for ER- breast cancer, the RR comparing highest to lowest quintiles was 0.79 (CI 0.60–1.03, trend 0.03) (after adjusting for potential confounders). The same score was applied to NIH-AARP cohort and was associated with a risk reduction of overall cancer mortality (0.83: CI 0.76–0.91) [189]. A meta-analysis of the health effects associated with adherence to a MedDiet *a priori* defined by MDS (where MDS, M-MDS and modified M-MDS were mixed) has been published [190]. The analyses showed a beneficial role for greater adherence to a MedDiet on incidence of, or mortality from, cancer (pooled RR 0.94: CI 0.92–0.96) (Figure 12.16). Adherence to the relative M-MDS (rMDS), a scoring system which reintroduced olive oil among the foods of the MDS, was associated with a significant reduction of gastric adenocarcinoma (HR 0.93: CI 0.89–0.99, after calibration of measurement errors) in the 485,044 subjects (144,577 men) aged 35–70y from 10 European countries in the EPIC study [191]. It is noteworthy that when each component of the rMDS was analysed separately, only the highest tertile of fruit was significantly associated with a risk reduction of gastric adenocarcinoma (HR 0.67: CI 0.51–0.87, trend 0.002) and the highest tertile of meat associated with an increased risk (HR 1.33: CI 1.03–1.72, trend: 0.033).

As has been discussed in relation to CVD (see Chapter 11), when analysing the relationship of diet with cancer, the original MDS cannot be applied to non-Mediterranean countries, thus requiring modifications. Also, since the MDS is based on median intakes within a population, consumption levels observed in study populations in non-Mediterranean countries may not correspond to the absolute amounts necessary for risk reduction as observed in a traditional Greek population. In addition, the *a priori* dietary pattern described by the MDS may be correlated with other nutritional or lifestyle factors with potential roles in risk reduction, and these may not be present in non-Mediterranean countries [192–194] (see also Chapter 11). Among these, one factor that might be especially important with regard to cancer is vitamin D. Mediterranean people enjoy abundant sunlight and this provides vitamin D (which is synthesised in the skin from 7-dehydro-cholesterol and converted into its active form in the liver). Vitamin D has been associated with protection from cancer in various studies (see Chapter 2). These various considerations may play a role in the health benefits of a MedDiet, and explain why most of the time the original MDS is associated with a higher risk reduction of cancer.

A posteriori approaches

Studies conducted in non-Mediterranean countries identified two dietary patterns by principal component analysis (PCA), namely prudent/plant-based and Western. The constant composition of the prudent diet is characterised by a high intake of vegetables, fruit, legumes fish/seafood and whole grains, and that of the Western diet by a high intake of red and processed meat, butter, potatoes, refined grains and high fat dairy products [195]. According to the different populations of the studies, other food groups can be found in the prudent diet (poultry, low fat dairy products, salad dressings, fruit juices and wine) or in the Western diet (sweets, French fries, high sugar drinks, pizzas, mayonnaise and margarine).

Results regarding the association between cancer and a prudent diet are not consistent. A multi-site, case-control study using factor analysis and several cancer sites (mouth and pharynx, oesophagus, stomach, colon, rectum larynx, lung, breast, prostate, bladder, kidney) was conducted in Uruguay [196]. The study included 3528 cases and 2532 controls. The PCA based on the food intake of the control group retained four factors per sex, labelled as prudent, drinker, traditional and Western. The prudent pattern (raw and cooked vegetables, fruit, fish and poultry) was mainly negatively associated with cancers of the upper aero-digestive tract in men (e.g. oesophagus: OR 0.27: CI 0.17–0.43, trend: <0.0001) and breast cancer in women (OR 0.6: CI 0.47–0.85, trend: 0.005).

The prudent diet pattern has been shown to be associated with a reduced risk for colon cancer in some, but not all, studies, whereas the Western pattern was more consistently associated with an increased risk [197–199]. A PCA using individual food data and aggregated cancer incidence from a Southern French population showed that a diet rich in raw and cooked vegetables, fruit, olive oil, light dairy products, herbs (thyme and rosemary) and a few emblematic Mediterranean foods like *ratatouille* and *tabouli*, was protective against all cancer incidence [200]. In a first analysis of the French EPIC cohort (E3N), the PCA was computed on 172 women with colorectal cancer (129 with colon and 43 with rectal cancer) and 67,312 colorectal cancer-free women [201]. Four patterns were identified: healthy, western, drinkers and meat eaters. The healthy pattern was characterised by a high consumption of raw and cooked vegetables, legumes, fruit, yogurt, fresh cheese, breakfast cereals, sea products, eggs and vegetable oils (olive oil and others) and by a low consumption of sweets. It was associated with a non-significant decreased RR of colorectal cancer (0.77: CI 0.49–1.20).

In two reports of dietary pattern analysis of the Nurses' Health Study, one in pre-menopausal [202], the other in post-menopausal women [187], there was no overall association between the prudent or Western pattern and breast cancer risk. However, in pre-menopausal women, there was a significant risk reduction in smokers with the highest score of the prudent diet. In post-menopausal women, a Western-type diet may elevate risk of breast cancer among smokers, and a prudent diet may protect against ER– tumours. Also in non-smokers, the association between a traditional "southern" dietary pattern and breast cancer was stronger than in the overall sample (40,559 post-menopausal women in the Breast Cancer Detection Demonstration Project, 1987–1998: 1868 of those women developed breast cancer)(HR 0.58: CI 0.36–0.94, trend 0.008 versus HR 0.78: CI 0.65–0.95, trend 0.003). Such an association was observed only in ER+ tumours. Curiously, a pattern of prudent diet (vegetable, fruit, fish/poultry) was not associated with breast cancer risk, the main difference between this dietary pattern and a traditional southern one being in intake of legumes.

A study of North Italian women (ORDET study) included a cohort of 8984 women with an average follow up of 9.5 years and 207 incident cases of breast cancer. Factor analysis identified four dietary patterns: salad vegetables (mainly consisting of raw vegetables and olive oil): western (mainly consisting of potatoes, red meat, eggs and butter): canteen (pasta and tomato sauce): and prudent (cooked vegetables, pulses, and fish, with negative loading on wines and spirits). After adjustment for potential confounders, only the salad vegetables + olive oil pattern was associated with a significantly lower breast cancer incidence (RR=0.66: CI 0.47–0.95 comparing highest with lowest tertile) with a significant linear trend (p=0.016) [203]. Women with a BMI<25 had an even greater risk reduction in the highest tertile of the salad vegetables + olive oil pattern (>50% less risk than the lowest tertile, RR=0.39: CI 0.22–0.69) with a significant trend (p=0.001): whereas women with a BMI ≥25 had no protective effect for the consumption of salad vegetables + olive oil.

Another analysis by sub-group based on HER2 status was done a few years later [25]. It showed that the inverse association of the dietary pattern salad vegetables + olive oil was significantly inversely associated with HER2+ breast cancer risk for the 2nd and 3rd tertiles (HR 0.33: CI 0.15–0.73 and HR 0.25: CI 0.10–0.64, respectively) with a significant linear relationship (p=0.001) whereas the association with the HER2- cancers was borderline significant only for the 3rd tertile of the salad vegetables + olive oil pattern (HR 0.71: CI 0.48–1.03, trend=0.072). This suggests that the components of this dietary pattern are especially efficient against HER2+ breast cancer. However, such an observation needs confirmation in several other studies, given that it was undertaken on only 40 patients HER-2+ compared with 198 HER2– patients and that categorisation induces chance findings (e.g. the mid-score "prudent" dietary patterns is associated with significant risk reduction in HER2+ cancers and increased risk in HER-2 cancers). However, if we compare the components of the different dietary pattern of this population, one notes that mixed vegetables in salads, raw tomatoes and leaf vegetables were present in the protective dietary pattern with a high loading factor[8] followed by olive oil (0.70 and 0.46, respectively), whereas they were absent from the prudent diet. Olive oil was present with a loading factor of 0.43 in another dietary pattern (canteen, mainly characterised by pasta and absence of vegetables), not associated with breast cancer.

Recently, food intake and breast cancer incidence data of 65,374 women of the E3N French EPIC cohort were analysed to study the relationship of post-menopausal invasive breast cancer (2381 cases) during a median 9.7 year follow-up (1993–2005) with scores for dietary patterns obtained by factor analysis [204]. Two dietary patterns were identified: alcohol/Western (essentially meat products, French fries, appetizers, rice/pasta, potatoes, pulses, pizza/pies, canned fish, eggs, alcoholic beverages, cakes, mayonnaise and butter/cream), and healthy/Mediterranean (essentially vegetables, fruit, seafood, olive oil and sunflower oil). This pattern was very comparable to the "healthy pattern" previously described by Kesse et al. [201], except that yogurt, fresh cheese and breakfast cereals were not present in the healthy/Mediterranean. The alcohol/Western pattern was positively associated with breast cancer risk (multivariable HR for the highest versus lowest quartile 1.20: CI 1.03–1.38, trend=0.007). The healthy/Mediterranean pattern was negatively associated with breast cancer risk (HR: 0.85: CI 0.75–0.95, trend=0.003). In ER+/PR+ and ER–/PR– the decrease was non-significant; the strongest effect was observed with ER+/PR– tumours (HR 0.65: CI 0.49–0.87, trend 0.001): when energy intake was less than the median 2037 Kcal/day, HR was 0.75 (CI 0.63–0.90: trend=0.002: significant interaction with energy (p:0.03) whereas the risk reduction was lower and the HR non-significant in women with energy intake >2037 Kcal/day. Although it is in line with the ORDET study, the French EPIC is the first one to show a significant effect of a complete MedDiet pattern on breast cancer, and also demonstrates that this pattern has to be limited by energy intake and/or energy balance. These results need confirmation, but are in line with the study of Benetou et al. [45] showing that the MDS was associated with a risk reduction for cancer in the Greek EPIC cohort. In this Greek cohort, MUFAs were essentially provided by olive oil, and the risk reduction was stronger in women (breast cancer is the major cancer in women). Similarly, Trichopoulou et al. showed that the MDS was marginally associated with a risk reduction for breast cancer in the Greek EPIC cohort [186].

In summary, the results are not fully conclusive with the prudent diet for cancers and the results are limited with regard to the incidence of cancers. However, it is interesting to note that when the prudent dietary pattern includes olive oil, and thus becomes very comparable to a MedDiet, there is a strong suggestion of a risk reduction for breast cancer, and this requires further investigation.

References

1. Davies, A.A. et al. Nutritional interventions and outcome in patients with cancer or preinvasive lesions: systematic review. *J Natl Cancer Inst*, 2006. **98**(14): 961–73.
2. Craig, W.J. Phytochemicals: guardians of our health. *J Am Diet Assoc*, 1997. **97**(10 Suppl 2): S199–204.

---

[8] Food groups with a positive loading are those that contribute directly to a dietary pattern and food groups with negative loading are inversely associated with a dietary pattern. Factor loadings can be considered as correlation coefficients between food groups and dietary patterns and take values between –1 and +1.

3. Chen, S., Parmigiani, G. Meta-analysis of BRCA1 and BRCA2 penetrance. *J Clin Oncol*, 2007. **25**(11): 1329–33.

4. Fearon, E.R., Vogelstein, B. A genetic model for colorectal tumorigenesis. *Cell*, 1990. **61**(5): 759–67.

5. Lippman, S.M. et al. Cancer prevention and the American Society of Clinical Oncology. *J Clin Oncol*, 2004. **22**(19): 3848–51.

6. Stolzenberg-Solomon, R.Z. et al. Folate intake, alcohol use, and postmenopausal breast cancer risk in the Prostate, Lung, Colorectal, and Ovarian Cancer Screening Trial. *Am J Clin Nutr*, 2006. **83**(4): 895–904.

7. Cole, B.F. et al. Folic acid for the prevention of colorectal adenomas: a randomized clinical trial. *Jama*, 2007. **297**(21): 2351–9.

8. Dashwood, R.H. et al. Dietary HDAC inhibitors: time to rethink weak ligands in cancer chemoprevention? *Carcinogenesis*, 2006. **27**(2): 344–9.

9. Knutson, M.D., Leeuwenburgh, C. Resveratrol and novel potent activators of SIRT1: effects on aging and age-related diseases. *Nutr Rev*, 2008. **66**(10): 591–6.

10. Aiyer, H.S. et al. Dietary berries and ellagic Acid prevent oxidative DNA damage and modulate expression of DNA repair genes. *Int J Mol Sci*, 2008. **9**(3): 327–41.

11. Halliwell, B. Oxidative stress and cancer: have we moved forward? *Biochem J*, 2007. **401**(1): 1–11.

12. Bear, W.L., Teel, R.W. Effects of citrus phytochemicals on liver and lung cytochrome P450 activity and on the in vitro metabolism of the tobacco-specific nitrosamine NNK. *Anticancer Res*, 2000. **20**(5A): 3323–9.

13. Ordovas, J.M. et al. Nutrition in the genomics era: cardiovascular disease risk and the Mediterranean diet. *Mol Nutr Food Res*, 2007. **51**(10): 1293–9.

14. Vincent-Baudry, S. et al. The Medi-RIVAGE study: reduction of cardiovascular disease risk factors after a 3-mo intervention with a Mediterranean-type diet or a low-fat diet. *Am J Clin Nutr*, 2005. **82**(5): 964–71.

15. Greenhough, A. et al. The COX-2/PGE2 pathway: key roles in the hallmarks of cancer and adaptation to the tumour microenvironment. *Carcinogenesis*, 2009. **30**(3): 377–86.

16. O'Leary, K.A. et al. Effect of flavonoids and vitamin E on cyclooxygenase-2 (COX-2) transcription. *Mutat Res*, 2004. **551**(1–2): 245–54.

17. Hanahan, D., Weinberg, R.A. The hallmarks of cancer. *Cell*, 2000. **100**(1): 57–70.

18. Colotta, F. et al. Cancer-related inflammation, the seventh hallmark of cancer: links to genetic instability. *Carcinogenesis*, 2009. **30**(7): 1073–81.

19. Aggarwal, B.B., Shishodia, S. Molecular targets of dietary agents for prevention and therapy of cancer. *Biochem Pharmacol*, 2006. **71**(10): 1397–421.

20. Oi, N. et al. Metabolic conversion of dietary quercetin from its conjugate to active aglycone following the induction of hepatocarcinogenesis in fisher 344 rats. *J Agric Food Chem*, 2008. **56**(2): 577–83.

21. William, W.N., Jr. et al. Molecular targets for cancer chemoprevention. *Nat Rev Drug Discov*, 2009. **8**(3): 213–25.

22. Solanas, M. et al. Effects of a high olive oil diet on the clinical behavior and histopathological features of rat DMBA-induced mammary tumors compared with a high corn oil diet. *Int J Oncol*, 2002. **21**(4): 745–53.

23. Menendez, J.A., Lupu, R. Mediterranean dietary traditions for the molecular treatment of human cancer: anti-oncogenic actions of the main olive oil's monounsaturated fatty acid oleic acid (18:1n-9). *Curr Pharm Biotechnol*, 2006. **7**(6): 495–502.

24. Menendez, J.A. et al. tabAnti-HER2 (erbB-2) oncogene effects of phenolic compounds directly isolated from commercial Extra-Virgin Olive Oil (EVOO). *BMC Cancer*, 2008. **8**: 377.

25. Sant, M. et al. Salad vegetables dietary pattern protects against HER-2-positive breast cancer: a prospective Italian study. *Int J Cancer*, 2007. **121**(4): 911–4.

26. He, S. et al. Red wine polyphenols for cancer prevention. *Int J Mol Sci*, 2008. **9**(5): 842–53.

27. Cowey, S., Hardy, R.W. The metabolic syndrome: A high-risk state for cancer? *Am J Pathol*, 2006. **169**(5): 1505–22.

28. Mantzoros, C.S. et al. Insulin-like growth factor 1 in relation to prostate cancer and benign prostatic hyperplasia. *Br J Cancer*, 1997. **76**(9): 1115–8.

29. Nimptsch, K. et al. Plasma insulin-like growth factor 1 is positively associated with low-grade prostate cancer in the Health Professionals Follow-up Study 1993–2004. *Int J Cancer*, 2010. **53** Supl2: S184–93.

30. Minich, D.M., Bland, J.S. Dietary management of the metabolic syndrome beyond macronutrients. *Nutr Rev*, 2008. **66**(8): 429–44.

31. Anderson, R.A. Chromium and polyphenols from cinnamon improve insulin sensitivity. *Proc Nutr Soc*, 2008. **67**(1): 48–53.

32. Juan, M.E. et al. Olive fruit extracts inhibit proliferation and induce apoptosis in HT-29 human colon cancer cells. *J Nutr*, 2006. **136**(10): 2553–7.

33. Khan, N. et al. Apoptosis by dietary factors: the suicide solution for delaying cancer growth. *Carcinogenesis*, 2007. **28**(2): 233–9.

34. Edwards, I.J., O'Flaherty, J.T. Omega-3 fatty acids and PPARgamma in cancer. *PPAR Res*, 2008. **2008**: 358052.

35. Sainis, I. et al. PPARgamma: The portrait of a target ally to cancer chemopreventive agents. *PPAR Res*, 2008. **2008**: p. 436489.

36. Bhat, T.A., Singh, R.P. Tumor angiogenesis–a potential target in cancer chemoprevention. *Food Chem Toxicol*, 2008. **46**(4): 1334–45.

37. Kawasaki, B.T. et al. Targeting cancer stem cells with phytochemicals. *Mol Interv*, 2008. **8**(4): 174–84.

38. Weinstein, I.B. Cancer. Addiction to oncogenes–the Achilles heal of cancer. *Science*, 2002. **297**(5578): 63–4.

39. Janne, P.A. et al. Factors underlying sensitivity of cancers to small-molecule kinase inhibitors. *Nat Rev Drug Discov*, 2009. **8**(9): 709–23.

40. Tosetti, F. et al. Metabolic regulation and redox activity as mechanisms for angioprevention by dietary phytochemicals. *Int J Cancer*, 2009. **125**(9): 1997–2003.

41. de la Lastra, C.A., Villegas, I. Resveratrol as an antioxidant and pro-oxidant agent: mechanisms and clinical implications. *Biochem Soc Trans*, 2007. **35**(Pt 5): 1156–60.

42. Loo, G. Redox-sensitive mechanisms of phytochemical-mediated inhibition of cancer cell proliferation (review). *J Nutr Biochem*, 2003. **14**(2): 64–73.

43. Trachootham, D. et al. Targeting cancer cells by ROS-mediated mechanisms: a radical therapeutic approach? *Nat Rev Drug Discov*, 2009. **8**(7): 579–91.

44. Jacobs, D.R., Jr., Tapsell, L.C. Food, not nutrients, is the fundamental unit in nutrition. *Nutr Rev*, 2007. **65**(10): 439–50.

45. Benetou, V. et al. Conformity to traditional Mediterranean diet and cancer incidence: the Greek EPIC cohort. *Br J Cancer*, 2008. **99**(1): 191–5.

46. Halliwell, B., et al. Health promotion by flavonoids, tocopherols, tocotrienols, and other phenols: direct or indirect effects? Antioxidant or not? *Am J Clin Nutr*, 2005. **81**(1 Suppl): 268S–276S.

47. Martinez-Gonzalez, M.A., Sanchez-Villegas, A. The emerging role of Mediterranean diets in cardiovascular epidemiology: monounsaturated fats, olive oil, red wine or the whole pattern? *Eur J Epidemiol*, 2004. **19**(1): 9–13.

48. Chou, T.C. Theoretical basis, experimental design, and computerized simulation of synergism and antagonism in drug combination studies. *Pharmacol Rev*, 2006. **58**(3): 621–81.

49. Ulrich-Merzenich, G. et al. New perspectives for synergy research with the "omic"-technologies. *Phytomedicine*, 2009. **16**(6–7): 495–508.

50. Segal, E. et al. From signatures to models: understanding cancer using microarrays. *Nat Genet*, 2005. **37 Suppl**: S38–45.

51. de Kok, T.M. et al. Mechanisms of combined action of different chemopreventive dietary compounds: a review. *Eur J Nutr*, 2008. **47 Suppl 2**: 51–9.

52. Auclair, S. et al. Catechin reduces atherosclerotic lesion development in apo E-deficient mice: a transcriptomic study. *Atherosclerosis*, 2009. **204**(2): e21–7.

53. Ulrich-Merzenich, G. et al. Synergy research: vitamins and secondary plant components in the maintenance of the redox-homeostasis and in cell signaling. *Phytomedicine*, 2009. **16**(1): 2–16.

54. van Breda, S.G. et al. Vegetables affect the expression of genes involved in anticarcinogenic processes in the colonic mucosa of C57BL/6 female mice. *J Nutr*, 2005. **135**(8): 1879–88.

55. Liu, R.H. Health benefits of fruit and vegetables are from additive and synergistic combinations of phytochemicals. *Am J Clin Nutr*, 2003. **78**(3 Suppl): 517S–520S.

56. Dragoni, S. et al. Red wine alcohol promotes quercetin absorption and directs its metabolism towards isorhamnetin and tamarixetin in rat intestine in vitro. *Br J Pharmacol*, 2006. **147**(7): 765–71.

57. Horie, N. et al. Synergistic effect of green tea catechins on cell growth and apoptosis induction in gastric carcinoma cells. *Biol Pharm Bull*, 2005. **28**(4): 574–9.

58. Wallig, M.A. et al. Synergy among phytochemicals within crucifers: does it translate into chemoprotection? *J Nutr*, 2005. **135**(12 Suppl): 2972S–2977S.

59. Brigelius-Flohe, R., Banning, A. Part of the series: from dietary antioxidants to regulators in cellular signaling and gene regulation. Sulforaphane and selenium, partners in adaptive response and prevention of cancer. *Free Radic Res*, 2006. **40**(8): 775–87.

60. Zhang, J. et al. Synergy between sulforaphane and selenium in the induction of thioredoxin reductase 1 requires both transcriptional and translational modulation. *Carcinogenesis*, 2003. **24**(3): 497–503.

61. Seeram, N.P. et al. In vitro antiproliferative, apoptotic and antioxidant activities of punicalagin, ellagic acid and a total pomegranate tannin extract are enhanced in combination with other polyphenols as found in pomegranate juice. *J Nutr Biochem*, 2005. **16**(6): 360–7.

62. de Beer, D. et al. Unravelling the total antioxidant capacity of pinotage wines: contribution of phenolic compounds. *J Agric Food Chem*, 2006. **54**(8): 2897–905.

63. Basu, A., Imrhan, V. Tomatoes versus lycopene in oxidative stress and carcinogenesis: conclusions from clinical trials. *Eur J Clin Nutr*, 2007. **61**(3): 295–303.

64. Shi, J. et al. Stability and synergistic effect of antioxidative properties of lycopene and other active components. *Crit Rev Food Sci Nutr*, 2004. **44**(7–8): 559–73.

65. Fini, L. et al. Chemopreventive properties of pinoresinol-rich olive oil involve a selective activation of the ATM-p53 cascade in colon cancer cell lines. *Carcinogenesis*, 2008. **29**(1): 139–46.

66. Kristal, A.R., Lippman, S.M. Nutritional prevention of cancer: new directions for an increasingly complex challenge. *J Natl Cancer Inst*, 2009. **101**(6): 363–5.

67. Howells, L.M. et al. Predicting the physiological relevance of in vitro cancer preventive activities of phytochemicals. *Acta Pharmacol Sin*, 2007. **28**(9): 1274–304.

68. Vastag, B. Nutrients for prevention: negative trials send researchers back to drawing board. *J Natl Cancer Inst*, 2009. **101**(7): 446–8, 451.

69. Theodoratou, E. et al. Dietary fatty acids and colorectal cancer: a case-control study. *Am J Epidemiol*, 2007. **166**(2): 181–95.

70. Gerber, M. Background review paper on total fat, fatty acid intake and cancers. *Ann Nutr Metab*, 2009. **55**(1–3): 140–61.

71. Prentice, R.L. et al. Low-fat dietary pattern and risk of invasive breast cancer: the Women's Health Initiative Randomized Controlled Dietary Modification Trial. *Jama*, 2006. **295**(6): 629–42.

72. Chlebowski, R.T. et al. Dietary fat reduction and breast cancer outcome: interim efficacy results from the Women's Intervention Nutrition Study. *J Natl Cancer Inst*, 2006. **98**(24): 1767–76.

73. Gerber, M. et al. Dietary fat, fatty acid composition and risk of cancer. *Eur J Lipid Sci Technol*, 2005. **107**: 540–559.

74. Wang, J. et al. Dietary fat, cooking fat, and breast cancer risk in a multiethnic population. *Nutr Cancer*, 2008. **60**(4): 492–504.

75. Thiebaut, A.C. et al. Dietary fat and postmenopausal invasive breast cancer in the National Institutes of Health-AARP Diet and Health Study cohort. *J Natl Cancer Inst*, 2007. **99**(6): 451–62.

76. Martin-Moreno, J.M. et al. Dietary fat, olive oil intake and breast cancer risk. *Int J Cancer*, 1994. **58**(6): 774–80.

77. Trichopoulou, A. et al. Consumption of olive oil and specific food groups in relation to breast cancer risk in Greece. *J Natl Cancer Inst*, 1995. **87**(2): 110–6.

78. Bessaoud, F. et al. Dietary factors and breast cancer risk: a case control study among a population in Southern France. *Nutr Cancer*, 2008. **60**(2): 177–87.

79. Garcia-Segovia, P. et al. Olive oil consumption and risk of breast cancer in the Canary Islands: a population-based case-control study. *Public Health Nutr*, 2006. **9**(1A): 163–7.

80. Gerber, M. Olive oil, monounsaturated fatty acids and cancer. *Cancer Lett*, 1997. **114**(1–2): 91–2.

81. Beauchamp, G.K. et al. Phytochemistry: ibuprofen-like activity in extra-virgin olive oil. *Nature*, 2005. **437**(7055): 45–6.

82. Rasmussen, O. et al. Differential effects of saturated and monounsaturated fat on blood glucose and insulin responses in subjects with non-insulin-dependent diabetes mellitus. *Am J Clin Nutr*, 1996. **63**(2): 249–53.

83. Thiebaut, A.C. et al. Dietary intakes of omega-6 and omega-3 polyunsaturated fatty acids and the risk of breast cancer. *Int J Cancer*, 2009. **124**(4): 924–31.

84. WCRF/AICR, World Cancer Research Fund/American Institute for Cancer Research. *Food, nutrition, physical activity, and the prevention of cancer: a global perspective.* 2007, AICR: Washington DC.

85. Mozaffarian, D. et al. Health effects of trans-fatty acids: experimental and observational evidence. *Eur J Clin Nutr*, 2009. **63 Suppl 2**: S5–21.

86. Bingham, S.A. et al. Dietary fibre in food and protection against colorectal cancer in the European Prospective Investigation into Cancer and Nutrition (EPIC): an observational study. *Lancet*, 2003. **361**(9368): 1496–501.

87. Schatzkin, A. et al. Dietary fiber and whole-grain consumption in relation to colorectal cancer in the NIH-AARP Diet and Health Study. *Am J Clin Nutr*, 2007. **85**(5): 1353–60.

88. Park, Y. et al. Dietary fiber intake and risk of colorectal cancer: a pooled analysis of prospective cohort studies. *Jama*, 2005. **294**(22): 2849–57.

89. Dahm, C.C. et al. Dietary fiber and colorectal cancer risk: a nested case-control study using food diaries. *J Natl Cancer Inst*, 2010. **102**(9): 614–26.

90. Bingham, S.A. et al. Are imprecise methods obscuring a relation between fat and breast cancer? *Lancet*, 2003. **362**(9379): 212–4.

91. Gerber, M. Fiber and breast cancer: another piece of the puzzle–but still an incomplete picture. *J Natl Cancer Inst*, 1996. **88**(13): 857–8.

92. Park, Y. et al. Dietary fiber intake and risk of breast cancer in postmenopausal women: the National Institutes of Health-AARP Diet and Health Study. *Am J Clin Nutr*, 2009. **90**(3): 664–71.

93. Perrin, P. et al. Only fibres promoting a stable butyrate producing colonic ecosystem decrease the rate of aberrant crypt foci in rats. *Gut*, 2001. **48**(1): 53–61.

94. Ziegler, R.G. et al. Nutrition and lung cancer. *Cancer Causes Control*, 1996. **7**(1): 157–77.

95. Peto, R. et al. Can dietary beta-carotene materially reduce human cancer rates? *Nature*, 1981. **290**(5803): 201–8.

96. Albanes, D. et al. Effects of alpha-tocopherol and beta-carotene supplements on cancer incidence in the Alpha-Tocopherol Beta-Carotene Cancer Prevention Study. *Am J Clin Nutr*, 1995. **62**(6 Suppl): 427S–1430S.

97. Omenn, G.S. et al. Risk factors for lung cancer and for intervention effects in CARET, the Beta-Carotene and Retinol Efficacy Trial. *J Natl Cancer Inst*, 1996. **88**(21): 1550–9.

98. Cook, N.R. et al. Effects of beta-carotene supplementation on cancer incidence by baseline characteristics in the Physicians' Health Study (United States). *Cancer Causes Control*, 2000. **11**(7): 617–26.

99. Gerber, M. et al. Re: Beta-carotene: a miss for epidemiology. *J Natl Cancer Inst*, 2000. **92**(12): 1014–6.

100. Omaye, S.T. et al. Beta-carotene: friend or foe? *Fundam Appl Toxicol*, 1997. **40**(2): 163–74.

101. Palozza, P. et al. Prooxidant activity of beta-carotene under 100% oxygen pressure in rat liver microsomes. *Free Radic Biol Med*, 1995. **19**(6): 887–92.

102. Touvier, M. et al. Dual association of beta-carotene with risk of tobacco-related cancers in a cohort of French women. *J Natl Cancer Inst*, 2005. **97**(18): 1338–44.

103. Blot, W.J. et al. Nutrition intervention trials in Linxian, China: supplementation with specific vitamin/mineral combinations, cancer incidence, and disease-specific mortality in the general population. *J Natl Cancer Inst*, 1993. **85**(18): 1483–92.

104. Hercberg, S. et al. The SU.VI.MAX Study: a randomized, placebo-controlled trial of the health effects of antioxidant vitamins and minerals. *Arch Intern Med*, 2004. **164**(21): 335–42.

105. Ezzedine, K. et al. Incidence of skin cancers during 5-year follow-up after stopping antioxidant vitamins and mineral supplementation. *Eur J Cancer*, 2010. **46** (18): 3316–22.

106. Hercberg, S. et al. Antioxidant supplementation increases the risk of skin cancers in women but not in men. *J Nutr*, 2007. **137**(9): 2098–105.

107. Meyer, F. et al. Antioxidant vitamin and mineral supplementation and prostate cancer prevention in the SU.VI.MAX trial. *Int J Cancer*, 2005. **116**(2): 182–6.

108. Saintot, M. et al. Oxidant-antioxidant status in relation to survival among breast cancer patients. *Int J Cancer*, 2002. **97**(5): 574–9.

109. Lippman, S.M. et al. Effect of selenium and vitamin E on risk of prostate cancer and other cancers: the Selenium and Vitamin E Cancer Prevention Trial (SELECT). *Jama*, 2009. **301**(1): 39–51.

110. Bougnoux, P. n-3 polyunsaturated fatty acids and cancer. *Curr Opin Clin Nutr Metab Care*, 1999. **2**(2): 121–6.

111. Knekt, P. et al. Dietary flavonoids and the risk of lung cancer and other malignant neoplasms. *Am J Epidemiol*, 1997. **146**(3): 223–30.

112. Wang, L. et al. Dietary intake of selected flavonols, flavones, and flavonoid-rich foods and risk of cancer in middle-aged and older women. *Am J Clin Nutr*, 2009. **89**(3): 905–12.

113. Touillaud, M.S. et al. Dietary lignan intake and postmenopausal breast cancer risk by estrogen and progesterone receptor status. *J Natl Cancer Inst*, 2007. **99**(6): 475–86.

114. Buck, K. et al. Meta-analyses of lignans and enterolignans in relation to breast cancer risk. *Am J Clin Nutr*, 2010. **92**(1): 141–53.

115. Saarinen, N.M. et al. Role of dietary lignans in the reduction of breast cancer risk. *Mol Nutr Food Res*, 2007. **51**(7): 857–66.

116. Brooks, J.D. et al. Supplementation with flaxseed alters estrogen metabolism in postmenopausal women to a greater extent than does supplementation with an equal amount of soy. *Am J Clin Nutr*, 2004. **79**(2): 318–25.

117. McCann, S.E. et al. Changes in 2-hydroxyestrone and 16alpha-hydroxyestrone metabolism with flaxseed consumption: modification by COMT and CYP1B1 genotype. *Cancer Epidemiol Biomarkers Prev*, 2007. **16**(2): 256–62.

118. Wynder, E.L. et al. Nutrition and prostate cancer: a proposal for dietary intervention. *Nutr Cancer*, 1994. **22**(1): 1–10.

119. Baron, J.A. et al. Calcium supplements for the prevention of colorectal adenomas. Calcium Polyp Prevention Study Group. *N Engl J Med*, 1999. **340**(2): 101–7.

120. Bonithon-Kopp, C. et al. Calcium and fibre supplementation in prevention of colorectal adenoma recurrence: a randomised intervention trial. European Cancer Prevention Organisation Study Group. *Lancet*, 2000. **356**(9238): 1300–6.

121. Ahn, J. et al. Dairy products, calcium intake, and risk of prostate cancer in the prostate, lung, colorectal, and ovarian cancer screening trial. *Cancer Epidemiol Biomarkers Prev*, 2007. **16**(12): 2623–30.

122. Raimondi, S. et al. Diet and prostate cancer risk with specific focus on dairy products and dietary calcium: a case-control study. *Prostate*, 2010. **70**(10): 1054–65.

123. Tavani, A. et al. Calcium, dairy products, and the risk of prostate cancer. *Prostate*, 2001. **48**(2): 118–21.

124. Baron, J.A. et al. Risk of prostate cancer in a randomized clinical trial of calcium supplementation. *Cancer Epidemiol Biomarkers Prev*, 2005. **14**(3): 586–9.

125. Gropper, S.S. et al. *Advanced nutrition and human metabolism.* 5th ed. 2009, Belmont, Calif.; London: Wadsworth/Thomson Learning.

126. Rizzoli, R. et al. Maximizing bone mineral mass gain during growth for the prevention of fractures in the adolescents and the elderly. *Bone*, 2009. **46**(2): 294–305.

127. Qin, L.Q. et al. Milk consumption and circulating insulin-like growth factor-I level: a systematic literature review. *Int J Food Sci Nutr*, 2009. **60 Suppl 7**: 330–40.

128. Takenaka, A. et al. Dietary restriction of single essential amino acids reduces plasma insulin-like growth factor-I (IGF-I) but does not affect plasma IGF-binding protein-1 in rats. *J Nutr*, 2000. **130**(12): 2910–4.

129. Itsiopoulos, C. et al. Can the Mediterranean diet prevent prostate cancer? *Mol Nutr Food Res*, 2009. **53**(2): 227–39.

130. Lippmann, S.M. et al. Effect of selenium and vitamin E on risk of prostate cancer and other cancers: The selenium and vitamin E cancer prevention trial (SELECT). *Jama*, 2009. **301**(1): 39–51.

131. Boehm, K. et al. Green tea (Camellia sinensis) for the prevention of cancer. *Cochrane Database Syst Rev*, 2009(3): CD005004.

132. Brausi, M.et al. Chemoprevention of human prostate cancer by green tea catechins: two years later. A follow-up update. *Eur Urol*, 2008. **54**(2): 472–3.

133. Yang, C.S. et al. Cancer prevention by tea and tea polyphenols. *Asia Pac J Clin Nutr*, 2008. **17 Suppl 1**: 245–8.

134. Yang, C.S. et al. Cancer prevention by tea: animal studies, molecular mechanisms and human relevance. *Nat Rev Cancer*, 2009. **9**(6): 429–39.

135. Gardner, E.J. et al. Black tea – helpful or harmful? A review of the evidence. *Eur J Clin Nutr*, 2007. **61**(1): 3–18.

136. Han, K.C. et al. Genoprotective effects of green tea (Camellia sinensis) in human subjects: results of a controlled supplementation trial. *Br J Nutr*, 2010: 1–8.

137. Tachibana, H. et al. A receptor for green tea polyphenol EGCG. *Nat Struct Mol Biol*, 2004. **11**(4): 380–1.

138. Tachibana, H. Molecular basis for cancer chemoprevention by green tea polyphenol EGCG. *Forum Nutr*, 2009. **61**: 156–69.
139. Cavin, C. et al. Cafestol and kahweol, two coffee specific diterpenes with anticarcinogenic activity. *Food Chem Toxicol*, 2002. **40**(8): 1155–63.
140. Je, Y. et al. Coffee consumption and risk of colorectal cancer: a systematic review and meta-analysis of prospective cohort studies. *Int J Cancer*, 2009. **124**(7): 1662–8.
141. Sieri, S. et al. Patterns of alcohol consumption in 10 European countries participating in the European Prospective Investigation into Cancer and Nutrition (EPIC) project. *Public Health Nutr*, 2002. **5**(6B): 1287–96.
142. Ferraroni, M. et al. Alcohol and breast cancer risk: a case-control study from northern Italy. *Int J Epidemiol*, 1991. **20**(4): 859–64.
143. Richardson, S. et al. Alcohol consumption in a case-control study of breast cancer in southern France. *Int J Cancer*, 1989. **44**(1): 84–9.
144. Bessaoud, F., Daures, J.P. Patterns of alcohol (especially wine) consumption and breast cancer risk: a case-control study among a population in Southern France. *Ann Epidemiol*, 2008. **18**(6): 467–75.
145. Tseng, M. et al. Mediterranean diet and breast density in the Minnesota Breast Cancer Family Study. *Nutr Cancer*, 2008. **60**(6): 703–9.
146. Gonzalez, C.A. The European Prospective Investigation into Cancer and Nutrition (EPIC). *Public Health Nutr*, 2006. **9**(1A): 124–6.
147. EPIC. *Key findings* [cited]. Available from: http://www.iarc.fr/epic/S.
148. Ferrari, P. et al. Lifetime and baseline alcohol intake and risk of colon and rectal cancers in the European prospective investigation into cancer and nutrition (EPIC). *Int J Cancer*, 2007. **121** (9): 2065–72.
149. Allen, N.E. et al. Moderate alcohol intake and cancer incidence in women. *J Natl Cancer Inst*, 2009. **101**(5): 296–305.
150. Li, Y. et al. Wine, liquor, beer and risk of breast cancer in a large population. *Eur J Cancer*, 2009. **45**(5): 843–50.
151. Tjonneland, A. et al. Alcohol intake and breast cancer risk: the European Prospective Investigation into Cancer and Nutrition (EPIC). *Cancer Causes Control*, 2007. **18**(4): 361–73.
152. Sutcliffe, S. et al. A prospective cohort study of red wine consumption and risk of prostate cancer. *Int J Cancer*, 2007. **120**(7): 1529–35.
153. Poschl, G., Seitz, H.K. Alcohol and cancer. *Alcohol Alcohol*, 2004. **39**(3): 155–65.
154. Jelski, W., Szmitkowski, M. Alcohol dehydrogenase (ADH) and aldehyde dehydrogenase (ALDH) in the cancer diseases. *Clin Chim Acta*, 2008. **395**(1–2): 1–5.
155. Lachenmeier, D.W., Sohnius, E.M. The role of acetaldehyde outside ethanol metabolism in the carcinogenicity of alcoholic beverages: evidence from a large chemical survey. *Food Chem Toxicol*, 2008. **46**(8): 2903–11.
156. Seitz, H.K., Maurer, B. The relationship between alcohol metabolism, estrogen levels, and breast cancer risk. *Alcohol Res Health*, 2007. **30**(1): 42–3.
157. Carruba, G. et al. A traditional Mediterranean diet decreases endogenous estrogens in healthy postmenopausal women. *Nutr Cancer*, 2006. **56**(2): 253–9.
158. Baglietto, L. et al. Does dietary folate intake modify effect of alcohol consumption on breast cancer risk? Prospective cohort study. *BMJ*, 2005. **331**(7520): 807.
159. Negri, E. et al. Re: dietary folate consumption and breast cancer risk. *J Natl Cancer Inst*, 2000. **92**(15): 1270–1.
160. Rohan, T.E. et al. Dietary folate consumption and breast cancer risk. *J Natl Cancer Inst*, 2000. **92**(3): 266–9.
161. La Vecchia, C. et al. Dietary folate and colorectal cancer. *Int J Cancer*, 2002. **102**(5): 545–7.
162. Navarro Silvera, S.A. et al. Dietary folate consumption and risk of ovarian cancer: a prospective cohort study. *Eur J Cancer Prev*, 2006. **15**(6): 511–5.
163. Bach-Faig, A. et al. Evaluating associations between Mediterranean diet adherence indexes and biomarkers of diet and disease. *Public Health Nutr*, 2006. **9**(8A): 1110–7.
164. Gerber, M. Biofactors in the Mediterranean diet. *Clin Chem Lab Med*, 2003. **41**(8): 999–1004.
165. Modun, D. et al. The increase in human plasma antioxidant capacity after red wine consumption is due to both plasma urate and wine polyphenols. *Atherosclerosis*, 2008. **197**(1): 250–6.
166. Nothlings, U. et al. Intake of vegetables, legumes, and fruit, and risk for all-cause, cardiovascular, and cancer mortality in a European diabetic population. *J Nutr*, 2008. **138**(4): 775–81.

167. Boffetta, P. et al. Fruit and vegetable intake and overall cancer risk in the European Prospective Investigation into Cancer and Nutrition (EPIC). *J Natl Cancer Inst*, 2010. **102**(8): 529–37.
168. Buchner, F.L. et al. Fruits and vegetables consumption and the risk of histological subtypes of lung cancer in the European Prospective Investigation into Cancer and Nutrition (EPIC). *Cancer Causes Control*, 2010. **21**(3): 357–71.
169. van Duijnhoven, F.J. et al. Fruit, vegetables, and colorectal cancer risk: the European Prospective Investigation into Cancer and Nutrition. *Am J Clin Nutr*, 2009. **89**(5): 1441–52.
170. Galeone, C. et al. Onion and garlic use and human cancer. *Am J Clin Nutr*, 2006. **84**(5): 1027–32.
171. Sivam, G.P. Protection against Helicobacter pylori and other bacterial infections by garlic. *J Nutr*, 2001. **131**(3s): 1106S–8S.
172. Kim, J.Y., Kwon, O. Garlic intake and cancer risk: an analysis using the Food and Drug Administration's evidence-based review system for the scientific evaluation of health claims. *Am J Clin Nutr*, 2009. **89**(1): 257–64.
173. Trichopoulou, A. et al. Anatomy of health effects of Mediterranean diet: Greek EPIC prospective cohort study. *BMJ*, 2009. **338**: b2337.
174. Gonzalez, C.A., Salas-Salvado, J. The potential of nuts in the prevention of cancer. *Br J Nutr*, 2006. **96 Suppl 2**: S87–94.
175. Kavanaugh, C.J. et al. The U.S. Food and Drug Administration's evidence-based review for qualified health claims: tomatoes, lycopene, and cancer. *J Natl Cancer Inst*, 2007. **99**(14): 1074–85.
176. Bosetti, C. et al. Fraction of prostate cancer incidence attributed to diet in Athens, Greece. *Eur J Cancer Prev*, 2000. **9**(2): 119–23.
177. Jenab, M. et al. Variations in lycopene blood levels and tomato consumption across European countries based on the European Prospective Investigation into Cancer and Nutrition (EPIC) study. *J Nutr*, 2005. **135**(8): 2032S–6S.
178. Bogani, P., Visioli, F. Antioxidants in the Mediterranean diets: an update. *World Rev Nutr Diet*, 2007. **97**: 162–79.
179. Fielding, J.M. et al. Increases in plasma lycopene concentration after consumption of tomatoes cooked with olive oil. *Asia Pac J Clin Nutr*, 2005. **14**(2): 131–6.
180. van Het Hof, K.H. et al. Dietary factors that affect the bioavailability of carotenoids. *J Nutr*, 2000. **130**(3): 503–6.
181. Schatzkin, A. et al. Lack of effect of a low-fat, high-fiber diet on the recurrence of colorectal adenomas. Polyp Prevention Trial Study Group. *N Engl J Med*, 2000. **342**(16): 1149–55.
182. Peters, U. et al. Dietary fibre and colorectal adenoma in a colorectal cancer early detection programme. *Lancet*, 2003. **361**(9368): 1491–5.
183. Pierce, J.P. et al. Influence of a diet very high in vegetables, fruit, and fiber and low in fat on prognosis following treatment for breast cancer: the Women's Healthy Eating and Living (WHEL) randomized trial. *Jama*, 2007. **298**(3): 289–98.
184. Rock, C.L. et al. Longitudinal biological exposure to carotenoids is associated with breast cancer-free survival in the Women's Healthy Eating and Living Study. *Cancer Epidemiol Biomarkers Prev*, 2009. **18**(2): 486–94.
185. Trichopoulou, A. et al. Adherence to a Mediterranean diet and survival in a Greek population. *N Engl J Med*, 2003. **348**(26): 2599–608.
186. Trichopoulou, A. et al. Conformity to traditional Mediterranean diet and breast cancer risk in the Greek EPIC (European Prospective Investigation into Cancer and nutrition) cohort. *Am J Clin Nutr*, 2010. doi: 10.3945/ajcn.2010.29619.
187. Fung, T.T. et al. Dietary patterns and the risk of postmenopausal breast cancer. *Int J Cancer*, 2005. **116**(1): 116–21.
188. Fung, T.T. et al. Diet quality is associated with the risk of estrogen receptor-negative breast cancer in postmenopausal women. *J Nutr*, 2006. **136**(2): 466–72.
189. Mitrou, P.N. et al. Mediterranean dietary pattern and prediction of all-cause mortality in a US population: results from the NIH-AARP Diet and Health Study. *Arch Intern Med*, 2007. **167**(22): 2461–8.
190. Sofi, F. et al. Adherence to Mediterranean diet and health status: meta-analysis. *BMJ*, 2008. **337**: a1344.
191. Buckland, G. et al. Adherence to a Mediterranean diet and risk of gastric adenocarcinoma within the European Prospective Investigation into Cancer and Nutrition (EPIC) cohort study. *Am J Clin Nutr*, 2010. **91**(2): 381–90.

192. Knoops, K.T. et al. Mediterranean diet, lifestyle factors, and 10-year mortality in elderly European men and women: the HALE project. *Jama*, 2004. **292**(12): 1433–9.
193. Naska, A. et al. Siesta in healthy adults and coronary mortality in the general population. *Arch Intern Med*, 2007. **167**(3): 296–301.
194. Tessier, S., Gerber, M. Comparison between Sardinia and Malta: the Mediterranean diet revisited. *Appetite*, 2005. **45**(2): 121–6.
195. Hu, F.B., Willett, W.C. Optimal diets for prevention of coronary heart disease. *Jama*, 2002. **288**(20): 2569–78.
196. De Stefani, E. et al. Dietary patterns and risk of cancer: a factor analysis in Uruguay. *Int J Cancer*, 2009. **124**(6): 1391–7.
197. Slattery, M.L. et al. Eating patterns and risk of colon cancer. *Am J Epidemiol*, 1998. **148**(1): 4–16.
198. Terry, P. et al. Prospective study of major dietary patterns and colorectal cancer risk in women. *Am J Epidemiol*, 2001. **154**(12): 1143–9.
199. Wu, K. et al. Dietary patterns and risk of colon cancer and adenoma in a cohort of men (United States). *Cancer Causes Control*, 2004. **15**(9): 853–62.
200. Siari, S. et al. Subregional variations of dietary consumption and incidences of cancer in Southern France. In: *Nutrition and lifestyle: opportunities for cancer prevention*, ed. E. Riboli and R. Lambert. 2002, Lyon: International Agency for Research on Cancer; Oxford: Oxford University Press [distributor], xiv.
201. Kesse, E. et al. Dietary patterns and risk of colorectal tumors: a cohort of French women of the National Education System (E3N). *Am J Epidemiol*, 2006. **164**(11): 1085–93.
202. Adebamowo, C.A. et al. Dietary patterns and the risk of breast cancer. *Ann Epidemiol*, 2005. **15**(10): 789–95.
203. Sieri, S. et al. Dietary patterns and risk of breast cancer in the ORDET cohort. *Cancer Epidemiol Biomarkers Prev*, 2004. **13**(4): 567–72.
204. Cottet, V. et al. Postmenopausal breast cancer risk and dietary patterns in the E3N-EPIC prospective cohort study. *Am J Epidemiol*, 2009. **170**(10): 1257–67.

13 Neurological and Other Disorders

Summary

- A few prospective studies have demonstrated that a MedDiet reduces the risk for Alzheimer's disease, and although the results of these studies need confirmation, the quality of the data is good. Constituents found in Mediterranean foods that may explain the reduced risk for pre-dementia or dementia include moderate amounts of alcohol and red wine, MUFAs and n-3 fatty acids, vitamin B12 and folates, and antioxidants.
- Studies on Parkinson's disease and depression are limited at present.
- The immunosuppressive effects of FAs in fish and olive oil may be of benefit in rheumatoid arthritis although epidemiological studies in relation to the MedDiet are limited. Vitamin D synthesis is a possible protective mechanism in sunny Mediterranean countries and warrants further study.
- Constituents in the MedDiet linked with possible protection against age-related macular degeneration include lutein, zeaxanthin and DHA, although epidemiological studies in relation to the MedDiet are very limited.
- Studies convincingly show that a MedDiet is associated with a reduced risk of all cause mortality, and MDS and M-MDS are consistently associated with reductions in all cause mortality, with a higher percentage reduction in Greece than when the M-MDS is applied to non-Mediterranean countries.

13.1 Introduction

Although the role of diet in neurological disorders has not received the same kind of attention given to cancer and heart disease, this is now changing. One reason for this is that current drug treatments are not very effective and so alternative approaches are needed in order to prevent and manage these disorders. There is increasing evidence that some foods are essential for normal brain function such as memory, and that poor nutrition contributes to neurological disorders such as dementias, attention-deficit hyperactivity disorder, dyslexia, depression, schizophrenia and Parkinson's disease [1]. In relation to the MedDiet, most studies have focussed on dementias, Parkinson's disease and, to a lesser extent, on depression. Neurological disorders are multifactorial, and other important factors include age, poor vascular conditions in the brain and genetic background.

For the other disorders discussed in this chapter, epidemiological information in relation to the Mediterranean dietary pattern is at present very limited, although

The Mediterranean Diet: Health and Science, First Edition. Richard Hoffman and Mariette Gerber.
© 2012 Richard Hoffman and Mariette Gerber. Published 2012 by Blackwell Publishing Ltd.

certain nutrients found in the MedDiet have shown positive benefits in experimental and epidemiological studies.

13.2   Dementias

13.2.1   Introduction

Dementia is a syndrome associated with impairment of memory and of other cognitive functions that are severe enough to cause significant decline from a previous level of social and occupational functioning. A loss of weight may also accompany Alzheimer's disease (AD), although it is not known whether this is an early symptom or whether it follows on from alteration in cerebral functions. Dementias affect about 1 in 20 people in the UK aged 65 and over and this figure rises significantly with increasing age [2]. One in three older people will end their life with a form of dementia, and the Alzheimer's Society estimates that there are currently over 700,000 people in the UK with dementia. Caring for someone with dementia also has a deep impact on the caregiver. As poignantly stated by the Alzheimer's Society: "dementia is not just a little bit of memory loss; it gradually robs people of their lives" [3].

The most common causes of dementia are AD, a neurodegenerative disorder in the brain accounting for about 70% of cases, and vascular dementia, a cerebro-vascular disorder accounting for about 15% of cases. Symptoms of AD include loss of memory, confusion and problems with speech and understanding. It is often difficult to distinguish between a normal decline in cognitive performance with ageing and decline which is a forerunner of disease (a so-called prodromal effect). Mild memory or cognitive impairment that cannot be accounted for by any recognised medical or psychiatric condition is sometimes referred to as mild cognitive impairment (MCI). MCI is thought to represent a predementia syndrome for AD [4]. Age-related cognitive decline (ARCD), on the other hand, is generally considered as a non-progressive syndrome, that is, as a part of normal ageing [4]. There is a strong genetic component to AD, subjects bearing the ε4 allele of the apolipoproteine E (apoE) being more at risk. But environmental factors should also be considered, and certain metals are suspected, especially aluminium.

13.2.2   Epidemiology

Studies examining the relationship between diet and dementias have used various end-points: preventing the development of MCI, prevention of the progression of MCI to full dementia and prevention of the development of AD. Epidemiological evidence suggests that the MedDiet is likely to be more effective at reversing MCI to normal cognitive function rather than reversing later stages of dementia. Since possession of the ε4 allele for the apoE gene is a risk factor for AD, this confounding factor is adjusted for in studies examining the relationship between diet and AD.

Wine and alcohol

A number of epidemiological studies have investigated the relationship between alcohol consumption and neurodegenerative disorders, with some studies suggesting a J-shaped relationship, i.e. moderate alcohol consumption is more beneficial than none, or excessive, intake [4]. Beneficial effects of moderate consumption have been seen in relation to reducing mild cognitive impairment (MCI) (a predementia state), progression of MCI to dementias and Parkinson's disease [4, 5]. Controlling for other sources of alcohol, moderate wine consumption was found to be significantly associated with a lower rate of progression to dementia in individuals with MCI although there may be residual confounding factors [6]. Of course, high intake of alcohol impairs some short-term brain functions such as psychomotor activity and information processing.

The mechanistic basis for the potential neuroprotective effects of moderate alcohol consumption are currently unknown but could be related to a reduction in risk factors for vascular disease and/or by increasing production of acetylcholine, a neurotransmitter important for memory performance [4]. Antioxidant phenolics in red wine may afford additional protection since oxidative stress is associated with several neurodegenerative disorders such as AD (see Section 13.2.3).

Dietary pattern

A limited number of prospective studies have examined the relationship between MDS and dementias. A study in the US (WHICAP, an ageing project in various counties of New York state) first considered the incidence of AD in a cohort of 2258 subjects for which a consensus diagnosis of AD was made after several cognitive tests [7]. There were 262 cases of AD during the course of four years of follow-up. Each additional unit of the non-modified MDS was associated with a 9–10% reduced risk of developing AD (HR 0.91: CI 0.83–0.98). Compared with subjects in the lowest MD-QI tertile, subjects in the highest tertile had an HR of 0.60 (CI 0.42–0.87) for AD (p for trend=0.007). The same authors then undertook an analysis on risk of mortality [8]. These analyses were restricted to 471 subjects diagnosed with AD at the baseline of the WHICAP evaluation. Of the subjects, 192 remained available for the final analyses after exclusion requirements. Eighty-five patients with AD (44%) died during the course of 4.4 years of follow-up. Higher adherence to the non-modified MDS, as assessed statistically by a continuous model using increments of one point in the MDS, was associated with lower mortality risk (HR 0.76: CI 0.65–0.89 in fully adjusted models). Compared with AD patients in the lowest non-modified MDS adherence tertile, those in the highest tertile had lower risk with a 3.91 year longer survival (HR 0.27: CI 0.10–0.69, p for trend=0.003). The results of these studies need confirmation, but are very impressive in relation to the quality of the data. In a continuation of this study, there was less risk of MCI progressing to AD in individuals who adhered to a MedDiet (45% and 48% less risk in the middle and upper tertiles respectively compared to the lowest tertile) [9]. Physical activity was also independently associated with a lower risk of developing AD in this study [10].

A second prospective study conducted in France produced different results. Higher adherence to the MedDiet was significantly associated with better global cognitive performances and episodic memory [11]. However, there was no association between adherence to a MedDiet and risk of dementia or AD. The authors of this study have discussed possible reasons for discrepancies between the US and French studies [12]. These include:

(a) a longer follow-up in the US study – the MedDiet may need to be consumed at least five years before the onset of clinical symptoms of dementia.

(b) French individuals in the lowest tertile of consumption of a MedDiet may correspond to the middle or upper tertile in the US study – hence the French may have had better protection against dementia from their diet.

13.2.3 Mechanisms

It is interesting that several studies have found that subjects at risk for dementia presented with several components of metabolic syndrome [13]. This suggests that common mechanisms may underlie these two disorders. Pre-disease states associated with both metabolic syndrome and dementia include inflammation, insulin resistance and adiposity [13]. This common ground also provides a framework for understanding why similar nutrients may afford protection against both disorders. In addition, the well-established protective effects of the MedDiet against CVD may also be important for protecting against vascular dementia. Constituents found in Mediterranean foods that have been linked to a reduced risk for MCI or dementia (mainly AD) include moderate amounts of alcohol and red wine, MUFAs and n-3 fatty acids, vitamin B12 and folates, and antioxidants [14]. Generally, the evidence for a benefit from individual constituents is weaker than when the whole dietary pattern is considered. AD is considered to be a multifactorial disease, and it has been argued that this can explain why a broad dietary regime, where nutrients can interact in additive and synergistic ways, is more effective than a single nutrient [15]. However, since current understanding of these interactions is limited, most of the following discussion is limited to individual nutrients.

Fatty acids

The Italian Longitudinal Study on Aging (ILSA) found that a high intake of MUFAs and PUFAs was associated with a significantly better cognitive performance in individuals with ARCD [4]. By contrast, animal studies indicate that SFAs may adversely affect cognitive function [4]. In the Greek cohort of the EPIC study there was evidence that polyunsaturated fats found in seed oils decreased cognitive performance [16].

Particular attention has focussed on the PUFA DHA, since this fatty acid comprises up to 60% of the total fatty acids in the phospholipids of neuronal cell membranes [17]. Numerous studies have found that individuals with a deficiency of DHA are at increased risk of cognitive decline and AD [18]. Intervention studies aimed at slowing or reversing cognitive decline or early stages of AD have examined consumption of fish – the major dietary source of DHA, or supplementation with DHA. Whereas there is good evidence that dietary fish is effective at reversing the decline in cognitive function, the evidence from studies with DHA supplementation are less consistent [18].

Several mechanisms have been proposed to explain the protective effects of DHA against dementias [18]:

1. Maintaining the correct fluidity of neuronal membranes. DHA is highly enriched in the phospholipid bilayer of neuronal membranes.
2. Reducing the production of amyloid-β (Aβ) peptide. Aβ is the major constituent of senile plaques. These accumulate in the brain in early stages of AD and are strongly implicated in the pathology of this disease.
3. Generating various neuroprotective metabolites from DHA (so-called docosanoids), especially neuroprotectin D1 (NPD1). NPD1 is produced by the

enzymatic oxidation of DHA. It reduces Aβ secretion and also has anti-apoptotic effects thus decreasing neuronal cell death.

4. Generating anti-inflammatory mediators (Chapter 9).
5. Maintaining a healthy cardiovascular system (Chapter 11).
6. Decreasing oxidative stress (see below).

Evolution, DHA and brain development

It has been hypothesised that having a good food source of DHA during hominid evolution played a key role in increasing the brain/body-mass ratio (a process known as encephalisation) [19]. Hence it is possible that a shore-based diet giving access to seafood rich in DHA was indispensable for hominid encephalisation. It is now considered that DHA is essential for brain development in children.

Anti-oxidants

Oxidative stress is thought to contribute to a wide range of neurological disorders including AD and Parkinson's disease [20]. Oxidative stress is found in the brain in early stages of cognitive decline related to dementia, and this is thought to be at least in part caused by the accumulation of Aβ. Hence, it has been proposed that various dietary antioxidants present in the MedDiet may help prevent these disorders.

One antioxidant that may help protect against oxidative stress is DHA [18]. However, DHA, being a PUFA, is also very prone to being oxidised by free radicals, a process termed lipid peroxidation. This is a non-enzymatic process, and is distinct from the *enzymatic* oxidation of DHA which can generate beneficial products such as NPD1. Some of the oxidation products of DHA generated by lipid peroxidation (known as neuroprostanes) are very damaging and have been implicated in the pathology of AD [21]. Hence it has been argued that DHA supplements may be more effective when given in combination with antioxidants [22]. In support of this proposal, one study found that cognitive functioning in elderly women was improved with a combination of DHA and the antioxidant carotenoid lutein [23]. Since the MedDiet is rich in antioxidants, these could conceivably help prevent adverse oxidation of DHA by free radicals.

In addition to DHA, several other antioxidants present in the MedDiet have been linked to improved cognitive function, including wine polyphenols, vitamin E, lipoic acid and flavonoids from berries [19]. These studies have mostly used individual antioxidants, and possible synergistic effects between antioxidants and DHA have not been evaluated – although this situation is relevant to the overall MedDiet. An additional consideration of importance in relation to the role of antioxidants in neurological disorders is establishing that the antioxidants cross the blood–brain barrier and reach the brain in sufficient quantities [24, 25]. Olive oil consumption is also linked with a reduced incidence of MCI and it has been suggested that it could be acting in combination with other dietary antioxidants [26].

Another anti-oxidant that has attracted a good deal of attention in the pathology of AD is melatonin [27]. Melatonin is more often thought of as a chemical in the brain produced at night that triggers sleep, but recent research has highlighted an important role in repairing oxidative damage to neurones. Patients with AD have low levels of melatonin, and melatonin supplementation shows promise for treating AD [27]. The MedDiet could potentially help redress a deficiency since many fruits and vegetables, seeds, walnuts and wine contain variable amounts of melatonin [28, 29].

Vitamins

There is a good correlation between folate intake and adherence to the MedDiet, and folate has been implicated as a possible protective factor in the MedDiet [30]. There are biologically plausible mechanisms to support a role for folate in the prevention of dementias. Folate is essential for normal methylation reactions in the brain, and is required for the synthesis of some neurotransmitters. In addition, folate, acting with vitamin B12, is required for the conversion of homocysteine to methionine. A deficiency in folate results in an increase in blood homocysteine levels. Homocysteine generates free radicals that can damage the endothelium and lead to a more prothrombotic state and this could contribute to vascular dementias [31].

Based on these mechanisms, it has been postulated that deficiencies in folate and vitamin B12 may contribute to the aetiology of both AD and vascular dementias. Despite an association between low folate status and all forms of dementia, there is no consistent evidence, based on current studies, that folic acid supplementation, with or without vitamin B12, improves cognitive function in unselected elderly people either with or without dementia [32, 33]. However, when elderly people with high levels of homocysteine are considered, there is some evidence that long-term use may improve cognitive function [32]. These studies suggest that the role of folates in the MedDiet may be more important in predementia situations, and by preventing blood homocysteine levels rising to pathologically dangerous levels. A possible example of the importance of interactions between dietary components comes from the suggestion that the benefits of folate are enhanced when levels of DHA are optimal [31]. This proposal is based on interlinking mechanisms of action between these two nutrients. For example, both folate and DHA enhance nitric oxide generation which in turn protects the endothelium and improves vascular function which in turn improves cognitive function [31].

Lifestyle factors

Exercise – a key aspect of the traditional Mediterranean lifestyle – was found to reduce the progression of cognitive impairment in Greek men and women [16] and this finding is supported by many other studies. A rich mental life may also be important. This conclusion is based on the observation that AD is less common in better educated individuals. This has led to the "cognitive reserve" hypothesis whereby increased mental capacity is hypothesised to compensate for loss of some neurological activity through disease [34]. However, more educated individuals also tend to have a better diet and so this is a possible confounding factor. The benefits of the overall Mediterranean dietary pattern have been summed up: "It may not be the direct effect of diet or specific nutrients that provide the protection, but healthy diets very similar to the Mediterranean dietary pattern may be an indicator of a complex set of favourable social and lifestyle factors." [35]

13.3 Parkinson's disease

13.3.1 Introduction

Parkinson's disease (PD) is characterised by a slowing in the ability to start and continue movements and impaired ability to adjust the body's position (bradykinesia), and by tremor and rigidity. As well as these defects in motor function, mental disorders such as depression or psychosis may occur. The prevalence of PD in various European countries has been compared, but these comparisons are difficult because of differences in diagnostic criteria between countries [36]. There is evidence that oxidative stress is important in the pathogenesis of PD, hence raising the possibility that a MedDiet might be of benefit.

13.3.2 Epidemiology

Gao et al. [37] analysed data from the Health Professionals Follow-Up Study (1986–2002) and the Nurses' Health Study (1984–2000) for the risk of PD associated with a modified MD-QI (modified by excluding from the score the requirement for moderate intake of dairy products, since in the US most people use skimmed milk and hence there is no necessity for a moderate intake) [38]. They documented 508 new PD cases after 16 y of follow-up. There was no association with PD in men and a borderline significant risk reduction in women (RR 0.66: CI 0.43–1.00, trend 0.09). When men and women were pooled, the RR was 0.75 (CI 0.57–1.00, trend 0.07). A high intake of fruit, vegetables and fish was inversely associated with PD in this analysis. Some, but not all, studies have found positive associations between coffee consumption and reduced risk of PD in both Mediterranean and non-Mediterranean populations, although some studies have only found this protective effect at high levels of consumption [39, 40].

13.3.3 Mechanisms

PD involves neurodegeneration of dopaminergic neurones in the substantia nigra. Oxidative stress promotes the aggregation of α-synuclein, and this is considered to be an important event in the pathogenesis of PD. In a meta-analysis, intake of vitamin E, an antioxidant present in almonds and other nuts, was inversely associated with risk of PD [41]. Vitamin C and β-carotene did not afford any protection. The activity of vitamin C may have been limited because, being water soluble, it requires active transport to enter the CNS. Folate may protect neurones by preventing the build up of homocysteine which has been shown to be neurotoxic [42]. Various mechanisms have been proposed for the protective effects of coffee. It is rich in antioxidants and, in addition, caffeine may protect dopaminergic neurons from excitotoxic factors by blocking adenosine A_{2A} receptors [40]. However, data are at present insufficient to support this hypothesis. Oestrogen may modify the effects of caffeine in women and this could explain the lack of protection against PD seen in some studies in women.

Data from the PREDIMED study found a correlation by multiple linear regression analysis significant only in men (R 0.047: CI 0.023–0.07, p < 0.001) between alcohol, and particularly wine consumption, and urinary hydroxytyrosol [43]. The authors of this study suggested that alcohol-generated hydroxytyrosol, which is a potent antioxidant (although one more usually associated with virgin olive oil), could be one mechanism for explaining the potential inverse association between alcohol consumption and a decreased risk of Parkinson's disease.

13.4   Depression

13.4.1   Introduction

The term "depression" covers a wide spectrum of moods, ranging from a normal feeling of unhappiness to an abnormal condition that is severe and incapacitating. Of course, many factors can contribute to depression including social factors (loneliness, lack of a social network, etc), a family history of depression, and lifestyle factors (e.g. drug use, lack of exercise), and establishing the role of diet in this mix is clearly a challenge. Age-standardised suicide rates are useful as an indirect indicator for the prevalence of severe depression. These rates tend to be lower in Mediterranean countries than North European countries [44], and hence there is interest in ascertaining whether a MedDiet and/or lifestyle factors associated with eating in Mediterranean countries may contribute to this reduced rate.

13.4.2   Epidemiology

A cross-sectional analysis of the association between intake of B vitamins and n-3 fatty acids and the prevalence of depression was performed in the SUN study [45]. Folate intake was inversely associated with depression among men, especially smokers, and vitamin B12 intake was inversely associated with depression among women. There was no significant association with intake of n-3 fatty acids. In the same cohort (10,094 subjects) longitudinally analysed after a follow-up of 4.4 years, 480 new cases of depression were diagnosed. Adherence to the overall Mediterranean dietary pattern was inversely associated with depression (HR 0.58: CI 0.44–0.77, p for trend <0.001), and inverse dose-response relationships were found for fruit and nuts, the MUFA/SFA ratio, and for legumes [46].

In the Greek cohort from the EPIC study, the role of dietary lipids was evaluated using a geriatric depression scale (GDS) of increasing depression [47]. GDS score was negatively associated with dietary intake of MUFAs and their main source, olive oil. The GDS was positively associated with intake of seed oils (rich in n-6 fatty acids) and, as with the first SUN report [45], there was no significant association with fish and seafood (rich in n-3 fatty acids). By contrast, in the MEDIS (Mediterranean Islands) study, there was an inverse correlation between the GDS score and fish consumption [48]. Overall, it can be concluded that further epidemiological studies for a role of the MedDiet in depression are required.

In these epidemiological studies using olive oil as a placebo control for examining the effects of n-3 fatty acids, these studies are compromised by the possible beneficial effects of the olive oil itself.

13.4.3   Mechanisms

Some mechanisms that have been postulated to explain how constituents in the MedDiet protect against depression overlap with mechanisms associated with protection against other disorders. A good example of this is in relation to the cerebral vasculature. Many constituents of the MedDiet, such as those with anti-inflammatory action, improve the function of vascular endothelial cells. Endothelial cells in the brain synthesise and secrete brain-derived neurotrophic factor (BDNF), a neuroprotective factor that improves synaptic plasticity, and has been reported to be reduced in individuals with depression. Hence, one possible way by which the MedDiet protects against depression is by maintaining a healthy cerebral endothelium and so improving BDNF production. Exercise is also thought to increase BDNF production.

B vitamins prevent excess accumulation of homocysteine and hence reduce vascular damage and so could also help maintain BDNF production. Folate is required for the conversion of homocysteine to methionine, and methionine is thought to be required for the synthesis of some neutrotransmitters including serotonin, dopamine and noradrenaline. Olive oil has also been linked to neurotransmitter function since it has been shown to enhance binding of serotonin to its receptors. Other possible mechanisms of action for olive oil are increased biosynthesis of the sleep-inducing substance oleamide and antioxidant properties of the phenolic substances present in the oil [49].

13.5 Rheumatoid arthritis

13.5.1 Introduction

Rheumatoid arthritis (RA) is an autoimmune disease that affects between 0.3% and 1.0% of the general population. The aetiology of RA is not known, but various infectious agents and smoking are associated with increased risk [50]. There is increasing evidence that, as for other autoimmune disorders, insufficient sunlight, and hence a lack of vitamin D, is an important contributory factor [51, 52]. Some studies have suggested that high meat or low fish intake increases the risk of acquiring RA, but the evidence is weak and conflicting. On the other hand, many people with established RA attempt to improve their condition by dietary means.

13.5.2 Epidemiology

A case-control study (145 cases, 188 controls) conducted in Southern Greece found that the risk of developing RA was significantly inversely associated with consumption of cooked vegetables (OR 0.39: CI 0.20–0.77, trend <0.001) and olive oil (OR 0.39: CI 0.19–0.82, trend 0.03), independently from other foods [53]. Rather than disease prevention, most epidemiological studies of dietary intervention for RA are based on reducing symptoms, and these studies were reviewed in a Cochrane report in 2009 [54]. Of these studies, only a few have examined an association between RA and the MedDiet. In a small study, standard hospital food was compared to a modified MedDiet (which included rapeseed oil-based margarine as well as olive oil, replacing dairy with low fat dairy but no overall reduction in amount, and replacing wine with tea) [55]. After 12 weeks there was a significant reduction in pain in the MedDiet group relative to the control group (p=0.004), although there was no statistically significant difference in morning stiffness between the two groups. A pilot study was conducted to examine the feasibility of modifying dietary lifestyle in female patients with RA living in areas of social deprivation in Glasgow [56]. There was a modest improvement in the pain score and early morning stiffness as reported by the patients, although clinical features did not improve as assessed by a 28-point disease assessment score.

Modest improvements are generally seen in patients taking fish oil supplements rich in n-3 fatty acids suggesting that oily fish may contribute to the benefits from consuming a MedDiet. Some additional benefits, such as reduced joint pain and improved handgrip strength, were seen when the fish oil intake was supplemented with extra virgin olive oil added to salads [57].

13.5.3   Mechanisms

EPA and DHA present in fish oils decrease the amount of arachidonic acid (AA) in cell membranes and reduce the production of pro-inflammatory eicosanoids from AA, and this has been discussed in Section 9.4.3.

One mechanism proposed for the protective effects of olive oil also involves modifying pro-inflammatory eicosanoids. The major MUFA in olive oil, oleic acid, is converted to eicosatrienoic acid (ETA; C20:3 n-9), and ETA in turn is converted to LTA3, which has been shown to inhibit the synthesis of the pro-inflammatory cytokine leukotriene B4 [58]. Olive oil also has a wide range of suppressive effects on the immune function and these may also contribute to beneficial effects of olive oil against RA and other autoimmune disorders. These effects include decreasing lymphocyte proliferation and decreasing the expression of various adhesion molecules in blood vessels [59]. Adhesion of white blood cells to the vascular wall is required prior to the cells leaving the vessel (a process known as extravasation) and contributing to an inflammatory reaction. Another possible benefit of extra virgin olive oil arises from the discovery of the anti-inflammatory, ibuprofen-like constituent oleocanthal, and this could conceivably contribute to the pain-relieving properties of extra virgin olive oil. In this context, the quality of the extra virgin olive oil would be important since there is wide variation in the oleocanthal content between olive oils (see Section 6.2.5). Rapeseed oil products would not be an equivalent substitute for extra virgin olive oil in this regard since rapeseed oil contains oleic acid but not oleocanthal.

13.6   Age-related macular degeneration

13.6.1   Introduction

Age-related macular degeneration (AMD), the late stage of age-related maculopathy (ARM), is a major cause of adult blindness in many developed countries, including Europe. There are two main types of AMD: dry, accounting for up to 90% of cases, and wet. In dry AMD, lipid deposits ("drusen") accumulate underneath the pigment-rich cells in the retina known as the retinal pigment epithelium (RPE), with later stages of dry AMD resulting in destruction of the central retinal area (geographic atrophy). In wet AMD, abnormal blood vessels grow under the RPE, a process known as neovascularisation, and this form of AMD is also known as neovascular AMD. These blood vessels become leaky, hence the term "wet". The prevalence of AMD increases significantly with age; almost 30% of people over the age of 75 years have early signs of AMD and 7% have late stage disease.

The macular region of the retina, which surrounds the fovea and has the highest level of visual acuity, is yellow because of a high concentration of the antioxidant carotenoids lutein and zeaxanthin. In addition, the human retina is rich in *n*-3 PUFAs, and in particular in DHA, which may play an important structural and protective role in the macula [60]. Clearly identified risk factors for maculopathies are smoking and polymorphisms in the genes for apolipoprotein E and Complement Factor, thus implicating lipid metabolism and inflammation in the aetiology of these disorders [61]. In animal models, a high fat diet, combined with human variants of apolipoproteins, leads to retinal lesions similar to those observed in AMD.

13.6.2 Epidemiology

A number of constituents found in the MedDiet have been associated with a reduced risk of AMD, although results are inconsistent. These include oily fish, and various dietary antioxidants, especially lutein and zeaxanthin [62, 63]. Results from studies with β-carotene and vitamin E are conflicting, with some recent studies indicating an increase in risk with increased intake [62]. Epidemiological data on the associations between dietary fat and ARM are scarce and partly inconsistent. In a study conducted in Southern France, high total, saturated and monounsaturated fat intake was associated with increased risk for ARM (OR 4.74: CI 1.32–17.0, trend 0.007; OR 2.70: CI 0.94–7.7, trend 0.04; and OR 3.50: CI 1.09–11.2 trend 0.03, respectively after multivariate adjustment) [64]. Total PUFA was not significantly associated with ARM. Total and white fish intake was not significantly associated with ARM, but fatty fish intake (more than once a month versus less than once a month) was associated with a 60% reduction in risk for ARM (OR 0.42, p=0.01). A number of other studies have found some evidence for a protective effect from diets rich in DHA [63, 65].

Some, but not all, epidemiological studies suggest a correlation between high dietary intake of lutein and zeaxanthin and a reduction in AMD, although these studies were not carried specifically in the context of the MedDiet. Maize is the richest source of zeaxanthin (named after the Latin for maize, *Zea mays*). Green leafy vegetables are also a good source of lutein and zeaxanthin, although the bioavailability of these carotenoids from egg yolks is several fold higher. There is no clear evidence that carotenoids taken as supplements can reduce the risk of AMD [66].

Visual impairment was assessed in six European countries in the European Eye (EUREYE) study. The prevalence of visual impairment was higher in the Mediterranean countries than the North European countries (with the exception of Estonia) [67]. The principal causes for the visual impairment were AMD or cataracts. Although a causal relationship between sunlight exposure and AMD has not been established, a significant association between sunlight (blue light) exposure and neovascular AMD was observed in individuals from the EUREYE study with low antioxidant status (especially low vitamin C, zeaxanthin, and vitamin E) (OR 3.7: CI 1.6–8.9), whereas there was no association with AMD when blue light exposure alone was considered [68]. Results from other studies that have examined an association between AMD and exposure to sunlight alone have been inconsistent.

No epidemiological studies have specifically investigated whether the MedDiet may mitigate against the effects of high levels of sun exposure in Mediterranean countries. However, the presence of high levels of putative protective factors in the

MedDiet, such as lutein, zeaxanthin and DHA, provides a rationale for such studies. An analysis of diet, environmental factors (including sun exposure) and medical factors of a small rural community in Italy found that age, hypertension and prior cataract surgery had the greatest impact on the risk of AMD, and a vegetable-based diet seemed to prevent early signs of AMD ($p=0.007$) [69].

13.6.3 Mechanisms

The retina is subject to significant oxidative stress due to its high consumption of oxygen and high rate of phagocytic activity by white blood cells (which produce reactive oxygen species due to the "respiratory burst"). Lipid peroxidation resulting from photochemical damage to DHA-rich retinal cell membranes will further compound the oxidative stress. Since most DHA in the body is thought to derive from dietary sources, this may explain why consumption of oily fish and DHA are associated with a reduced risk of AMD [63]. Lutein and zeaxanthin are thought to protect the eye by filtering out blue light and these antioxidant carotenoids may also help prevent peroxidation of DHA in the retina [70]. Hence, if there are insufficient levels of lutein and zeaxanthin in the diet, this may lead to injury to the RPE.

RPE injury results in an inflammatory response which is associated with the formation of drusen and deposition of complement components. Predisposing genes are implicated in the pathogenesis of AMD since individuals with single nucleotide polymorphisms in complement factors (which renders these proteins ineffective) are at an increased risk of AMD. The multifactorial nature of AMD, including complex gene-environment interactions, indicates that many factors probably contribute to the pathogenic process.

Current trials are examining the efficacy of using supplements of carotenoids and *n*-3 fatty acids in combination (in a study called the Age-Related Eye Disease Study 2). Although no studies have specifically looked at an association between the MedDiet and AMD, a MedDiet – which is naturally rich in carotenoids and *n*-3 fatty acids – would, based on current understanding, seem to be a good insurance policy against oxidative damage associated with AMD.

AMD and neovascularisation

Inhibitors of neovascularisation (so-called anti-angiogenic agents) are used clinically to treat wet AMD. The MedDiet is rich in anti-angiogenic substances (see Chapter 12), and the wine phenolic resveratrol has been demonstrated to reverse the abnormal formation of blood vessels in the retinas of mice [71]. Hence, it is of interest to ascertain if dietary anti-angiogenic substances may help delay the vascularisation process associated with wet AMD.

13.7 All cause mortality

CVD mortality and cancers are the main causes of mortality in Western and industrialised countries. Until recently, few studies had looked specifically at all cause mortality, and most of these studies used *a priori* and *a posteriori* dietary patterns based on data in relation to CVD and cancers. However, the relationship between all cause mortality and other diseases is now being considered.

13.7.1   Fruit and vegetables

Fruit and vegetables were found to be inversely related to all cause mortality in diabetic participants of the EPIC study [72]. An increment in intake of 80 g/d of total vegetables, legumes and fruit was associated with a RR of death from all causes of 0.94 (CI 0.90–0.98). This risk reduction was mainly associated with vegetables and legumes.

13.7.2   Alcohol

The cumulative evidence from many studies suggests that moderate alcohol consumption (of any type) is associated with a reduced risk of all cause mortality compared to either no consumption or to high levels of consumption. This relationship between alcohol consumption and all cause mortality is described by a J-shaped curve [73]. As consumption increases the beneficial effect is lost, and this occurs more quickly for women than for men. For both sexes, the precise shape of the J-shaped curve is modified when other confounding factors are taken into consideration.

13.7.3   Wine

In the Greek population of the EPIC study higher adherence to the MedDiet was associated with a statistically significant reduction in total mortality (adjusted mortality ratio per two unit increase in score 0.864: CI 0.802–0.932). Moderate consumption of alcohol (mainly wine with a meal) was the highest contributor to this association (23.5%) followed by moderate intake of meat and meat products (16.6%), high vegetable consumption (16.2%), high fruit and nut consumption (11.2%), high monounsaturated-to-saturated lipid ratio (10.6%), and high legume consumption (9.7%) [74]. However, the authors of this report emphasised the importance of the overall dietary pattern driving the association of high Mediterranean diet score with low mortality [74].

In a prospective cohort study conducted on healthy middle-aged men from Eastern (non-Mediterranean) France, moderate wine drinkers (those who consumed <60 g alcohol/day and no beer) had lower risks of death (drinkers in mean quartiles of systolic blood pressures of 158±12.72, 139±2.47, 129±2.32 or 116±5.96 mm Hg had reductions in all cause mortality of 23%, 27%, none, and 37%, respectively, compared to abstainers [75]). However, as well as the inconsistency of the effect, this study did not control for diet. For middle-aged men taking part in the Zutphen Study, long-term consumption of low amounts of wine (on average, less than half a glass per day) was inversely associated with all cause mortality (HR 0.73: CI 0.62–0.87) and CHD (HR 0.61: CI 0.41–0.89) and CVD (HR 0.68: CI 0.53–0.86) [76]. Much of the reduction of overall mortality resulting from moderate wine/alcohol drinking with a meal is due to a reduction in CVD [77], and specific mechanisms to explain this are discussed in Chapter 11.

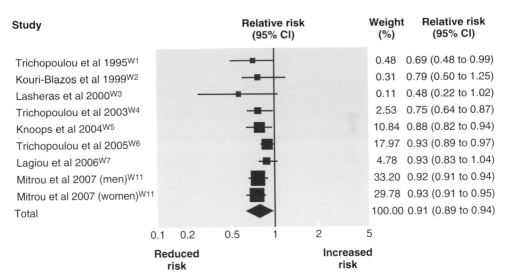

Study	Relative risk (95% CI)	Weight (%)	Relative risk (95% CI)
Trichopoulou et al 1995[W1]		0.48	0.69 (0.48 to 0.99)
Kouri-Blazos et al 1999[W2]		0.31	0.79 (0.50 to 1.25)
Lasheras et al 2000[W3]		0.11	0.48 (0.22 to 1.02)
Trichopoulou et al 2003[W4]		2.53	0.75 (0.64 to 0.87)
Knoops et al 2004[W5]		10.84	0.88 (0.82 to 0.94)
Trichopoulou et al 2005[W6]		17.97	0.93 (0.89 to 0.97)
Lagiou et al 2006[W7]		4.78	0.93 (0.83 to 1.04)
Mitrou et al 2007 (men)[W11]		33.20	0.92 (0.91 to 0.94)
Mitrou et al 2007 (women)[W11]		29.78	0.93 (0.91 to 0.95)
Total		100.00	0.91 (0.89 to 0.94)

0.1   0.2   0.5   1   2   5

Reduced risk   **Increased risk**

Figure 13.1 Risk of all cause mortality associated with 2-point increase in adherence score for Mediterranean diet [80]. Squares represent effect size; extended lines show confidence intervals; diamond represents total effect size. With permission from BMJ Publishing Group Ltd.

13.7.4   Dietary pattern

With regard to the overall MedDiet, adherence to the MDS by elderly Greeks showed a 25% reduction in all causes of death (adjusted HR 0.75: CI 0.64–0.87) [38]. When the M-MDS was applied to all EPIC cohorts, the overall HR showed that a 2-unit increment in the M-MDS was associated with a modest decrease in risk of mortality (HR 0.92: CI 0.88–0.96). However, this was essentially due to the Greek cohort (HR 0.70: CI 0.56–0.88) and to a lesser extent to the Spanish cohort (HR 0.81: CI 0.63–1.05); none of the other cohorts showing a significant risk reduction in all cause mortality [78]. This once again supports the specificity of the MDS for Mediterranean populations, and is in line with the various arguments supporting this assertion and discussed in previous chapters. Rather, the MDS needs adapting for other populations, as in the alternate MDS (see Chapter 8) to show comparable effects to the MDS in Mediterranean countries [79]. Sofi et al. computed a meta-analysis on all studies for all cause mortality and obtained a pooled RR of 0.91 (CI 0.89–0.94) (Figure 13.1) [80].

The *a posteriori* dietary pattern reveals more an effect of "healthy" or "prudent" or "plant-based" diets rather than of a true MedDiet. However, the principal component analysis (PCA) computed in the EPIC cohorts is of interest with respect to the MedDiet. A "plant-based diet" was defined as the first component of the PCA: it is a diet rich in plant foods such as vegetables and vegetable oils, fruit, pasta/rice/other grains and legumes, but poor in potatoes, margarine and non-alcoholic beverages [81]. An increase in the adherence to the plant-based diet was associated with a lower overall mortality, a one standard deviation increment corresponding to a statistically significant reduction (RR 0.89: CI 0.79–0.99). In country-specific analyses the apparent association was stronger in Greece (RR 0.55: CI 0.36–0.85) and the Netherlands (RR 0.70: CI 0.52–0.96). The plant-based diet is very close to the food groups of the M-MDS, with high consumption of fruit and vegetables, and increasing plant-based dietary intake was accompanied by a reduction in the intakes of food groups of which high consumption may be considered non-beneficial, such as meat and dairy products. While the factor loading of each group is not given in the report, it is interesting to note that wine consumption increases from the first tertile of plant-based diet to the third (32.56±58.67 to 98.31±165.25 g/day), whereas other alcoholic beverages and non-alcoholic beverages decrease (167.63±325.40 to 31.84±102.18 and 1488.51±707.77 to 551.70±591.48, respectively). Thus, this dietary pattern is very close to the MedDiet. Nevertheless, the overall correlation between modified M-MDS and the plant-based dietary score was only 0.621, indicating that the M-MDS and the main principal component extracted from the foods consumed by the study participants capture partially (but not fully) overlapping beneficial aspects of a MedDiet.

13.8   General conclusions

MDS and M-MDS are consistently associated with a reduction in all cause mortality, with a higher percentage reduction in Greece than when the M-MDS is analysed specifically by country. In addition, the MDS is associated with risk reduction of CVD and cancer mortality, and also of cancer incidence. The MDS or M-MDS applied to Mediterranean countries like Greece shows a stronger correlation with disease prevention than when an M-MDS is applied to North European countries. This might be because adapting the score to other population samples alters its properties, or because other protective variables are correlated to the MDS in the Mediterranean populations but not in other populations. Olive oil – which is primarily used in Mediterranean countries – might be the food that makes the difference. But it might be another food or food group not identified in the questionnaires, such as herbs and spices, which contributes to the beneficial effects, and which is correlated to the MDS only in Mediterranean countries. Other behaviours related to food consumption such as meal structures and daily organisation, absence of snacking and communal eating are variables associated with the MDS in Mediterranean countries, and are less commonly found in some other countries. In addition, other conditions (such as sun exposure) or behaviours (such as siesta) might be beneficial players, and are correlated with a MedDiet.

A prudent diet, comparable to most components to the MedDiet, is consistently associated with a risk reduction of all cause mortality and mortality from CHD. With regard to weight loss and maintenance, metabolic disorders or other pathological conditions further research is needed to confirm the effect of a MedDiet, including the role of other risk factors and behaviours. Although results are more limited for cancer incidence, when this prudent diet moves towards a MedDiet by the inclusion of olive oil in the pattern, several studies have shown a risk reduction of breast cancer. Is it the association of olive oil with another food item, or a confounding factor related to this consumption that plays a role? This question remains to be answered, and opens up new research perspectives, both in biological sciences and in anthropological and cultural sciences.

References

1. Dauncey, M.J. New insights into nutrition and cognitive neuroscience. *Proc Nutr Soc*, 2009. 68(4): 408–15.
2. Matthews, F., Brayne, C. The incidence of dementia in England and Wales: findings from the five identical sites of the MRC CFA Study. *PLoS Med*, 2005. 2(8): e193.
3. Alzheimer's Society. http://www.alzheimers.org.uk/Facts_about_dementia/index.htm.[cited]

4. Solfrizzi, V. et al. Lifestyle-related factors in predementia and dementia syndromes. *Expert Rev Neurother*, 2008. **8**(1): 133–58.
5. Ganguli, M. et al. Alcohol consumption and cognitive function in late life: a longitudinal community study. *Neurology*, 2005. **65**(8): 1210–7.
6. Solfrizzi, V. et al. Alcohol consumption, mild cognitive impairment, and progression to dementia. *Neurology*, 2007. **68**(21): 1790–9.
7. Scarmeas, N. et al. Mediterranean diet and risk for Alzheimer's disease. *Ann Neurol*, 2006. **59**(6): 912–21.
8. Scarmeas, N. et al. Mediterranean diet and Alzheimer disease mortality. *Neurology*, 2007. **69**(11): 1084–93.
9. Scarmeas, N. et al. Mediterranean diet and mild cognitive impairment. *Arch Neurol*, 2009. **66**(2): 216–25.
10. Scarmeas, N. et al. Physical activity, diet, and risk of Alzheimer disease. *Jama*, 2009. **302**(6): 627–37.
11. Feart, C. et al. Adherence to a Mediterranean diet, cognitive decline, and risk of dementia. *Jama*, 2009. **302**(6): 638–48.
12. Feart, C. et al. Mediterranean diet and cognitive function in older adults. *Curr Opin Clin Nutr Metab Care*, 2010. **13**(1): 14–8.
13. Yaffe, K. *Metabolic syndrome and cognitive disorders: is the sum greater than its parts? Alzheimer Dis Assoc Disord*, 2007. **21**(2): 167–71.
14. Scarmeas, N. et al. Mediterranean diet, Alzheimer disease, and vascular mediation. *Arch Neurol*, 2006. **63**(12): 1709–17.
15. Panza, F. et al. Mediterranean diet and cognitive decline. *Public Health Nutr*, 2004. **7**(7): 959–63.
16. Psaltopoulou, T. et al. Diet, physical activity and cognitive impairment among elders: the EPIC-Greece cohort (European Prospective Investigation into Cancer and Nutrition). *Public Health Nutr*, 2008: 1–9.
17. Lukiw, W.J., Bazan, N.G. Docosahexaenoic acid and the aging brain. *J Nutr*, 2008. **138**(12): 2510–4.
18. Cunnane, S.C. et al. Fish, docosahexaenoic acid and Alzheimer's disease. *Prog Lipid Res*, 2009. **48**(5): 239–56.
19. Gomez-Pinilla, F. Brain foods: the effects of nutrients on brain function. *Nat Rev Neurosci*, 2008. **9**(7): 568–78.
20. Barnham, K.J. et al. Neurodegenerative diseases and oxidative stress. *Nat Rev Drug Discov*, 2004. **3**(3): 205–14.
21. Montine, T.J., Morrow, J.D. Fatty acid oxidation in the pathogenesis of Alzheimer's disease. *Am J Pathol*, 2005. **166**(5): 1283–9.
22. Cole, G.M. et al. Omega-3 fatty acids and dementia. *Prostaglandins Leukot Essent Fatty Acids*, 2009. **81**(2–3): 213–21.
23. Johnson, E.J. et al. Cognitive findings of an exploratory trial of docosahexaenoic acid and lutein supplementation in older women. *Nutr Neurosci*, 2008. **11**(2): 75–83.
24. Singh, M. et al. Challenges for research on polyphenols from foods in Alzheimer's disease: bioavailability, metabolism, and cellular and molecular mechanisms. *J Agric Food Chem*, 2008. **56**(13): 4855–73.
25. Spencer, J.P. Beyond antioxidants: the cellular and molecular interactions of flavonoids and how these underpin their actions on the brain. *Proc Nutr Soc*, 2010. **69**(2): 244–60.
26. Solfrizzi, V. et al. Dietary fatty acids intake: possible role in cognitive decline and dementia. *Exp Gerontol*, 2005. **40**(4): 257–70.
27. Srinivasan, V. et al. Melatonin in Alzheimer's disease and other neurodegenerative disorders. *Behav Brain Funct*, 2006. **2**: 15.
28. Iriti, M., Faoro, F. Grape phytochemicals: a bouquet of old and new nutraceuticals for human health. *Med Hypotheses*, 2006. **67**(4): 833–8.
29. Reiter, R.J. et al. Melatonin in edible plants (phytomelatonin): Identification, concentrations, bioavailability and proposed functions. *World Rev Nutr Diet*, 2007. **97**: 211–30.
30. Bach-Faig, A. et al. Evaluating associations between Mediterranean diet adherence indexes and biomarkers of diet and disease. *Public Health Nutr*, 2006. **9**(8A): 1110–7.
31. Das, U.N. Folic acid and polyunsaturated fatty acids improve cognitive function and prevent depression, dementia, and Alzheimer's disease – but how and why? *Prostaglandins Leukot Essent Fatty Acids*, 2008. **78**(1): 11–9.

32. Malouf, R., Grimley, E.J. Folic acid with or without vitamin B12 for the prevention and treatment of healthy elderly and demented people. *Cochrane Database of Systematic Reviews* 2008(4); p. Art. No.: CD004514. doi:10.1002/14651858.CD004514.pub2.
33. Aisen, P.S. et al. High-dose B vitamin supplementation and cognitive decline in Alzheimer disease: a randomized controlled trial. *Jama*, 2008. **300**(15): 1774–83.
34. Stern, Y. Cognitive reserve. *Neuropsychologia*, 2009. **47**(10): 2015–28.
35. Panza, F. et al. Mediterranean diet, mild cognitive impairment, and Alzheimer's disease. *Exp Gerontol*, 2007. **42**(1–2): 6–7; author reply 8–9.
36. von Campenhausen, S. et al. Prevalence and incidence of Parkinson's disease in Europe. *Eur Neuropsychopharmacol*, 2005. **15**(4): 473–90.
37. Gao, X. et al. Prospective study of dietary pattern and risk of Parkinson disease. *Am J Clin Nutr*, 2007. **86**(5): 1486–94.
38. Trichopoulou, A. et al. Adherence to a Mediterranean diet and survival in a Greek population. *N Engl J Med*, 2003. **348**(26): 2599–608.
39. Dorea, J.G., da Costa, T.H. Is coffee a functional food? *Br J Nutr*, 2005. **93**(6): 773–82.
40. Saaksjarvi, K. et al. Prospective study of coffee consumption and risk of Parkinson's disease. *Eur J Clin Nutr*, 2008. **62**(7): 908–15.
41. Etminan, M. et al. Intake of vitamin E, vitamin C, and carotenoids and the risk of Parkinson's disease: a meta-analysis. *Lancet Neurol*, 2005. **4**(6): 362–5.
42. Lipton, S.A. et al. Neurotoxicity associated with dual actions of homocysteine at the N-methyl-D-aspartate receptor. *Proc Natl Acad Sci USA*, 1997. **94**(11): 5923–8.
43. Schroder, H. et al. Alcohol consumption is associated with high concentrations of urinary hydroxytyrosol. *Am J Clin Nutr*, 2009. **90**(5): 1329–35.
44. Chishti, P. et al. Suicide mortality in the European Union. *Eur J Public Health*, 2003. **13**(2): 108–14.
45. Sanchez-Villegas, A. et al., Mediterranean diet and depression. *Public Health Nutr*, 2006. **9**(8A): 1104–9.
46. Sanchez-Villegas, A. et al. Association of the Mediterranean dietary pattern with the incidence of depression: the Seguimiento Universidad de Navarra/University of Navarra follow-up (SUN) cohort. *Arch Gen Psychiatry*, 2009. **66**(10): 1090–8.
47. Kyrozis, A. et al. Dietary lipids and geriatric depression scale score among elders: the EPIC-Greece cohort. *J Psychiatr Res*, 2009. **43**(8): 763–9.
48. Bountziouka, V. et al. Long-term fish intake is associated with less severe depressive symptoms among elderly men and women: the MEDIS (MEDiterranean ISlands Elderly) epidemiological study. *J Aging Health*, 2009. **21**(6): 864–80.
49. Logan, A.C. Omega-3 and depression research: hold the olive oil. *Prostaglandins Leukot Essent Fatty Acids*, 2005. **72**(6): 441.
50. Kobayashi, S. et al. Molecular aspects of rheumatoid arthritis: role of environmental factors. *Febs J*, 2008. **275**(18): 4456–62.
51. Adorini, L., Penna, G. Control of autoimmune diseases by the vitamin D endocrine system. *Nat Clin Pract Rheumatol*, 2008. **4**(8): 404–12.
52. Cutolo, M. Vitamin D and autoimmune rheumatic diseases. *Rheumatology (Oxford)*, 2009. **48**(3): 210–2.
53. Linos, A. et al. Dietary factors in relation to rheumatoid arthritis: a role for olive oil and cooked vegetables? *Am J Clin Nutr*, 1999. **70**(6): 1077–82.
54. Hagen, K.B. et al. Dietary interventions for rheumatoid arthritis. *Cochrane Database Syst Rev*, 2009(1): CD006400.
55. Skoldstam, L. et al. An experimental study of a Mediterranean diet intervention for patients with rheumatoid arthritis. *Ann Rheum Dis*, 2003. **62**(3): 208–14.
56. McKellar, G. et al. A pilot study of a Mediterranean-type diet intervention in female patients with rheumatoid arthritis living in areas of social deprivation in Glasgow. *Ann Rheum Dis*, 2007. **66**(9): 1239–43.
57. Berbert, A.A. et al. Supplementation of fish oil and olive oil in patients with rheumatoid arthritis. *Nutrition*, 2005. **21**(2): 131–6.
58. James, M.J. et al. Dietary polyunsaturated fatty acids and inflammatory mediator production. *Am J Clin Nutr*, 2000. **71**(1 Suppl): 343S–8S.
59. Wahle, K.W. et al. Olive oil and modulation of cell signaling in disease prevention. *Lipids*, 2004. **39**(12): 1223–31.
60. SanGiovanni, J.P., Chew, E.Y. The role of omega-3 long-chain polyunsaturated fatty acids in health and disease of the retina. *Prog Retin Eye Res*, 2005. **24**(1): 87–138.

61. Ehrlich, R. et al. Age-related macular degeneration and the aging eye. *Clin Interv Aging*, 2008. **3**(3): 473–82.
62. Johnson, E.J. Age-related macular degeneration and antioxidant vitamins: recent findings. *Curr Opin Clin Nutr Metab Care*, 2010. **13**(1): 28–33.
63. Augood, C. et al. Oily fish consumption, dietary docosahexaenoic acid and eicosapentaenoic acid intakes, and associations with neovascular age-related macular degeneration. *Am J Clin Nutr*, 2008. **88**(2): 398–406.
64. Delcourt, C. et al. Dietary fat and the risk of age-related maculopathy: the POLANUT study. *Eur J Clin Nutr*, 2007. **61**(11): 1341–4.
65. Chiu, C.J. et al. Does eating particular diets alter the risk of age-related macular degeneration in users of the Age-Related Eye Disease Study supplements? *Br J Ophthalmol*, 2009. **93**(9): 1241–6.
66. Rhone, M., Basu, A. Phytochemicals and age-related eye diseases. *Nutr Rev*, 2008. **66**(8): 465–72.
67. Seland, J.H. et al. Visual Impairment and quality of life in the Older European Population, the EUREYE study. *Acta Ophthalmol*, 2009. Published online: 19 NOV 2009, DOI: 10.1111/j.1755–3768.2009.01794.x
68. Fletcher, A.E. et al. Sunlight exposure, antioxidants, and age-related macular degeneration. *Arch Ophthalmol*, 2008. **126**(10): 1396–403.
69. Carresi, C. et al. Montelparo study: risk factors for age-related macular degeneration in a little rural community in Italy. *Clin Ter*, 2009. **160**(3): e43–51.
70. Thurnham, D.I. Macular zeaxanthins and lutein – a review of dietary sources and bioavailability and some relationships with macular pigment optical density and age-related macular disease. *Nutr Res Rev*, 2007. **20**(2): 163–79.
71. Khan, A.A. et al. Resveratrol regulates pathologic angiogenesis by a eukaryotic elongation factor-2 kinase-regulated pathway. *Am J Pathol*, 2010. **177**(1): 481–92.
72. Nothlings, U. et al. Intake of vegetables, legumes, and fruit, and risk for all-cause, cardiovascular, and cancer mortality in a European diabetic population. *J Nutr*, 2008. **138**(4): 775–81.
73. Di Castelnuovo, A. et al. Alcohol dosing and total mortality in men and women: an updated meta-analysis of 34 prospective studies. *Arch Intern Med*, 2006. **166**(22): 2437–45.
74. Trichopoulou, A. et al. Anatomy of health effects of Mediterranean diet: Greek EPIC prospective cohort study. *BMJ*, 2009. **338**: b2337.
75. Renaud, S.C. et al. Moderate wine drinkers have lower hypertension-related mortality: a prospective cohort study in French men. *Am J Clin Nutr*, 2004. **80**(3): 621–5.
76. Streppel, M.T. et al. Long-term wine consumption is related to cardiovascular mortality and life expectancy independently of moderate alcohol intake: the Zutphen Study. *J Epidemiol Community Health*, 2009. **63**(7): 534–40.
77. Opie, L.H., Lecour, S. The red wine hypothesis: from concepts to protective signalling molecules. *Eur Heart J*, 2007. **28**(14): 1683–93.
78. Trichopoulou, A. et al. Modified Mediterranean diet and survival: EPIC-elderly prospective cohort study. *BMJ*, 2005. **330**(7498): 991.
79. Mitrou, P.N. et al. Mediterranean dietary pattern and prediction of all-cause mortality in a US population: results from the NIH-AARP Diet and Health Study. *Arch Intern Med*, 2007. **167**(22): 2461–8.
80. Sofi, F. et al. Adherence to Mediterranean diet and health status: meta-analysis. *BMJ*, 2008. **337**: a1344.
81. Bamia, C. et al. Dietary patterns and survival of older Europeans: the EPIC-Elderly Study (European Prospective Investigation into Cancer and Nutrition). *Public Health Nutr*, 2007. **10**(6): 590–8.

14 Public Health Issues

Summary

- Public health in western countries faces important challenges, especially in relation to obesity and chronic degenerative diseases (mainly CVDs and cancers), and nutritional recommendations can have an important impact on public health as illustrated by successful campaigns in Finland.
- A framework exists that is able to translate scientific knowledge about the MedDiet into nutritional and lifestyle guidelines for Mediterranean people and other populations, including a UK population. This includes: giving the largest place to diversified and seasonal plant foods (including fruit and vegetables, herbs and spices, unrefined cereals and legumes), preferring fish to meat, and olive oil to other added and cooking fats; changing patterns of alcohol consumption, especially in the young.
- Individual help through dietary advice tailored to the individual is helpful for changing food habits in the home, which is especially important, but should be accompanied by community and government campaigns.
- Community and government campaigns could include: public television programmes; supermarket displays of Mediterranean produce emphasising the whole diet; local food production, preferably organic; revising the Common Agricultural Policy towards one that encourages the production of healthier foods with lower environmental impacts.

14.1 Introduction

The first appearance of an organisation responsible for Public Health was in the UK, where a Public Health Ministry was created in 1848. After the great flu pandemics in 1918, the Nations Society subsequently decided to create the World Health Organisation. Public health is now a major objective in most countries in the world, and reflects the concern for health at the population level. Public health has been important for decades in Northern Europe, and several countries used the results of epidemiological studies to implement prevention guidelines. Two British epidemiologists, Richard Doll and Richard Peto, must be named for their seminal work on the harmful effects of tobacco, and on cholesterol as a marker for CVD [1, 2], and these studies opened up the way for important public health recommendations on cancers and CVD. In addition, the analysis by Marmot on the impact of social factors on health has been very helpful when proposing public health recommendations [3].

14.1.1   Public health and its objectives

Public health is a complex, multidisciplinary undertaking that is focussed on practical implementation. Its major challenge is to understand lifestyle, sociological and environmental factors that are determinants of health, and to identify those that can be modified and translated into guidelines for the general population. Thus, the first specific objective of public health is to observe the state of health of a population, and to collect data about factors related to the observed pathologies, when they are known, or to make hypotheses and verify them when they are unknown. General recommendations can be made when factors are convincingly or probably related to a disease, are widely present in a population, and are able to be modified.

In our society, obesity and chronic degenerative diseases (CDDs) are the major threats to public health. Some of the causal factors of CDDs are well known and can be taken into account when establishing recommendations. A good illustration of this is the successful Finnish campaign of nutritional recommendations for reducing CVD. This was implemented in the 1980s after the publication of the Seven Countries study. At that time, there was a high incidence of CVD in Finland, a high hypercholesterolaemia in the population, and a high consumption of saturated fatty acids (around 17% of total energy intake). The recommendation to decrease saturated fat and to increase plant-based foods led to a strong decrease in the incidence of CVD [4]. A comparable observation has now been made for colorectal cancer [4, 5].

Although nutritional recommendations have a major role for the prevention of chronic diseases, one must not forget other lifestyle and societal factors which might also play a role. Some of these are well understood, such as physical activity, tobacco, alcohol, low socio-economic status, but others are still under investigation.

14.1.2   The challenges of public health in Europe

Cardiovascular diseases

CVDs are the most common causes of mortality in Europe and have the highest standardised mortality rates (SMRs) in Europe among the non-communicable diseases (354 versus 144 for cancers), except in France where the cancer SMR is higher (142 versus 118 for CVD) [6]. However, this global figure hides strong disparities within Europe where there exists a clear north–east to south–west gradient in mortality from CVDs. The use of mortality as an indicator implies that many more factors other than just lifestyle factors are taken into account, such as care access and socio-economic level. Having said this, except for Greece, a clear advantage is illustrated for men living in Southern Europe, especially Mediterranean countries, with regard to ischaemic heart disease (IHD) (Figure 14.1). When looking at the SMRs, the only countries to present SMR values <100 for both sexes are France (65: CI 59–71), Portugal (87: CI 80–94), Italy (91: CI 84–98) and Spain (92: CI 85–99). Mortality from IHD has been continuously decreasing in most West European countries over the last few decades. By contrast, IHD mortality increased during the 1970s and 1980s in most Central and East European countries, and only started to decline in the early to mid-1990s. Despite the recent decrease, mortality rates are still considerably higher in most Central and East European countries compared with West European countries. Some countries, such as the Ukraine, have one of the highest rates in the world. Although most Central and East European countries appear to have reached

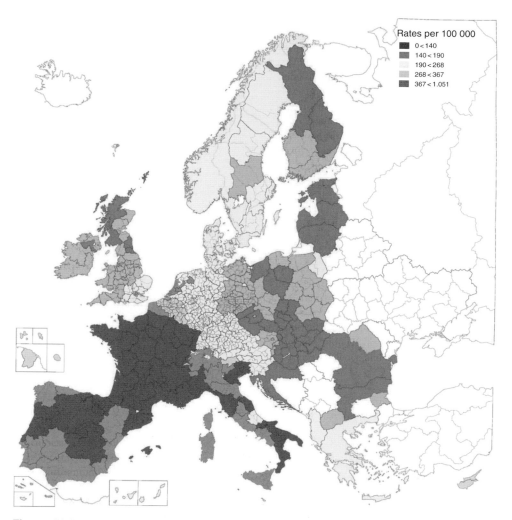

Figure 14.1 Age-standardised mortality from ischaemic heart disease in European regions (men; age group 45–74 years; year 2000) [7]. With permission from Oxford University Press.

their peak in cardiovascular mortality, the majority of them can clearly still be classified as high-risk countries and deserve special preventive strategies. Within the UK, in 2000, some parts of Scotland, Wales and England were among the European regions with the highest mortality rates with SMRs (men+women/100000) of 175 (CI 166–185) for Scotland and 202 (CI 191–212) for England and Wales.

Cancers

With an estimated 2.9 million new cases (54% occurring in men, 46% in women) and 1.7 million deaths (56% in men, 44% in women) each year, cancer remains an important public health problem in Europe, and the ageing of the European population will cause these numbers to continue to grow even if age-specific rates remain constant [8]. There were over two million (2,060,400) cases of cancer in 2004 in the European Union (EU) and over one million cancer deaths (1,161,300). Prostate

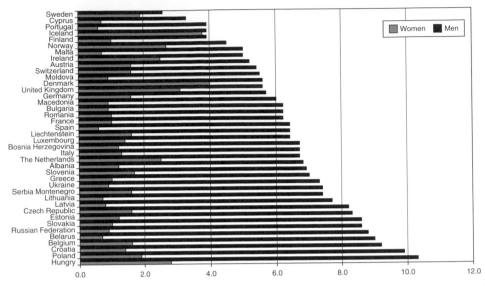

Figure 14.2 Cumulative lifetime (age 0–74 years) risk (percent) of lung cancer in men and women in Europe [8]. With permission from Oxford University Press.

cancer was the most frequent form of cancer in men with an estimated 202,100 new cases (18.1% of all cases). Lung cancer was a very close second with 196,100 cases (17.6 %), then colorectal cancer (149,400 cases, 13.4 %) and bladder cancer (91,000 cases, 8.2%). In women, breast cancer is the most common cancer with 275,000 cases (29%), followed by colorectal cancer (129,800 cases, 13.7%). Lung cancer incidence is rising in women with 62,000 cases (6.5%) in 2004.

Lung cancer continued to be the most common cause of cancer death in men in the EU, with 178,400 deaths estimated in 2004 (27.3% of all cancer deaths), and the lifetime risk of dying of 5.5%. Colorectal cancer ranked second (72,300 deaths, 11.1%), followed by prostate cancer (68,200, 10.4%). In women, breast cancer is the leading cause of death in the EU (88,400 deaths, 17.4% of total), colorectal cancer was the second most common cause of cancer death (67,000, 13.2%), with lung cancer clearly established as the third most frequent cause of cancer deaths in women (55,900 deaths, 11%) [8].

When considering the cumulative lifetime risk of lung cancer in men and women in Europe[1], it is to be noted that whereas men from Eastern Europe countries have the highest cumulative risk of lung cancer compared to other European men, women in North European countries have the highest risk relative to other European women (Figure 14.2). This observation illustrates the importance of taking into account not only sex but also cultural and lifestyle factors when setting prevention guidelines.

In the UK, prostate cancer was the most common cancer in men with 27,463 new cases and 9834 deaths (IARC data, 2002). Lung cancer was second with 24,300 new cases in 2002 but was first for mortality (21,959 deaths). Colorectal cancer was third with 19,407 new cases and 8912 deaths. In the same year, there were 49,298 new cases of breast cancer in women, and 13,303 died, and 16,562 new colorectal

---

[1] EU + Iceland, Liechtenstein, Norway, Switzerland, Bulgaria, Belarus, Moldova, Romania, Macedonia, Serbia, Montenegro, Albania, Bosnia and Herzegovina, Russian Federation, Ukraine.

cancer cases were diagnosed in women and 8278 deaths were observed. Lung cancer is getting close to colorectal cancer for incidence in women (15,424 new cases) and is the leading cause of death (13,390).

Other diseases

About 150 million women suffer from osteoporosis in the world. Osteoporosis is a disease that occurs mainly in post-menopausal women, and it has been estimated that about 40% of women in Europe might be affected compared with only 8% of men, and one woman in three might suffer a bone fracture related to this pathology after the age of 50 years.

Few statistics are available for other degenerative diseases in which diet might be implicated. The incidence of Alzheimer's disease (AD) is higher in industrialised countries, where life expectancy is long, with the noticeable exception of Japan. In Europe, incidence is expected to increase from 2 million cases to 4 million in 50 years. In Belgium and France about 20% of persons over 80 years are affected by AD.

The incidence of age-related macular degeneration (AMD) is rising and is the major cause of vision loss in people over 65 years. In Belgium, one in three people present signs of AMD after 75 years of age.

Dietary prevention

The potential role of diet as a tool in public health can be illustrated using cancer as an example. Death rates from cancer in the US decreased very little in the 25 years up to the new millennium, and this is in stark contrast with the dramatic fall in mortality from heart disease seen over the same period (Figure 14.3). Despite major advances in understanding the biology of cancer, new treatment strategies have at present had only a minor effect on overall mortality rates. The reductions in mortality that have occurred for a few specific cancers (such as stomach cancer) are mainly due to better hygiene and screening strategies.

As previously mentioned, obesity is a major threat to public health, and one important aspect of this is the association between obesity and the increased risk of various cancers [10]. It is noteworthy that the incidence of the most common cancers in the EU, including the UK, can be reduced not only by lifestyle factors, mainly through tobacco eradication, but also through nutritional prevention by the MedDiet as discussed in Chapter 12. Overall, the composition of the MedDiet, along with other aspects of the Mediterranean lifestyle, is broadly in line with the cancer prevention strategy proposed in the 2007 report from the WCRF/AICR [11].

WCRF/AICR 2007 Cancer Prevention Strategy [11]

Be as lean as possible within the normal range of body weight
Be physically active as part of everyday life
Limit consumption of energy-dense foods and avoid sugary drinks
Eat mostly foods of plant origin
Limit intake of red meat and avoid processed meat
Limit alcoholic drinks
Limit consumption of salt and avoid mouldy cereals (grains) or pulses (legumes)
Aim to meet nutritional needs through diet alone

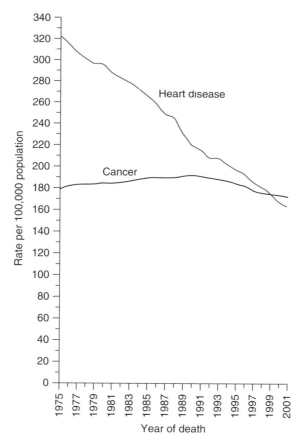

Figure 14.3   Death rates from cancer and heart disease in US (<85 years old) [9].

As shown in previous chapters, the MedDiet has the potential to prevent, decrease or postpone not only cancer but also the incidence of CVD, and hence of overall mortality since these diseases are among the major causes of death. Neurodegenerative diseases and AMD might also be favourably influenced by the MedDiet, and these diseases are important disability burdens on individuals and society. Thus, recommending the MedDiet could have a major impact on the prevention of major CDDs, and would be highly rewarding in terms of public health.

14.2   Which MedDiet?

The diversity of dietary patterns in countries around the Mediterranean has been discussed in Chapter 1. These have been a matter of debate between nutritional anthropologists and nutritionists. Nutritional anthropologists evoke the subtle differences in diets among the countries around the Mediterranean that result from geographical, agricultural and cultural specificities, whereas nutritional epidemiologists and nutritionists, observing the same health benefits in these countries, tend to pinpoint the common features of the various diets to set up a model of a dietary pattern beneficial for health. Although recognising the value of the anthropological approach, we will focus on describing "the nutritionist model" of the MedDiet that we expect to be beneficial in terms of health, first by components, then by integrating them in the MedDiet pattern.

14.3 Which constituents are important in the MedDiet?

14.3.1 Olive oil

Olive oil is the most commonly-used fat in most Mediterranean countries, and it was the first component identified by Ancel Keys as being an important factor for reducing the risk of CVD [12]. Olive oil is from a fruit, whereas most other used vegetable oils are made from seeds. This origin explains the content of phenolic compounds of the olive oil which, together with the high content of oleic acid, a *cis*-MUFA, are the two characteristics of olive oil.

In spite of the quasi-constant presence of olive oil in dietary patterns associated with a reduction of risk of CDD, epidemiological studies cannot convincingly relate olive oil to a decreased risk in CDD, because this effect can be confounded by other constituents of the MedDiet (especially vegetables and fish, which are significantly correlated with olive oil intake in Mediterranean countries). However, experimental studies provide support to this observation, with mechanistic explanations emphasising the role of the various phenolic compounds of olive oil (see Chapters 11 and 12).

In terms of public health, two aspects are particularly important: (a) the relative proportion of oleic acid with regard to other FAs and (b) the absolute intake of this FA.

(a) The beneficial effects of oleic acid have been observed in certain conditions peculiar to the MedDiet, namely: (i) olive oil as the major source of MUFA intake over a lifetime; (ii) concomitant low intake of SFA; (iii) sufficient intake of PUFA, especially *n*-3 FAs. These conditions are recognised as important by the scientific and public health authorities.

   (i) When MUFAs from sources other than olive oil replace SFA there is no benefit with regard to CVD, as was observed in a pooled analysis of studies conducted in the US and Northern Europe where the source of MUFAs is essentially meat and dairy products, consumed within a Western dietary pattern [13]. These animal sources of MUFAs are kept to moderate levels in the MedDiet.

   (ii) The dietary reference values proposed by the European Food Safety Authority (EFSA) recommend keeping SFA as low as possible, and WHO/FAO (World Health Organisation and Food and Agriculture Organisation) set 10% of total energy intake (TEI) as the upper limit of the acceptable macronutrient distribution range (AMDR) of SFA.

   (iii) A certain amount of PUFAs is recognised as necessary, not only because linoleic acid and α-linolenic acid are essential FAs but also with regard to prevention of CDD. EFSA set an adequate intake (AI) for linoleic acid of 4% TEI, and WHO/FAO an AMDR of 2.5–9% TEI. For *n*-3 FAs, EFSA set an AI of 0.5%TEI, and WHO/FAO ≥0.5% TEI of α-linolenic acid, with an intake of absolute amount of LC-PUFA, an AI of 250 mg/day for

       EFSA, and an AMDR of 250mg–2g/day for WHO/FAO according to physiological and pathological conditions.

(iv)   WHO/FAO acknowledge that the convenient proportion of MUFAs in the diet will be obtained by substitution of SFA and PUFAs, that is to say around 20% TEI.

Thus, the lipid characteristics of the MedDiet are in line with European and international recommendations.

(b)   Oleic acid, as for other lipids, provides 9kcal/g, thus it is highly correlated to energy intake. Because it is necessary to keep a balance between energy intake and expenditure, the absolute amount of olive oil intake must be balanced with the other energy providers in the diet and in the organism (other FAs and carbohydrates), and with physical activity. It should be kept in mind that the traditional MedDiet was in use in a frugal and physically active society (e.g. farmers and shepherds).

Nowadays olive oil remains the principal fat source in Mediterranean countries as long as industrially transformed food is not in use. Most of the time, olive oil is still used for salads, but other less expensive oils or fats are used for cooking. Thus, a return to the use of olive oil in cooking is advisable.

14.3.2 Cereals and legumes

As discussed earlier (Chapter 5), cereals have been the staple food for providing energy in Mediterranean countries since antiquity. Each country or culture developed particular preferences, usually wheat or rice, or, less commonly, corn. This food was complemented by legumes, and the association of cereals with legumes provides the satisfactory range of amino acids, which is important in order to supplement the moderate consumption of animal proteins. In addition to being energy providers and sources of proteins, legumes and unrefined cereals typical of the traditional MedDiet are rich in micronutrients (Chapter 5).

Consumption of unrefined cereals and legumes is the aspect of the MedDiet that has disappeared the most from food habits. This should be translated into actual public health recommendations so as to favour the consumption of complex carbohydrates at the expense of simple carbohydrates, and to include ancient cultivars of wheat (hard wheat varieties and spelt), and legumes such as lentils, various cultivars of dry beans, and chick-peas, since fibre is known to be associated with a reduced risk of CVD and some cancers. Cereal products should retain a large part of the grain envelope, which contains most of the micronutrients. In relation to this, organically-grown cereals are to be preferred since most of pesticides are concentrated in the envelope. Although the contaminants content of each batch is kept at tolerated levels, the effects of accumulation with time and of synergy with other contaminants are unknown.

14.3.3 Fruit and vegetables

Consumption of fruit and vegetables is the most widespread characteristic of the MedDiet, and many countries have set consumption of at least five portions of fruit and vegetables a day as part of their public health guidelines. A supplementary recommendation is to consume seasonal fruit and vegetables because UV light exposure is partly responsible for the content in micronutrients (many plant foods raised in glasshouses have lower amounts of phenolic compounds than field-raised ones – see Chapter 3). Thus it is better to use preserved tomatoes in winter than fresh ones. This was the case in the traditional MedDiet, for example in Italy which used a sterilised "tomata" product prepared with the summer tomatoes and olive oil. This not only consisted of tomatoes with a high carotenoid content, but the bioavailability of phytochemicals was increased due to the addition of lipids to the preparation.

A last characteristic of vegetables in the MedDiet is their variety. It is generally believed that the main Mediterranean vegetables are tomatoes, courgettes (zucchini), aubergines (egg-plants), cucumbers and sweet peppers. Certainly, these are the ones found in summer and autumn, and these are the ones that are consumed by summer visitors to Mediterranean countries. But winter and spring vegetables such as leeks, turnips, carrots, all kinds of cabbage (green and red), broccoli, cauliflower, green peas and fava beans, etc, are part of the winter and spring diet in Mediterranean countries and should be preferred to supposedly typical vegetables that have been grown in greenhouses, or vegetables such as aubergines, zucchini, green peppers and green beans that have been imported from more southerly countries. This ensures a larger variety and quantity of micronutrients and microconstituents, since the nutritional and organoleptic qualities of greenhouse-grown vegetables are mostly inferior to those grown in the field.

A large variety of fresh fruit is also part of the MedDiet, especially in summer and autumn (apricots, peaches, nectarines, plums, grapes, cantaloupe melons, honey-dew melons and water-melons) compared to winter. However, apples, pears and a wide range of citrus fruits provide a significant part of the vitamin and micronutrient intake in winter, followed in the spring by cherries and strawberries. Besides fresh fruit, dried fruit and nuts are an important component of the MedDiet, and are to be recommended. Dried fruits are highly calorific and should be included in dietary patterns respecting the overall energy balance, but they are also rich in fibre (especially dates and figs), minerals (calcium in dates and magnesium in almonds and pistachios), in micronutrients (phenolic compounds in dates, figs, raisins) and n-3 PUFAs (almonds and pistachios) and n-6 PUFAs (walnuts).

The consumption of fruit is nowadays generally better maintained than that of other plant foods, whereas the variety of consumed vegetables has decreased considerably. Consumption of vegetables needs to be revitalised in Mediterranean countries, together with an increased consumption of nuts and dry fruits.

14.3.4   Herbs and spices

Thyme, rosemary, parsley, basil, mint, cinnamon, nutmeg and saffron are an integral part of the MedDiet. It has been shown experimentally that these plants are rich in various compounds, such as phenolics (Chapter 5), which in *in vitro* or animal models have properties expected to be beneficial to human health (Chapter 9). It might be argued that the small amounts of these plants in the diet will reduce the likelihood of any health benefits. However, daily consumption might help to maintain a plateau of microconstituents in plasma by accumulation. Another important aspect is that they improve the taste of most foods, especially vegetables.

14.3.5   Meat and dairy products

Meat and dairy products are consumed in moderation in the MedDiet. This moderation not only has positive health benefits (by contributing to the low intake of SFA), but can also have a major positive impact in relation to the environment and sustainable development by decreasing greenhouse gas emissions [14]. Yogurt and fresh cheeses are the main daily dairy products in the MedDiet whereas hard cheese consumption is less frequent. Moreover, goats and sheep are the major sources of milk and meat in the majority of Mediterranean countries, with the exception of Italy where cow milk and cheese are also popular. One hundred grams of goat and ewe cheeses provide about 0.11 g of ALA which represents about 10% of the recommended ALA intake (0.5% total energy) [15]. Another area of interest is the relatively high content of <12C SFAs, which are less atherogenic, in goat and sheep cheeses. Thus, there is a strong justification for recommending meat and dairy products from ovine (sheep) and caprine (goat) species.

14.3.6   Wine and tea

It is interesting to note that wine and tea, two beverages traditionally consumed around the Mediterranean basin, are rich in phenolics and may have beneficial effects for human health (Chapter 7). Although these beverages are still consumed today, there are changes to these drinks and/or the way in which they are consumed, and this is a cause for some concern.

Traditionally, wine was the beverage consumed with meals. It was generally rather low in alcohol (around 10% v/v) and it was not unusual to dilute it with water. Men also drank other alcoholic beverages (most often containing anise) from time to time and at fiestas. Women drank very little wine, and other alcoholic beverages even less frequently. The wine consumed was not of a high quality and could neither be kept for years nor commercialised. Thus, a trend towards producing better wines with a higher alcohol content developed, both for better quality and for pleasure. However, this wine should be consumed in moderation and with a meal, given that having a drink before or after the meal strongly increases the amount of alcohol that is absorbed by the body. However, many young people in Mediterranean countries now ignore wine at meals, preferring Coca-cola or beer, and also drink other types of alcoholic beverages, sometimes binge-drinking on an empty stomach. It was shown that young people in Southern France who drank wine also had a good MedDiet quality index [16, 17]. This opens up a debate on the relevance of encouraging adolescents to drink a low amount of wine with meals.

There is another type of concern with tea. Tea is traditionally consumed around the Mediterranean, most often with mint and sometimes with pine kernels, and this is concordant with benefits related to the MedDiet. However, it is also traditional to add a lot of sugar. This was probably not too damaging when the diet was poor in refined carbohydrates, namely when cola drinks and other sodas were practically unknown. But with the nutritional transition in these countries, attention should now be paid to the overall content of carbohydrates, and especially of sugars, in the diet [18].

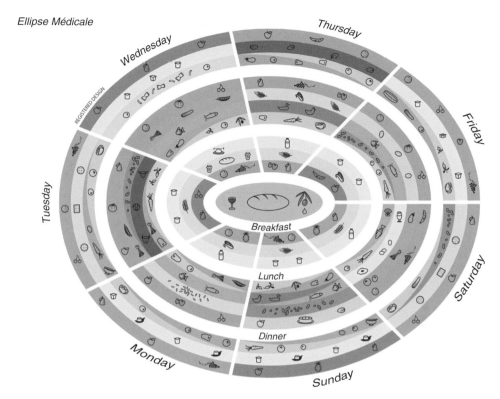

Figure 14.4   A day-by-day Mediterranean food pattern [20].

14.3.7   How can the Mediterranean dietary pattern be implemented?

As can be seen from the above discussion, each component of the MedDiet has its place in terms of nutritional recommendations and for the prevention of CDD. But listing each one is not in itself sufficient to implement guidelines. Rather, they must be organised in a real dietary pattern with three structured meals a day, and on a day-by-day basis. Such a Mediterranean nutritional model has been devised for an intervention study, the Medi-Rivage study, for people at risk of CVD [19]. This model is based on a seven-day pattern that takes into account all the elements and integrates them into a pattern to ensure a balanced diet (Figure 14.4).

In the centre of this pattern are displayed foods that are consumed daily and as part of the principal meals of the day, namely wholemeal or semi-wholemeal bread, olive oil and a small quantity of wine. The other beverage is simply water, still or sparkling; sweet sodas are avoided. Then, a suggestion is made meal by meal for each day of the week. At breakfast, a fruit is always included, and this is better than a fruit juice – even home-made – because it retains fibre and phenolic compounds. The beverage will be tea or coffee, depending upon the Mediterranean country, and there will be wholemeal bread with fresh cheese or yogurt, preferably made from goat or ewe milk and, once a week, butter if wished. Other type of raw cereals might be used with low-fat milk.

In Mediterranean countries, the principal meal is lunch. This consists of:

- an entrée – mostly raw vegetables, less often cooked vegetables or legumes, and sometimes seafood
- a main dish with an animal food, mostly fish and less often poultry, and eggs or red meat about once or twice a week,. It is accompanied by vegetables, a cereal product or legumes
- fruit as a dessert, a pastry as a treat on Sunday or another celebratory day.

The evening meal includes a plant food-based dish, such as soup, noodles, green pie or salad, and is completed with cheese or yogurt most of the time, or biscuits, and fresh or dry fruit depending upon the calorific intake of the day.

Generally there is no snacking, although a snack in the afternoon might be recommended for children or aged and frail people. Also, the evening meal will be higher in calories for adolescents and persons with high physical activity, and will include another dish made of animal food or cereals and legumes.

This dietary pattern ensures an adequate intake of all the beneficial components of the MedDiet. It is in line also with the observations made regarding other characteristics of the MedDiet, namely structured meals, lunch as the main meal, and no snacking [21]. However, it does not reflect another reported important aspect of the MedDiet, namely sharing meals with members of the family or colleagues (conviviality). This might have an effect both on the speed of eating and on the amount of food consumed. The possible effects on health of such a habit has been suspected for some time, and has now been demonstrated in recent studies since obesity is less prevalent in children sharing their meals with the family compared to those having their meals by themselves or watching TV [22–24].

It is important to emphasise some aspects discussed previously which are an integral part of the MedDiet, such as preferring seasonal vegetables and fruit to out-of-season produce that is either grown in greenhouses or imported from more southerly countries. Mediterranean populations could easily readopt such a food pattern, even though there is a tendency, especially by the young, to lose the MedDiet [17, 25]. It is very important to take action to revive the MedDiet in Mediterranean countries, especially in countries where obesity plagues young people, often to levels comparable to those in the US. In addition, recommendations on dietary patterns have to be accompanied with other lifestyle factors including physical activity, and low alcohol intake and tobacco use.

Another point of current importance is that the MedDiet is a sustainable diet: (1) it maintains and emphasises biodiversity through the recommendation of a diversity of plant-foods; (2) it reduces energy consumption by advocating seasonal and field-grown products use; (3) it recommends a moderate amount of meat, thus keeping the environmental impact of livestock at acceptable levels [14]. One point of debate is the recommended large intake of seafood products in spite of decreasing marine resources: this recommendation requires the implementation of sustainable seafood and fish farming of high quality.

14.4 Transferring the Mediterranean dietary pattern

In 1995 James commented that "Mediterranean diets can now be recognized as both limited in toxicity and abundant in nutrient and non-nutrient protective factors, but a coherent evaluation of these diets will be needed to shift the current [post-war] simplified views of dietary needs in Western societies" [26]. It was shown in chapters 10–13 that there now exists a coherent evaluation of this diet. However, it was also shown that a dietary pattern composed of the components encompassed by the Mediterranean diet score (MDS) was not as protective in other countries as it was in Greece, either because the amount of intake was different or because some factors, correlated to the MDS in Greece, were absent in other countries. This suggests that it is necessary to adapt the MedDiet in order for it to be implemented in culturally diverse populations, especially North European populations, and also to reflect changes in society.

Learning from observations on populations losing the MedDiet might help identify some features that should be compensated for or modified in order to render the MedDiet more attractive. Studies by Scott's group provide important obser-vations with regard to the possible implementation of a MedDiet in Northern Europe [27, 28]. A cross-sectional survey of eating habits before and after moving from Greece to Scotland (Glasgow) was conducted on a sample of 80 post-graduate Greek students. After moving to Glasgow, significant decreases were reported in the frequency of consuming fresh fruit, raw vegetables, fish, legumes, meat, poultry and fresh fruit juice. The frequency of eating biscuits, savoury snacks, soft-fizzy drinks, alcoholic drinks and mayonnaise, dips and sauces increased. The estimated median daily consumption of fruit and vegetables decreased from 363 g in Greece to just 124 g in Glasgow. Although this can be qualified as "acculturation", especially with respect to the increase in biscuits, savoury snacks, soft-fizzy drinks, mayonnaise, dips and sauces intake, the main perceived barriers to maintaining customary eating habits were the price of food, the greater availability of convenience food and the limited variety of food available in Glasgow, when compared to Greece. These are factors that should be taken into account when designing campaigns to promote the MedDiet. These authors refined their results by comparing Greek students living away from home but still in Greece with Greek students living in Scotland and showed that some of these changes were the result of living away from the family home where someone else was taking care of the cooking [27]. The way Greek students away from their family, but still remaining in Greece, modified their customary eating habits suggests a simplification of the way they prepare and cook food: they eat less vegetables cooked from raw, less legumes and less fish ie all foodstuff that need preparation and more elaborate cooking. Thus, these studies provide some clues about how to approach the widespread adoption of a MedDiet by Western populations.

The same group also set up an internet-based intervention promoting the MedDiet in Scotland. 53 women were recruited for the experimental group and 19 women as controls. Following a baseline dietary and psychosocial assessment, the control group received a minimal amount of tailored feedback and three brochures with general recommendations. By contrast, the experimental group received a tailored dietary feedback identifying areas for dietary improvement in comparison with MedDiet, and an emphasis on four key components of the MedDiet, namely vegetables (excluding potatoes), fruit (including nuts and seeds), legumes and the ratio of MUFA:SFA. During the 6-month intervention, participants completed four on-line validated short FFQs. The experimental group received tailored dietary feedback after each evaluation. They had access to a Mediterranean eating website which included articles describing the constituents and benefits of the MedDiet, recipes, cooking and buying tips, food nutrients and food safety. At the end of the 6 months, the web site was judged informative, trustworthy, attractive and encouraging. The recipe section was the most visited, and the participants found them rather easy to prepare and the ingredients generally easy to find [29]. At the end of the 6 months, the intervention group had increased consumption of the four key components; however, this increase was not statistically significant for legumes and fruit. The CVD risk markers tended also to improve [30]. A MDS was computed for the 8 traditional components of a MedDiet (fish was not included), using as cut-offs the means of consumption as computed originally for an elderly Greek population. However, the MDS did not even reach 4, although there was a slight increase in the score in the intervention group (from 3.21 to 3.64, p=0.013) [30].

Thus, this study showed the possibility that a Northern population could adopt some components of a MedDiet. And we can learn from it. For example, providing recipes is an important aspect, and this has also been shown in the Medi-Rivage study [31]. Working closely with people to keep them cooking and eating a MedDiet so that it becomes a normal and spontaneous way of cooking and eating also appears to be necessary. A website might be helpful. However, in the first study by Papadaki and Scott, it was shown that lack of time was a strong barrier to regularly consulting the site [29]. Moreover, the results of the MDS in the study strongly suggest that these subjects are far from showing a true adherence to the MedDiet since their food intake was far from encompassing the entirety of a MedDiet. There is insufficient data from the study to completely appreciate the degree of adequacy to a MedDiet. For example, was the source of MUFA olive oil? Was wine the source of alcohol? How was it consumed? Were the cereals whole-grain? Fish was not taken into account. A small pilot trial, albeit with low statistical power, suggests that behavioural counselling tends to improve the adoption of a MedDiet [32]. Although such a method of dietary advice cannot be applied to a large scale, it could be valuable if applied to groups at risk.

In sum, these studies tend to demonstrate that individual help only results in limited implementation, and emphasises the need for a global approach to public health nutrition. Besides information and education, other means to influence individual choices and attitudes have to be designed, and government and community approaches, as well as family and individuals ones, are necessary in order to implement all the essential characteristics of a MedDiet.

14.4.1   Public health recommendations and education

Based on the knowledge accumulated over several decades, the Mediterranean dietary pattern, together with the usual nutritional recommendations, can be proposed as a pleasant way to achieve public health recommendations, as well as enhancing their effectiveness. This implies not only *campaigns of promotion* with public television programmes providing the health arguments, but also the means to adopt a MedDiet pattern such as recipes and weekly menu organisation that change with the seasons. Basic information should be provided, such as variations that occur in micronutrient content with changes in ripeness (for example, vitamin C decreases and carotenoids increase in tomatoes with increasing ripeness), changes in degree of freshness (vitamin C decreases in cabbages with time after harvest), and effects of different cooking techniques (for example, the nutritive value of fruits and vegetables is reduced by cooking if the main micronutrient is vitamin C, whereas it is the opposite in the case of carotenoids, since these will be concentrated, especially if the preparation contains lipids). Recipes might include dishes which are not strictly from a traditional MedDiet, as long as they respect the principles of the MedDiet, namely the importance of plant foods (fruit and vegetables raw and cooked, fresh and dried), of unsaturated oils, preferably olive oil, fish rather than red or processed meat, fresh cheese rather than hard ones, and cheeses that are made mainly from ewe and goat milk rather than cow's milk.

Programmes should be specifically targeted to different groups. These programmes can be diffused on the web, and in schools where information should be adapted to the different levels of scholarly capabilities giving progressively more scientific insight. At the university level, specific teaching should be directed to dietitians, who have a key role in promoting the MedDiet. Journalists are responsible for much of the information delivered to the public. To avoid nutritional cacophony, they should be provided with prompts to read scientific articles in order to deliver sound evidence-based data in all types of media, rather than "scoops" based on one result that might distract people from the simple and effective MedDiet pattern. Moreover, advances in the field of nutritional prevention, e.g. the potential beneficial effect of vitamin D, should be placed within the context of a MedDiet pattern (fish intake, physical activity outdoors in the sun) to increase the feeling of coherence. Experts and scientists should also help to diffuse recommendations, and be prepared to answer the public demands of information, which is part of their mission.

14.4.2   Governments' and communities' food policies

A major objective of food policy in relation to diffusion of the MedDiet is to *help the consumer* select appropriate foods. A first approach might lie in food labelling. This can provide information on the content of the food and, if EU nutritional profiling is applied, on its nutritional quality. However, one food cannot encompass all the benefits of a MedDiet, and any type of Mediterranean logo on one food could lull the consumer into a false sense about the quality of his or her diet. Therefore, it is preferable to work on a *large display of most Mediterranean products*. The MedDiet won't be diffused throughout the population if the food items remain absent from the retail stores, or if they are too expensive. Thus, various policies should be implemented to help the population to comply with the MedDiet pattern.

Local production is to be encouraged because shortening the time between harvest and consumption results in a higher content and quality of micronutrients and microconstituents, and also decreases their environmental impact. Many traditional Mediterranean plant foods that readily grow in the British climate are currently under-represented in the UK and their seasonal cultivation could be encouraged (Table 14.1). These plants should preferably be grown outdoors, and hence be

Table 14.1 Some plant foods associated with the MedDiet that are under-represented in the UK.

Plant food	Eating seasons
Salad greens that are micronutrient-rich, e.g. cos and lollo rosso lettuces rather than iceberg	spring–autumn
Cultivated "wild" greens such as wild rocket and purslane	spring–autumn
Kale (various cultivars)	autumn–spring
Swiss chard (various cultivars)	summer–autumn
Tomato varieties suitable for outdoor cultivation	summer–autumn
Fresh outdoor-grown herbs	year-round according to the herb
Globe artichokes	summer–autumn

consumed according to the season, since this favours micronutrient production. Cultivars should be used that are adapted to local growing conditions and/or are known for their high content in micronutrients. (For example, one study found that Burbank tomatoes generally had higher levels of quercetin, kaempferol, total phenolics, and ascorbic acid compared to Ropreco tomatoes [33].) Cultivar selection is an important aspect for consideration by agronomic research institutions. In addition, climate change is already having a major impact on agriculture in the UK with increasing numbers of vineyards and, moreover, some fruits such as peaches and kiwi fruits, more traditionally associated with Mediterranean countries, are likely to be grown in increasing amounts in the UK in the near future [34].

With regard to the microconstituent component of the MedDiet, the question of the superiority of organic plant foods is still a matter of debate. It is difficult to ascertain whether or not organic foods have a higher nutritional quality [35], although the presence of a higher nutritional density (more phenolics and antioxidants) is often reported [36, 37]. The content of chemicals (nitrates and pesticides) is lower in organic plant foods than in conventional ones, whereas the level of some mycotoxins (e.g. ochratoxins in wine) or some atmospheric pollutants (e.g. dioxin in dairy products) has been found to be comparable [36, 37]. The EU promotes the production of foods using fewer pesticides, and governments in several countries have introduced laws to increase land-use for organic agriculture and to encourage organic food in cafeterias and school canteens. The debate regarding the level of greenhouse gases produced by organic agriculture is ongoing, but it looks probable that the combination of locally-produced food and organic agriculture practices might decrease their production. Organic agriculture also favours biodiversity and preserves water resources and soil structure. Therefore, in terms of food quality and environmental issues, governments and communities will be well-advised to recommend consumption of locally-produced organic food or food that minimises harm to the environment.

With regard to the specific promotion of a MedDiet, it is interesting to note that current opinion is supporting a change of the Common Agricultural Policy (CAP) towards promoting foods more in agreement with the principles of the MedDiet [38]. It proposes *key recommendations and general principles for a healthier CAP*: subsidising health-promoting food production; achieving global food security; environmental sustainability; protecting rural economies including those in developing countries. It also proposes specific reforms to achieve these goals, and among these reforms quite a few correspond to the characteristics of the MedDiet. These include: phasing out sugar beet production from whole farm payments; phasing out whole farm payments for milk and beef production except for grass-only fed methods, which are better for both health and for the environment; encouraging agricultural rather than livestock production by only including cereals for human consumption within whole farm payments; encouraging production which is good for health, such as fruit and vegetables, pulses, olive and seed oils. National governments should support such reforms and implement them in their country.

Another limit to MedDiet food choice might be the *price*. Several studies have shown that low income is a barrier to buying healthy food, especially fruit and vegetables [39, 40]. National governments should *specifically help low income families* to get MedDiet foods such as fruit and vegetables, unsaturated oils, fish, cereals and pulses. This could be done by a voucher distribution. Another aspect to be looked at by government agencies is the retail price in the supermarket. A survey conducted in French supermarkets showed that the margin taken by the retail store for an organic product is up to twice that for the same but conventional product, thus reducing the comparative advantage of quality products and penalising food quality.

Retail stores and the food industry could also play a part in promoting Mediterranean food. Retail stores could organise displays of the various foods of the Mediterranean dietary pattern to give the consumers a real picture of the pattern, since all consumers are sensitive to the stimulating environment of a food store [40]. The food industry could contribute by processing ready-to-use dishes with quality Mediterranean ingredients, seasonally harvested, and labelled with the origins of the ingredients. They should also reorganise their production towards developing this type of food and progressively reducing the production of less healthy products.

Finally, Mediterranean dietary patterns should penetrate cafeterias in schools and companies. It has been observed in the European multi-centre study, EPIC, that over 25% of Europeans, mostly young and educated, eat out [41, 42]. Eating out correlated with higher energy and sweets intake. Therefore, a massive effort should be put in catering to promote a MedDiet. In many catering organisations, dietitians are in charge of menu planning, which underlines the importance of having the characteristics and benefits of the MedDiet as part of their teaching programme.

14.4.3 Individual choices and attitudes

Family attitudes towards implementing a MedDiet are of paramount importance because it is in the home where information and education about the MedDiet will be translated into food habits. This assumes that parents will be informed of the beneficial effects of the MedDiet, and are able to reproduce this pattern, not only with its nutritional quality but also with its organoleptic ones and its social characteristics (food production, preparation and conviviality). Some steps towards achieving these goals are:

- At home, every day and through the week, the principles of the MedDiet should be applied. Every meal should be shared by all the family members present; this should follow the MedDiet pattern when the components of the meal are chosen, and in such a way that there becomes a natural rhythm to meal structures, their daily organisation, and through the seasons.
- Parents should educate their children from infancy. It is now well known that this early inculcation sets later attitudes and choices. Even before this, in the hospital, mothers should receive advice such as breast-feeding as much as possible, to avoid any sugar-added drink. Then, at six months, when food diversification starts to be implemented, it is advisable to give various types of vegetables, then fruit. It is better, as much as is possible, to prepare the vegetable puree at home rather than to buy it: the genuine taste of the vegetables will be better preserved and will inform the taste of the child.
- Later on, the growing child should be associated with a Mediterranean food pattern, including aspects of food shopping and preparation. Transmission of recipes and culinary *savoir-faire* set the scene for an adult not only conscious of the importance of food for health, but also with the pleasure of preparing and sharing food with beloved people.

- Finally, progressively, the child can be introduced to food production, meeting people and visiting places. Doing so, he or she will comprehend socio-economic and environmental aspects of food safety and security, all parts of sustainable environmental concern. Thus the child will feel that not only is eating with conscience an important part of personal wellbeing, but also that it is good for society.

References

1. Doll, R, Peto, R. Mortality in relation to smoking: 20 years' observations on male British doctors. *BMJ*, 1976. **2**: 1525–36.
2. Peto, R. et al. Plasma cholesterol, coronary heart disease, and cancer. *BMJ*, 1989. **298**: 1249.
3. Marmot, M.G. Status syndrome: a challenge to medicine. *Jama*, 2006. **295**: 1304–7.
4. Vartiainen, E., et al. Cardiovascular risk factor changes in Finland, 1972–1997. *Int J Epid*, 2000. **29**: 49–56.
5. Puska, P. The North Karelia Project: 30 years successfully preventing chronic diseases. *Diabetes Voice*, 2008. **53** (Special issue):26–9
6. WHO. WHO statistics: http://www.who.int/whosis/whostat/2006
7. Muller-Nordhorn, J. et al. An update on regional variation in cardiovascular mortality within Europe. *Eur Heart J*, 2008. **29**: 1316–26.
8. Boyle, P., Ferlay, J. Cancer incidence and mortality in Europe, 2004. *Ann Oncol.* 2005.**16**: 481–8.
9. Jemal, A. et al. Cancer statistics, 2005. *Cancer J Clin*, 2005. **55**: 10–30.
10. Calle, E.E. et al. Overweight, obesity, and mortality from cancer in a prospectively studied cohort of U.S. adults. *N Engl J Med*, 2003. **348**: 1625–38.
11. WCRF/AICR. World Cancer Research Fund/American Institute for Cancer Research. *Food, nutrition, physical activity, and the prevention of cancer: a global perspective.* Washington DC: AICR, 2007.
12. Keys, A. et al. The diet and 15-year death rate in the seven countries study. *Am J Epidemiol*, 1986. **124**: 903–15.
13. Jakobsen, M.U. et al. Major types of dietary fat and risk of coronary heart disease: a pooled analysis of 11 cohort studies. *Am J Clin Nutr*, 2009. **89**: 1425–32.
14. Steinfeld, H. et al. *Livestock's long shadow*. FAO 2006.
15. Berta, I. pers. comm. Ciqual ANSES 2010.
16. Scali, J. et al. [Alcohol consumption by young adults from three cities in Southern France]. *Revue d'epidemiologie et de sante publique*, 2002. **50**: 357–69.
17. Scali, J. Ret al. Diet profiles in a population sample from Mediterranean southern France. *Pub Health Nutr*, 2001. **4**: 173–82.
18. Issa, C. et al. A Mediterranean diet pattern with low consumption of liquid sweets and refined cereals is negatively associated with adiposity in adults from rural Lebanon. *Int J Obes*, 2010. **35**(2): 251–8.
19. Vincent-Baudry, S. et al. The Medi-RIVAGE study: reduction of cardiovascular disease risk factors after a 3-mo intervention with a Mediterranean-type diet or a low-fat diet. *Am J Clin Nutr*, 2005. **82**: 964–71.
20. Gerber, M. *Santé et alimentation Méditerranéenne au quotidien*. Aix-en-Provence: Édisud, 2004.
21. Tessier, S., Gerber, M. Comparison between Sardinia and Malta: the Mediterranean diet revisited. *Appetite*, 2005. **45**: 121–6.
22. Dubois, L. et al. Social factors and television use during meals and snacks is associated with higher BMI among pre-school children. *Public Health Nutr*, 2008. **11**: 1267–79.
23. Gable, S. et al. Television watching and frequency of family meals are predictive of overweight onset and persistence in a national sample of school-aged children. *J Am Diet Assoc*, 2007. **107**: 53–61.
24. Utter, J. et al. Relationships between frequency of family meals, BMI and nutritional aspects of the home food environment among New Zealand adolescents. *Int J Behav Nutr Phys Act*, 2008. **5**: 50.

25. Sanchez-Villegas, A. et al. Gender, age, socio-demographic and lifestyle factors associated with major dietary patterns in the Spanish Project SUN (Seguimiento Universidad de Navarra). *Eur J Clin Nutr*, 2003. **57**: 285–92.

26. James, W.P. Nutrition science and policy research: implications for Mediterranean diets. *Am J Clin Nutr*, 1995. **61**: 1324S–8S.

27. Kremmyda, L.S. et al. Differentiating between the effect of rapid dietary acculturation and the effect of living away from home for the first time, on the diets of Greek students studying in Glasgow. *Appetite*, 2008. **50**: 455–63.

28. Papadaki, A., Scott, J.A. The impact on eating habits of temporary translocation from a Mediterranean to a Northern European environment. *Eur J Clin Nutr*, 2002. **56**: 455–61.

29. Papadaki, A., Scott, J.A. Process evaluation of an innovative healthy eating website promoting the Mediterranean diet. *Health Ed Res*, 2006. **21**: 206–18.

30. Papadaki, A., Scott, J.A. Follow-up of a web-based tailored intervention promoting the Mediterranean diet in Scotland. *Patient Ed Counselling*, 2008. **73**: 256–63.

31. Vincent, S. et al. The Medi-RIVAGE study (Mediterranean Diet, Cardiovascular Risks and Gene Polymorphisms): rationale, recruitment, design, dietary intervention and baseline characteristics of participants. *Public Health Nutr*, 2004. **7**: 531–42.

32. Logan, K.J. et al. Adoption and maintenance of a Mediterranean diet in patients with coronary heart disease from a Northern European population: a pilot randomised trial of different methods of delivering Mediterranean diet advice. *J Hum Nutr Diet*, 2009. **23**: 30–7.

33. Chassy, A.W. et al. Three-year comparison of the content of antioxidant microconstituents and several quality characteristics in organic and conventionally managed tomatoes and bell peppers. *J Agric Food Chem*, 2006. **54**: 8244–52.

34. Anon. Kiwis and peaches to be grown in England due to climate change. *Daily Telegraph* online 2010; http://www.telegraph.co.uk/earth/environment/climatechange.

35. Dangour, A.D. et al. Nutritional quality of organic foods: a systematic review. *Am J Clin Nutr*, 2009. **90**: 680–5.

36. Afssa (French Agency for Food Security). Bénéfices et risques des aliments issus de l'Agriculture Biologique. 2003.

37. Lairon, D. Nutritional quality and safety of organic food. A review. Available online at wwwagronomy-journalorg 2009.

38. Health FoP. The Common Agricultural Policy, a position statement, October 2009. wwwfphorguk, 2009.

39. Locher, J.L. et al. Food choice among homebound older adults: motivations and perceived barriers. *J Nut Health Aging*, 2009. **13**: 659–64.

40. Webber, C.B. et al. Shopping for fruits and vegetables. Food and retail qualities of importance to low-income households at the grocery store. *Appetite*, 2009. **54**: 297–303.

41. Orfanos, P. et al. Eating out of home and its correlates in 10 European countries. The European Prospective Investigation into Cancer and Nutrition (EPIC) study. *Public Health Nutr*, 2007. **10**: 1515–25.

42. Orfanos, P. et al. Eating out of home: energy, macro- and micronutrient intakes in 10 European countries. The European Prospective Investigation into Cancer and Nutrition. *Eur J Clin Nutr*, 2009. **63** Suppl 4: S239–62.

Section 3
APPENDICES

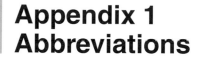

Appendix 1
Abbreviations

AA	Arachidonic acid
AD	Alzheimer's disease
ADH	Alcohol dehydrogenase
AI	Adequate intake
ALA	α-linolenic acid
ALDH	Acetaldehyde dehydrogenase
AMD	Age-related macular degeneration
AMDR	Acceptable macronutrient distribution range
BAC	Blood alcohol concentration
BMI	Body mass index
CDD	Chronic degenerative disease
CHD	Coronary heart disease
CI	Confidence interval (95% in this book, unless stated otherwise)
CLA	Conjugated linoleic acid
CO	Corn oil
COX	Cyclo-oxygenase
CRP	C reactive protein
CVD	Cardiovascular disease
CYP	Cytochrome P450
DHA	Docosahexaenoic acid
DW	Dry weight
ECG	Epicatechin-3-gallate
EFSA	European Food Safety Authority
EGCG	Epigallocatechin-3-gallate
EPA	Eicosapentaenoic acid
EVOO	Extra-virgin olive oil
FA	Fatty acid
FAO	Food and Agriculture Organisation
FW	Fresh weight
GI	Glycaemic index
GSH	Glutathione (reduced form)
GSSG	Glutathione (oxidised form)
HDL	High density lipoprotein
HDL-C	High density lipoprotein-cholesterol
HR	Hazards ratio
IGF-1	Insulin-like growth factor-1
IHD	Ischaemic heart disease

LC-PUFA	Long chain polyunsaturated fatty acid
LDL	Low density lipoprotein
LDL-C	Low density lipoprotein-cholesterol
LOX	Lipoxygenase
LT	Leukotrienes
MDS	Mediterranean diet score
MedDiet	Mediterranean diet
MI	Myocardial infarct
M-MDS	Modified-Mediterranean diet score
MUFA	Monounsaturated fatty acid
OA	Oleic acid
OO	Olive oil
OR	Odds ratio
ox-LDL	Oxidised low density lipoprotein
PAR	Population attributable risk
PC	Phosphatidylcholine
PCA	Principal component analysis
PD	Parkinson's disease
PG	Prostaglandin
PL	Phospholipid
PLA_2	Phospholipase A_2
PPAR	Peroxisome proliferator-activated receptor
PUFA	Polyunsaturated fatty acid
RR	Relative risk
SFA	Saturated fatty acid
SMR	Standardised mortality rate
SNP	Single nucleotide polymorphism
SOD	Superoxide dismutase
TAC	Total antioxidant capacity
TEI	Total energy intake
TFA	Trans fatty acid
TX	Thromboxane
VLDL	Very low density lipoprotein
VOO	Virgin olive oil
WHO	World Health Organisation

Appendix 2
Epidemiological Studies

ATTICA

The ATTICA study, randomly recruited 4056 inhabitants (of whom 3042 agreed to participate) from the Attica province of Greece (Athens and surrounding area) during May 2001 to December 2002. The aims of the study were to evaluate the prognostic significance of a range of risk factors for CVD (such as blood lipids, inflammatory markers) and several socio-economic, lifestyle and psychological characteristics of the participants, on the incidence of CHD through periodic follow-up examinations at 1, 5 and 10 years after entry into the study.

EPIC

The EPIC study (European Prospective Investigation into Cancer and Nutrition) is a prospective cohort study investigating the role of biological, dietary, lifestyle and environmental factors in the aetiology of cancer and other chronic diseases. Most volunteers were recruited between 1992 and 1998, and included 366,521 women and 153,457 men (total 519,978; 29.4% men), mostly aged 35–70, from 23 centres in 10 European countries (Denmark, France, Germany, Greece, Italy, the Netherlands, Norway, Spain, Sweden and the United Kingdom). It is the Greek cohort (28,572 participants) that has predominantly been used in relation to studies on the MedDiet. A validated, semi-quantitative, food-frequency questionnaire, which included 150 foods and beverages and several recipes, was used to assess usual intake during the year preceding enrolment.

HALE

The HALE study (Healthy Ageing: a Longitudinal Study in Europe) was a cohort study conducted between 1988 and 2000 in 11 European countries. It included 1507 apparently healthy men and 832 women, aged 70 to 90 years, who were enrolled in the SENECA study (see below) and elderly individuals in the so-called FINE study (which recruited populations in Finland, Italy and the Netherlands).

MEDIS

The MEDIS study (**Med**iterranean **Is**lands) evaluates clinical, lifestyle, behavioural and dietary characteristics of 1486 elderly people living in Mediterranean islands (Cyprus, and various Greek islands). All participants were without any clinical evidence of CVD or cancer in their medical history at the start of the study.

Medi RIVAGE

The Medi-RIVAGE study (Mediterranean Diet, Cardiovascular Risks and Gene Polymorphisms) is an intervention study conducted on 169 volunteers at cardiovascular risk from Marseille, France. A Mediterranean-type diet is being compared to a low fat diet. The study is assessing a range of clinical factors for arteriosclerosis (changes in plasma concentration of glucose, insulin, total cholesterol, LDL cholesterol, HDL cholesterol, triacylglycerols, fatty acids, carotenoids, vitamin B12, folates, apo E, apo A-I, apo B, and apo C-III, and insulin resistance by HOMA) as well as some genetic polymorphisms that influence lipoprotein metabolism and homeostasis.

PREDIMED

The PREDIMED (Prevencion con Dieta Mediterránea) study was initiated in 2003 and is an ongoing, multi-centre, randomised, primary prevention trial conducted on a population at high-risk of CVD (type 2 diabetics or individuals having three or more risk factors for CVD). This study is assessing the effects of three healthy diets (a low fat diet, a MedDiet rich in olive oil, a MedDiet rich in nuts) on cardiovascular outcomes.

SENECA

SENECA (Survey in Europe on Nutrition and the Elderly: a Concerted Action) recruited 631 men and 650 women, 70–75 years old, from Belgium, Denmark, Italy, The Netherlands, Portugal, Spain and Switzerland. The study began in 1988–1989, when diet, health status and lifestyle habits were obtained, and consisted of a 10-year survival follow-up. This study investigated the effects on survival of non-smoking, being physically active, and having a high-quality diet.

Seven Countries study

The Seven Countries Study was prompted by the low rates of CVD observed during the 1950s and 1960s in some Mediterranean countries. It was the first study that investigated the relationship between eating habits and the long-term incidence and mortality from cancer, CHD and stroke in various populations (25 year follow-up). Sixteen cohorts, comprising a total of 12,763 middle-aged men (aged 40–59), from seven countries (the US, Finland, The Netherlands, Italy, former Yugoslavia, Greece and Japan) were examined in relation to socio-demographic factors, clinical factors, lifestyle, dietary information and vital status.

SUN

The SUN study (Seguimiento Universidad de Navarra-Follow-up University of Navarra, Spain) began in 1999 on a population of Spanish university graduates and is an on-going prospective cohort study investigating the association between dietary and lifestyle factors with various diseases. It is based on self-reported data on obesity, hypertension, and physical activity and a validated semi-quantitative food frequency questionnaire.

Zutphen

This is a prospective cohort study of 1373 men born between 1900 and 1920 living in the industrial town of Zutphen in the Netherlands who were examined repeatedly between 1960 and 2000.

Index

Page numbers in *italics* refer to figures; those in **bold** refer to tables; those <u>underlined</u> indicate the main entry.

Keep up with critical fields

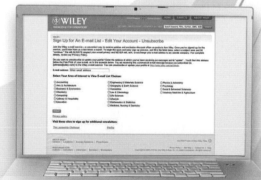

Would you like to receive up-to-date information on our books, journals and databases in the areas that interest you, direct to your mailbox?

Join the **Wiley e-mail service** - a convenient way to receive updates and exclusive discount offers on products from us.

Simply visit **www.wiley.com/email** and register online

We won't bombard you with emails and we'll only email you with information that's relevant to you. We will ALWAYS respect your e-mail privacy and NEVER sell, rent, or exchange your e-mail address to any outside company. Full details on our privacy policy can be found online.

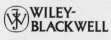